Biodynamics

Circulation

Y. C. Fung

Biodynamics
Circulation

With 189 Illustrations

Springer-Verlag
New York Berlin Heidelberg Tokyo

Y. C. Fung
Professor of Bioengineering
  and Applied Mechanics
University of California, San Diego
La Jolla, CA 92093
U.S.A.

Library of Congress Cataloging in Publication Data
Fung, Y. C. (Yuan-cheng), 1919–
  Biodynamics: circulation.
  Continues: Biomechanics.
  Includes bibliographies and index.
  1. Hemodynamics. 2. Blood—Circulation. I. Title.
QP105.F85   1984   599'.0113   83-14519

Typeset by Asco Trade Typesetting Ltd., Hong Kong.
Printed and bound by Halliday Lithograph, West Hanover, Massachusetts.
Printed in the United States of America.

9 8 7 6 5 4 3 2 1

ISBN 0-387-90867-6 Springer-Verlag New York Berlin Heidelberg Tokyo
ISBN 3-540-90867-6 Springer-Verlag Berlin Heidelberg New York Tokyo

Preface

This book is a continuation of my *Biomechanics*. The first volume deals with the mechanical properties of living tissues. The present volume deals with the mechanics of circulation. A third volume will deal with respiration, fluid balance, locomotion, growth, and strength. This volume is called *Biodynamics* in order to distinguish it from the first volume. The same style is followed. My objective is to present the mechanical aspects of physiology in precise terms of mechanics so that the subject can become as lucid as physics.

The motivation of writing this series of books is, as I have said in the preface to the first volume, to bring biomechanics to students of bioengineering, physiology, medicine, and mechanics. I have long felt a need for a set of books that will inform the students of the physiological and medical applications of biomechanics, and at the same time develop their training in mechanics. In writing these books I have assumed that the reader already has some basic training in mechanics, to a level about equivalent to the first seven chapters of my *First Course in Continuum Mechanics* (Prentice Hall, 1977). The subject is then presented from the point of view of life science while mechanics is developed through a sequence of problems and examples. The main text reads like physiology, while the exercises are planned like a mechanics textbook. The instructor may fill a dual role: teaching an essential branch of life science, and gradually developing the student's knowledge in mechanics.

The style of one's scientific approach is decided by the way one looks at a problem. In this book I try to emphasize the mathematical threads in the study of each physical problem. Experimental exploration, data collection, model experiments, in vivo observations, and theoretical ideas can be wrapped together by mathematical threads. The way problems are formulated, the kind of questions that are asked, are molded by this basic thought.

Much of the book can be read, however, with little mathematics. Those passages in which mathematics is essential are presented with sufficient details to make the reading easy.

This book begins with a discussion of the physics of blood flow. This is followed by the mechanics of the heart, arteries, veins, microcirculation, and pulmonary blood flow. The coupling of fluids and solids in these organs is the central feature. How morphology and rheology are brought to bear on the analysis of blood flow in organs is illustrated in every occasion. The basic equations of fluid and solid mechanics are presented in the Appendix. The subject of mass transfer, the exchange of water, oxygen, carbon dioxide, and other substances between blood and red cells and between capillary blood vessels and extravascular space, is deferred to the third volume, *Biodynamics: Flow, Motion, and Stress*, in order to keep the three volumes at approximately the same size.

Circulation is a many-sided subject. What we offer here is an understanding of the mechanics of circulation. We present methods and basic equations very carefully. The strengths and weaknesses of various methods and unanswered questions are discussed fully. To apply these methods to a specific organ, we need a data base. We must have a complete set of morphometric data on the anatomy, and rheological data on the materials of the organ. Unfortunately, such a data base does not exist for any organ of any animal. A reasonably complete set has been obtained for the lungs of the cat. Hence the analysis of the blood flow in the lung is presented in detail in Chapter 6. We hope that a systematic collection of the anatomical and rheological data on all organs of man and animals will be done in the near future so that organ physiology can be elevated to a higher level.

Blood circulation has a vast literature. The material presented here is necessarily limited in scope. Furthermore, there are still more things unknown than known. Progress is very rapid. Aiming at greater permanency, I have limited my scope to a few fundamental aspects of biomechanics. For handbook information and literature survey, the reader must look elsewhere. Many exercises are proposed to encourage the students to formulate and solve new problems. The book is not offered as a collection of solved problems, but as a way of thinking about problems. I wish to illustrate the use of mechanics as a simple, reliable tool in life science, and no more. A reasonably extensive bibliography is given at the end of each chapter, some with annotations from which further references can be found. Perhaps the author can be accused of quoting frequently papers and people familiar to him; he apologizes for this personal limitation and hopes that he can be forgiven because it is only natural that an author should talk about his own views. I have tried, however, never to forget mentioning the existence of other points of view.

I wish to express my thanks to many authors and publishers who permitted me to quote their publications and reproduce their figures and data in this book. I wish to mention especially Drs. Michael Yen, Sidney Sobin, Jen-Shih

Lee Benjamin Zweifach, Paul Patitucci, Geert Schmid-Schoenbein, William Conrad, Lawrence Talbot, H. Werlé, John Maloney, Paul Stein, and John Hardy who supplied original photographs for reproduction. I wish also to thank many of my colleagues, friends, and former students who read parts of the manuscripts and offered valuable suggestions. To Virginia Stephens I am grateful for typing the manuscript. Finally, I wish to thank the editorial and production staff of Springer-Verlag for their care and cooperation in producing this book.

In spite of great care and effort on my part, I am sure that many mistakes and defects remain in the book. I hope you will bring these to my attention so that I can improve in the future.

La Jolla, California   YUAN-CHENG FUNG

Contents

CHAPTER 1

Physical Principles of Circulation

1.1 The Conservation Laws

Blood flow must obey the principles of conservation of mass, momentum, and energy. Applied to any given region of space, the principle of conservation of mass means that whatever flows in must flow out. If flow is confined to blood vessels, then we obtain a rule similar to Kirchhoff's law of electric circuits: At any junction the summation of current flowing into a junction must be equal to the sum of the currents flowing out of that junction. In a single tube of variable cross section, a steady flow implies that the local velocity is inversely proportional to the local cross-sectional area.

Conservation of momentum means that the momentum of matter cannot be changed without the action of force. If there is force acting on a body, then according to the Newton's law of motion, the rate of change of momentum of the body is equal to the force.

Everyone knows these principles. Don't let familiarity breed contempt. Think of this: We are able to fly to the moon precisely because we know Newton's law. The ancient Greeks, with their superior knowledge about anatomy of the heart and blood vessels, were robbed of the glory of discovering blood circulation because they did not think of the principle of conservation of mass! The Western world had to wait for William Harvey (1578–1657) to establish the concept of circulation. Harvey remembered the principle of conservation of mass, all he needed was to show that in every heart beat there is a net flow of blood out of the heart!

There is nothing more cost-effective than learning the general principles and remembering to apply them.

1

1.2 The Forces that Drive or Resist Blood Flow

What are the forces that drive the blood flow? They are the gravitational force and the pressure gradient. The pressure in a blood vessel varies from point to point. The rate of change of pressure with distance is the pressure gradient. Pressure itself does not cause the blood to move; the pressure gradient does.

What are the forces that oppose blood flow? They are the shear stresses due to viscosity of the blood and turbulences.

We use the term "stress" to mean the force acting on a surface divided by the area of the surface. In the International System of Units the unit of stress is Newton per square meter, or Pascal. The stress acting on any surface can be resolved into two components: the shear stress, which is the component tangent to the surface, and the normal stress, which is the component perpendicular (i.e., normal) to a surface. Pressure is a normal stress. A

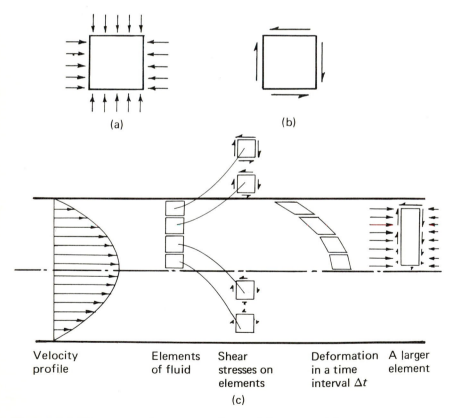

(a)   (b)

Velocity   Elements   Shear   Deformation   A larger
profile   of fluid   stresses on   in a time   element
                              elements   interval Δt

(c)

Figure 1.2:1 The concept of pressure gradient and divergence of shear stresses as motive forces for motion.

positive pressure is regarded as a negative normal stress. A positive normal stress is a tensile stress.

Figure 1.2:1(a) shows a small rectangular element of blood subjected to equal pressure on all sides. The element remains in equilibrium.

Figure 1.2:1(b) shows an element subjected to shear stresses that are equal on all sides. The element will be distorted by the shear stresses, but there will be no tendency to accelerate.

Figure 1.2:1(c) shows a steady flow of a fluid in a tube. The velocity distribution is indicated on the left. To its right, a series of fluid elements is shown. The shear stresses acting on these elements are indicated by the arrows, with their magnitude proportional to their lengths. These shear stresses will distort the elements, whose shapes after a certain interval of time are shown. If these elements are stacked together as shown by the larger rectangular element on the right, we see that the horizontal shear force (= stress × area) at the top is larger than the shear force on the bottom. The resultant of these shear forces is the force that resists the motion of this element. The resultant of the vertical shear forces acting on the two sides of the element is zero. On the other hand, the pressure on the left hand side of the element is larger than that on the right hand side. The difference of pressure per unit axial distance is the pressure gradient. The resultant pressure force (= pressure × area) is the force that drives the fluid to flow. In a blood vessel, the pressure and shear forces coexist and balance each other. If, together with the gravitational force, an exact balance is achieved, then the flow is steady. If the forces are out of balance, then the fluid either accelerates or decelerates.

1.3 Newton's Law of Motion Applied to a Fluid

Newton's law states that

$$\text{Mass} \times \text{acceleration} = \text{force}.$$

Applied to a fluid, it takes the following form, which will be explained in detail below:

Density × (transient acceleration + convective acceleration)
    = −pressure gradient + divergence of normal and shear stresses   (1)
    + gravitational force.

Here *density* refers to the density of blood, the *transient acceleration* refers to the rate of change of velocity with respect to time, and the *convective acceleration* refers to the rate of change of velocity of a fluid particle caused by the motion of the particle from one place to another in a nonuniform flow field. *Pressure gradient* has been explained in Sec. 1.2. The *divergence of normal and shear stresses* refers to the rate of change of those stresses arising from fluid viscosity and turbulences. The word "divergence" is a mathematical term refering to certain process of differentiation explained in detail in the Appendix at the end of this book. *Gravitational force* means weight per unit volume of the fluid, i.e., the density of the fluid multiplied by the gravitational acceleration.

Transient and convective accelerations exist in most problems of interest to biomechanics. Figure 1.3:1 shows a record of the velocity of flow in the center of the canine ascending aorta. It is seen that the velocity changes with time. In fact, the velocity record changes from one heart beat to another. An average of a large number of records is called an *ensemble average.* The difference between the velocity history of a specific record and the ensemble average is considered to be turbulence. Figure 1.3:1 shows the turbulence velocity of a specified record, and the root mean square values of the turbulence velocity of all records of the ensemble. The *partial derivative* of the velocity with respect to time is the transient acceleration at any given point in a fluid.

Convective acceleration also exists in most problems in bioengineering because interesting flow fields are usually nonuniform. See, for example, Figs. 1.5:1 and 2.5:5 for the closure of the mitral valve, Fig. 3.2:3 for entry flow in a tube, Fig. 3.7:2 for a pulsatile flow, and Fig. 3.17:1 for a flow separation from a solid wall. In each case, we can calculate the partial derivatives of the nonuniform velocity components with respect to the spatial coordinates. This set of partial derivatives forms a velocity gradient tensor. The product of the velocity vector and the velocity gradient tensor (by a process called *contraction*) gives us the convective acceleration. Detailed mathematical expressions of these products are given in Section A.2 of the *Appendix* at the end of this book.

Gravitational force is important. If our blood were to stop flowing, then blood pressure would vary with height just as water pressure in a swimming pool does. The blood pressure at any point in the body is the sum of the static pressure due to gravity and the pressure due to the pumping action of the heart and the frictional loss in the blood vessels. Hence the blood pressure in our body is a continuous variable which changes from place to place and from time to time.

In a soft, tenuous organ such as the lung, the effect of gravity is particularly evident. Due to the lung weight, in an upright posture the lung tissue at the apex of the lung is stretched much more than that at the base. As a consequence, the alveoli at the apex of our lungs are larger than those above the diaphragm, whereas the capillary blood vessels at the apex are much narrower than those at the base. The static pressure of blood at the apex is less than that at the base by an amount equal to the height of the lung times the specific weight of the blood. Since pulmonary capillary blood vessels are very compliant, the lumen size varies with this static pressure. As a result, blood flow in the lung varies with the height. In an upright position there could be virtually no blood flow in the apex region and full flow at the base, whereas in the middle region there is flow limitation. This example points

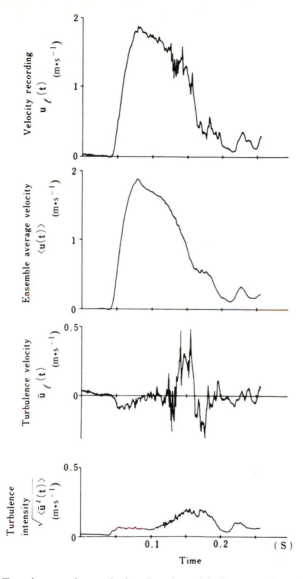

Figure 1.3:1 Transient motion: velocity changing with time at a given location. The partial derivative of velocity with respect to time while the location is fixed is the transient acceleration. The example shown here is from a paper by Yamaguchi, T., Kikkawa, S., Yoshikawa, T., Tanishita, K., and Sugawara, M,: Measurement of turbulent intensity in the center of the canine ascending aorta with a hot-film anemometer. *J. Biomechanical Engineering* **105**: 177–187, 1983. The first panel shows a recording of blood velocity history. The second panel gives an ensemble average of many experiments. The third panel is a sample of turbulence velocity history. The fourth panel gives the root-mean-square of the turbulence velocity, or the so-called turbulence intensity.

out another basic physical principle of blood flow: The blood vessel dimension is a function of the blood pressure, and the feedback influence between these two variables can have dramatic effects at times.

The other two terms in the equation of motion, Eq. (1), the gradient of pressure and the divergence of normal and shear stresses, have been discussed earlier. The shear stresses are proportional to the coefficient of viscosity of the fluid and the rate of change of strains.

Shear stresses are strongly influenced by turbulences, if any. In a fluid, turbulences are random motions whose statistical characteristics can be predicted, but for which the exact value of the velocity of any particle at a particular instant of time and at a given point in space is unpredictable.

1.4 The Importance of Turbulence

Turbulence dissipates energy. If a laminar flow in a tube turns turbulent, the resistance to flow may be increased greatly. The shear stress acting on the blood vessel endothelium may be increased many times when a laminar flow becomes turbulent.

We may think of an axisymmetric flow of blood in a blood vessel as the

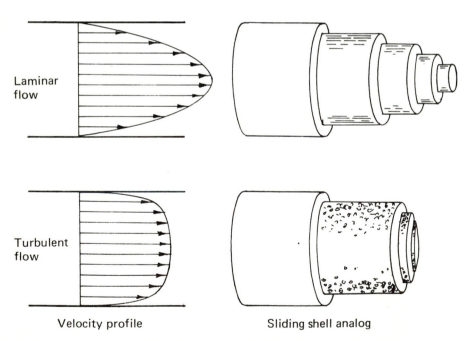

Figure 1.4:1 Schematic representation of fully developed laminar and turbulent flows in a tube at the same flow rate. The time-averaged velocity vectors are plotted in this figure as functions of spatial coordinates.

sliding of a series of concentric tubes of fluid as illustrated in Fig. 1.4:1. Then the differences between laminar and turbulent flows in the tube are twofold. First, the velocity profiles are different: the laminar flow has a parabolic profile, the turbulent flow has a profile which is much blunter at the central portion of the tube, and much sharper at the wall. Hence, the shear strain rate at the tube wall is much higher in the turbulent case as compared with a laminar flow of the same rate of volume flow. Secondly, the coefficients of friction or viscosity between the concentric tubes are different in these two cases. The "effective" or "apparent" coefficient of friction for the turbulent case is much higher than that of the laminar case. This is indicated by a smooth shading of the surfaces of the sliding cylinders in the laminar case and the rough appearance in the turbulent case. The viscosity, or friction, in the laminar case is due to molecular motion between the sliding cylinders. The friction in the turbulent case comes from two sources: the molecular transport which is usually the smaller part, and the convection of the turbulent "eddies" which is often the greater part. The shear stress in a fluid being equal to the product of the coefficient of viscosity and the shear strain rate, it is easy to see that the wall friction can become much larger if a laminar flow becomes turbulent. Turbulence is controllable to a certain degree, and the success of many medical devices depends on such control through good engineering design.

Turbulence in blood flow is strongly implicated in atherogenesis. Atherosclerotic plaques are often found at sites of turbulence in the aorta.

Associated with the velocity fluctuations in a turbulent flow are pressure fluctuations. Pressure fluctuations can excite vibrations in the ear drum and cochlea and can be heard if the frequencies are in the audible range. We can hear the howling of wind because the wind is turbulent. We can hear jet noise if the jet flow is turbulent. The Korotkov sound at systole is the sound of jet noise of the rushing blood. A heart murmur is a turbulent noise. Flow separation at a site of stenosis in an artery often causes turbulence in the separated region; making it possible to detect a stenosis by listening to the noise in the blood flow with a stethoscope.

1.5 Deceleration as a Generator of Pressure Gradient

If there is no turbulence and if the gravitational and frictional forces are small enough to be ignored, then Eq. (1) of Sec. 1.3 becomes

$$\text{Density} \times \text{acceleration} = -\text{pressure gradient}. \qquad (2)$$

Hence if the acceleration is negative (i.e., decelerating), then the left-hand side of Eq. (2) is negative and the right-hand side yields a positive pressure gradient. In other words, in a decelerating fluid the pressure increases in the direction of flow. This mechanism is used effectively in our bodies to operate the heart valves and the valves in the veins and lymphatics.

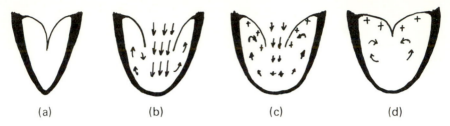

Figure 1.5:1 The operation of the mitral valve. (a) End of systole; (b) Mitral valve wide open, jet rushing in; (c) toward end of diastole, jet being broken. The deceleration creates a pressure gradient that tends to close the valve. (d) Mitral valve closed.

The Principle of Heart Valve Closure

Figure 1.5:1 shows the operation of the mitral valve. The mitral valve is composed of two very flexible, thin membranes. These membranes are pushed open at a stage of diastole when the pressure in the left atrium exceeds that of the left ventricle. Then a jet of blood rushes in from the left atrium into the left ventricle, impinges on the ventricular wall, and is broken up there. Thus, the blood stream is decelerated in its path and a positive pressure gradient is created. Toward the end of diastole the pressure acting on the ventricular side of the mitral valve membranes becomes higher than that acting on the side of the membranes facing the jet. The net force acts to close the valve. In a normal heart, closure occurs *without* any backward flow or regurgitation. The papillary muscles play no role at all in the opening and closing of the valve. They serve to generate systolic pressure in the isovolumetric condition by pulling on the membranes, and to prevent inversion of the valves into the atrium in systole.

   The same principle applies to the aortic valve (Fig. 2.5:4, p. 44) as well as the valves of the veins and lymphatics. Deceleration is the essence, not backward flow.

1.6 Pressure and Flow in Blood Vessels—Generalized Bernoulli's Equation

If we know the pressure and velocity of blood at one station in the blood vessel and wish to compute the pressure and velocity at another station, we may integrate Eq. (1) along a streamline, or more directly, we may consider the balance between the changes in kinetic, potential, and internal energies and the work done on the blood by forces acting on it. Consider a system of blood vessels, as illustrated in Fig. 1.6:1. Let the distance along a blood vessel be denoted by a variable x. Consider blood in the vessel between two stations, 1 and 2, located at $x = 0$ and $x = x$. Then we can derive the following equation from Eq. (1) (see Sec. 1.11 for details):

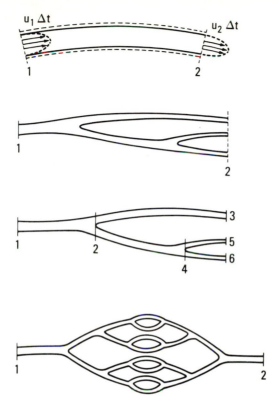

Figure 1.6:1 Two arbitrary stations, 1 and 2, in a blood vessel system. The energy equation (3) and that derived in Sec. 1.11 are applicable to any one of the systems illustrated here. In the uppermost figure the solid lines show the instantaneous boundary of the fluid in the vessel between stations 1 and 2 at an instant of time t; the dotted lines show the boundary at a time Δt later; u_1 and u_2 are the velocities of flow at stations 1 and 2.

Pressure at station 0 − pressure at station x

$$= \tfrac{1}{2} \cdot \text{density} \cdot (\text{velocity at } x)^2 - \tfrac{1}{2} \cdot \text{density} \cdot (\text{velocity at } 0)^2$$
$$+ (\text{specific weight}) (\text{height difference of station } x \text{ and station } 0)$$
$$+ \text{rate of change of the kinetic energy of blood between stations}$$
$$x \text{ and } 0 \tag{3}$$
$$+ \text{integrated frictional loss between stations } x \text{ and } 0.$$

If the last two lines can be ignored, then we have the famous *Bernoulli's equation*. It says that pressure can be converted from kinetic energy of motion and potential energy of height, provided that the flow is steady and the fluid is inviscid. Pressure rises when the velocity of flow is slowed down, and vice versa. Bernoulli's equation is useful to analyze pressure and flow in a tube in steady condition, and is used very often to calibrate flow-measuring instruments, pressure transducers, and flow meters.

For flow in blood vessels it is usually necessary to include more terms of Eq. (3) than are in the Bernoulli's equation. For flow in normal aorta and vena cava, the last term in Eq. (3) can be neglected, but all the other terms must be retained.

For flow in small blood vessels, the last term of Eq. (3) is not negligible. The smaller the blood vessel, the more significant the frictional loss becomes. In microcirculation, in blood vessels with diameters 100 μm and less, the last term of Eq. (3) becomes the predominant term on the right-hand side of the equation. In the capillary blood vessels the pressure drop balances the frictional loss exclusively.

1.7 Analysis of Total Peripheral Flow Resistance

If we read the Generalized Bernoulli's Equation (3) of the preceding section by putting station $x = 0$ in the aorta at the aortic valve and station x in the vena cava at the right atrium, then the velocities of flow at the two stations are approximately equal and the heights of these two stations are the same, so that the first two lines on the right-hand side of Eq. (3) vanish. Furthermore, if we make measurements of average pressure and flow over a period of time extended over several cycles of oscillation, then the third line on the right-hand side of Eq. (3) will average out to zero because it oscillates on the positive and negative sides equally. In this case Eq. (3) becomes

$$\text{Average pressure at aortic valve} - \text{average pressure at right atrium} = \text{integrated frictional loss.} \tag{4}$$

This is often written as

$$\text{Systemic arterial pressure} = \text{flow} \times \text{resistance.} \tag{5}$$

Here the *systemic arterial pressure* is the difference between the pressure at the aortic valve and that at the vena cava at the right atrium, the flow is the *cardiac output*, and the resistance is the *total peripheral vascular resistance*. Hence, writing in greater detail, we have

$$\text{Pressure at aortic valve} - \text{pressure at right atrium} = (\text{cardiac output}) \times (\text{total peripheral vascular resistance}). \tag{6}$$

The last term in Eq. (4) represents the sum of the pressure drops due to the friction loss along all segments of blood vessels. Since there are millions of capillary blood vessels in the body, there are millions of pathways along which one can integrate Eq. (1) to obtain Eqs. (3) and (4); the final result (Eq. (4)) is useful only if the pressures at the aortic valve and right atrium are uniform no matter which path of integration is used. Fortunately, this is true.

Thus, if we define

$$\text{Total peripheral vascular resistance} = \frac{\text{integrated frictional loss}}{\text{cardiac output}} \tag{7}$$

then Eq. (5) or (6) is obtained. Hence, the systemic arterial pressure is equal to the product of cardiac output and total peripheral vascular resistance.

The integrated frictional loss is the sum of frictional losses in all segments of vessels of the circuit. To compute the frictional loss of a segment let us consider first a steady laminar flow (i.e., one that is not turbulent) in a long, rigid, circular, cylindrical tube. Such a flow is governed by the famous *Hagen–Poiseuille Law* (or more commonly, *Poiseuille's law*), which states that the flow $\dot{Q}$ (short for "flow rate" or "volume flow rate," i.e., the volume of fluid flowing through a vessel in unit time) is related to the pressure drop Δp by the equation:

$$\dot{Q} = \frac{\pi d^4}{128} \frac{\Delta p}{\mu L}. \tag{8}$$

Here d is the diameter of the vessel, μ is the coefficient of viscosity of the fluid, and L is the length of the segment of vessel over which the pressure drop Δp is measured. Equation (8) can be written as

$$\Delta p = \text{laminar resistance in a tube} \times \text{flow in the tube}, \tag{9}$$

from which we obtain the resistance of a steady laminar flow in a circular cylindrical tube:

$$\text{Laminar resistance in a tube} = \frac{128 \mu L}{\pi d^4}. \tag{10}$$

If the nth generation of a vascular tree consists of N identical vessels in parallel, then the

Pressure drop in the nth generation of vessels
$$= \text{resistance in } N \text{ parallel tubes} \times \text{total flow in } N \text{ tubes} \tag{11}$$
$$= \frac{\text{resistance in one tube}}{N} \times \text{cardiac output}.$$

Note that according to Eq. (10) the laminar flow resistance is proportional to the coefficient of viscosity μ and the length of the vessel L, and *inversely proportional to the fourth power of the diameter, d.* Obviously the vessel diameter d is the most effective parameter to control the resistance. A reduction of diameter by a factor of 2 raises the resistance 16-fold, and hence leads to a 16-fold pressure loss. In peripheral circulation the arterioles are muscular and they control the blood flow distribution by changing the vessel diameters through contraction or relaxation of the vascular smooth muscles.

Equation (10) gives the resistance to a Poiseuillean flow in a pipe and is the minimum of resistance of all possible flows in a pipe. If the flow becomes turbulent, the resistance increases. If the blood vessel bifurcates, the local disturbance at the bifurcation region raises resistance. In these deviations from the Poiseuillean flow the governing parameter is a dimensionless number called the *Reynolds number* (in honor of Osborne Reynolds), which is the ratio of the inertia force to the viscous force in the flow:

$$\text{Reynolds number} = N_R = \frac{\text{inertia force}}{\text{viscous force}}$$

$$= \frac{\text{velocity of flow} \times \text{vessel diameter}}{\text{kinematic viscosity of fluid}}. \tag{12}$$

The kinematic viscosity is defined as the coefficient of viscosity divided by the density of the fluid. The flow in a vessel usually becomes turbulent when the Reynolds number exceeds a critical value of approximately 2300 (with exact value depending on the pulse rate and on whether the flow rate is increasing or decreasing). If a flow is turbulent, then

Resistance of a turbulent flow in a vessel
$$= (\text{laminar resistance}) \cdot (0.005 \ N_R^{3/4}). \tag{13}$$

Thus, if the Reynolds number is 3000, the resistance of a turbulent flow is over two times that of the laminar resistance. In the ascending and descending aorta of man and dog the peak Reynolds number does exceed 3000.

1.8 The Importance of Blood Rheology

For large blood vessels the resistance to flow is a function of the Reynolds number as discussed in the preceding section. For smaller blood vessels, the Reynolds numbers are smaller. Somewhere at the level of the smallest arteries and veins the Reynolds number becomes 1. Microvessels with further reduction of diameter will have a Reynolds number less than 1. From the definition of Reynolds number given in Eq. (12) we see that in these microvessels the viscous force dominates the scene. In capillary blood vessels, the Reynolds number is of the order of 10^{-2} or smaller, the inertia force becomes unimportant, and the flow is controlled almost entirely by the viscous force and pressure. Blood rheology then plays a vital role. This is because the coefficient of viscosity of blood, μ, figures importantly in Eqs. (8), and (10).

We have discussed blood rheology quite thoroughly in the book *Biomechanics: Mechanical Properties of Living Tissues* (Fung, 1981). For flow in the microvessels, we speak of the *apparent coefficient of viscosity* of blood to take into account the interactions of blood cells, plasma, and blood vessel wall. The apparent coefficient of viscosity is the value of μ that keeps Eq. (8) valid. It is obtained experimentally by measuring $\dot{Q}$, d, Δp, and L and using Eq. (8) to compute μ. The apparent coefficient of viscosity of blood in microvessels can be greatly increased under the following conditions:

(a) Existence of large leucocytes or exceptionally large erythrocytes with diameters greater than that of the capillary blood vessel. The vessel may be occluded by these cells.

(b) The smooth muscle in the arterioles or in the sphinctors of the capillaries may contract so that the diameters of these vessels are greatly reduced, causing the effect described in (a) to take place. The contraction of the smooth muscle may be initiated by nerves, by metabolites, or by mechanical stimulation. The vascular smooth muscle has a peculiar property to respond to a stretching by contraction.

(c) The leucocytes have a tendency to adhere to the blood vessel wall. If they do, they increase resistance to blood flow. The thrombocytes may be activated, causing clotting and increasing resistance.

(d) Cell flexibility may be changed. Hardening of the red blood cell, as in sickle cell disease, increases the coefficient of viscosity of the blood.

The effects (b) and (c), besides controlling the apparent coefficient of viscosity, effectively controls the vessel diameter. Since the vessel diameter appears in Eqs. (8) and (10) in fourth power, its importance is obvious.

1.9 The Mechanics of Circulation

The brief analysis presented in the preceding sections demonstrates how some very important results can be obtained by applying the laws of conservation of mass and momentum to the circulatory system. From a few pieces of information about the anatomy of the heart and blood vessels, we were able to derive the pressure-flow relationship which furnishes the basic principle for the understanding of the perfusion of organs, the control of blood pressure, and the operation of heart valves. These results are characterized by their simple and precise quantitative nature. From these examples we can anticipate that when more specific information about the physical properties of the circulation system is added, more penetrating specific results will be obtained. Some of them will help clarify the physiology and pathology of the organs, others will lead to diagnostic and clinical tools. The rest of this book will develop this theme.

1.10 A Little Bit of History

In Western culture, the concept of blood circulation was established by William Harvey (1578–1657). It was surprisingly late in history. In the early history of Greek physiology, there was a great error in the notion that the heart was the focus of respiration, as well as the center of the vascular system. Thus, it is not a coincidence that the original meaning of the Greek word "arteria" was "windpipe." Aristotle (384–322 B.C.) considered the heart as the focus of the blood vessels, but he made no distinction between arteries and veins and showed no signs of any knowledge of the cardiac valves. Aristotle's conception was an enormous improvement over the most famous of the earlier treatises of the "Hippocratic" corpus, *the Sacred Disease* (i.e., epilepsy), which regards the head as the starting point of the main blood vessels.

At the beginning of the third century B.C., if not earlier, Praxagoras found that the two separate great trunks of blood vessels—still all called veins— are different. One is about six times thicker than the other. In a corpse the veins collapse if emptied of blood, the arteries do not. Praxagoras insisted that the arteries contain no blood but only air. This mistaken idea of Praxagoras, more than any other single factor, prevented the ancients from arriving at the discovery of the circulation of the blood. How did Praxagoras reach such a conclusion? According to Harris (1980), it was probably based on the observation that when he cut open the chest of the animal which he dissected, the main arteries were found to be empty and full of air. Recently, Fåhraeus (1957) explained this phenomenon by the dilation of small arteries after death. Fåhraeus measured the pressures in the carotid or femoral artery in corpses at least 24 hours after death, and found them to be negative, varying from a few mm to 1 cm Hg. If one begin an autopsy and open the thoracic cage at that time, the pressure would rise to zero by sucking air into the arteries. Fåhraeus believes that the negative pressure arises due to dilation of the arterial system. He reasoned that this dilation cannot take place in the large arteries; it must therefore be the little arteries that dilate and draw a certain amount of blood from the large arteries. He found that the phenomenon varies with the age of the person. The height of the negative pressure increases sharply from the age of 18 to 70 and then remains relatively constant. Nor is it instantaneous at the moment of death. Perhaps this may also explain why the author of *De Corde* found the ventricle, but not the aorta, empty, (Harris, 1980).

The picture that evolved to the Greeks was that the arteries provide organs with pneuma, veins provide them with blood, and nerves endow muscles with the power of contraction.

In China, the concept of circulation was stated very clearly in one of the oldest books on medicine, the *Nei Jing* (內經), or "Internal Classic." The authorship of this book was attributed to Huang Ti (黃帝) or the *Yellow Emperor* (2697–2597 B.C., according to the dictionary 辭源). But most Chinese scholars believe that it was written by anonymous authors in the *Warring Period* (戰國時代, 475–221 B.C.). It was written in the style of conversations between the Emperor and his officials, discussing medicine and its relationship to heaven, earth, climate, seasons, day, and night. It has 18 chapters; the first 9 are called *Su Wen* (素問), or "Plain Questions," the second 9 are called *Ling Shu* (靈樞), or "Miraculous Pivot." In the chapter 脉要精微論篇 in Su Wen, it states that "the blood vessels are where blood is retained" (夫脉者, 血之府也). In the chapter 五臟生成篇 in Su Wen, it states that "all blood in the vessels originates from the heart" (諸血者, 皆屬於心). In *Ling Shu* 營衛生會第十八, it states that "(the blood and *Chi*) circulate without stopping. In fifty steps they return to the starting point. Yin succeeds Yang, and vice versa, like a circle without an end" (營周不休, 五十而復大會, 陰陽相貫, 如環之無端).

Chi (氣) is a concept not familiar to Western thinking, but it was central to the Chinese idea of life. In the Chinese language Chi means gas; but it may also mean spirit (精氣). When a man would rather die than surrender, you say he has Chi Tsi (氣節). When a person is willing to labor or suffer for his friend without a thought about compensation, you say he has Yi Chi (義氣). The physiological concept of Chi was derived from ancient Chinese's experimentation on acupuncture. The Chi circulates along the "meridional lines" (經絡), on which the acupunctural "points" (穴位) are located. The "points" are where the needle should be inserted. What Chi is, exactly, is not clear even today, but the thought is that it is something that circulates.

1.11 The Energy Balance Equation

Equation (3) in Sec. 1.6 is a very important one. It is especially useful in studying complex situations, such as the blood flow in the aortic arch or air flow in the trachea, in which the pressure gradient in the radial direction can be as large as the pressure gradient in the axial direction. In such a situation an accurate measurement of the pressure field is beyond the state of the art. On the other hand, current technology does permit a detailed measurement of the velocity field. Then the use of Eq. (3) of Sec. 1.6 would enable us to compute the pressure p.

Because of its importance, let us consider the derivation of this equation in detail in order to obtain a deeper insight, and therefore gain greater confidence in using it.

Consider the blood in a portion of the blood vessel system between two stations, 1 and 2 (Fig. 1.6:1). Since the rate of gain of energy (the sum of the kinetic, potential, and internal energies) must be equal to the sum of the rate at which work is done on the system and the heat transported in, the energy balance of the blood may be stated by the following equation:

(Rate at which pressure force at station 1 does work on blood)   (1)

+ (rate at which pressure force at station 2 does work on blood)   (2)

+ (rate at which pressure and shear on vessel wall do work on blood)   (3)

+ (rate at which heat is transported into the system)   (4)

= (rate of change of the kinetic energy of blood in the volume)   (5)

+ (rate at which kinetic energy is carried by particles leaving
the vessel at station 2)   (6)

− (rate at which kinetic energy is carried by particles
entering the vessel at station 1)   (7)

+ (rate at which kinetic energy is carried across the blood
vessel wall)   (8)

+ (rate of gain of potential energy of blood against gravity)   (9)

+ (rate of change of internal energy in the volume).   (10)

This equation is long, but obvious, except for the signs of the terms (6), (7), and (8). To explain these signs, we must remember that this equation is written for the *fluid particles* which occupy the volume in the blood vessel between stations 1 and 2 instantaneously. But these fluid particles are moving, so that in an infinitesimal time interval Δt later, the boundary of the space occupied by the fluid particles is no longer the original vessel wall and cross sections 1 and 2, but has become the new vessel wall and the curved surfaces, as illustrated in the uppermost figure in Fig. 1.6:1. Hence the change of kinetic energy (K.E.) of the *fluid particles* is equal to the change of K.E. in the *original volume* (bounded by the solid lines in the figure *plus* the K.E. of the particles that entered into the shaded area in the figure. The term (5) represents the rate of change of K.E. in the original volume; (6) represents the K.E. in the shaded area at the right; (7) represents the K.E. in the shaded area at the left, which does *not* belong to the original group of fluid particles, and hence has to be subtracted. The term (8) represents the K.E. in the shaded area bounding the vessel wall. The sum of (5), (6), (7), (8) is the rate of change of the K.E. of the fluid particles in the vessel between stations 1 and 2.

Let us translate this statement into a mathematical expression. Let us first identify the various rates listed in the equation above. First, the rate at which the pressure force acting on a small area dA does work on a fluid flowing across that surface with velocity u is equal to $pudA$, where u is the velocity component normal to the surface dA. Thus the rate at which the pressure force does work on the fluid passing station 1 is given by an integral over the cross section A_1:

$$\int_{A_1} pudA. \tag{1'}$$

A similar expression is obtained at station 2, except that a negative sign is needed because the pressure and u act in opposite directions. The expression for the work done on the vessel wall is also similar, and can be written as

$$\int_{S} \overset{v}{T}_i u_i dA, \tag{3'}$$

where $\overset{\scriptscriptstyle v}{T}_i$ is the stress vector acting on the surface of the vessel wall of area dA and normal v (with components $i = 1, 2, 3$ in the directions of a rectangular cartesian coordinate system x_1, x_2, x_3), and u_i is the velocity vector with components u_1, u_2, u_3. The integration is taken over the entire surface of contact between the blood and the vessel wall, S. Repetition of the index i means summation over i from 1 to 3.

The kinetic energy per unit volume of a small fluid element is $\frac{1}{2}\rho q^2$, where ρ is the density of the fluid and q is the speed of the element, i.e., $q^2 = u_1^2 + u_2^2 + u_3^2$. The rate at which kinetic energy is changing at any given place is given by its partial derivative with respect to time. Hence the rate of change of the K.E. in the volume V is

$$\int_V \frac{\partial}{\partial t}\left(\frac{1}{2}\rho q^2\right) dv. \tag{5}'$$

The rate at which the K.E. is carried out by particles crossing the instantaneous boundary at station 2 is

$$\int_{A_2} \frac{1}{2}\rho q^2 u\, dA. \tag{6}'$$

That at station 1 is given by a similar integral. The K.E. carried out of the instantaneous boundary by particles at the blood vessel wall is given by an expression similar to Eq. (3)', with $\overset{\scriptscriptstyle v}{T}_i$ replaced by $\frac{1}{2}\rho q^2$, and u_i replaced by the component of velocity normal to the vessel wall.

As it was explained earlier, the sum of (5), (6), (7), and (8) is the rate of change of the K.E. of all fluid particles that occupy instantaneously the space in the blood vessel between stations 1 and 2. Mathematically, it is represented by the so-called *material derivative* of the kinetic energy, and is denoted by the symbol D/Dt:

$$(5) + (6) + (7) + (8) = \frac{D}{Dt}\int \frac{1}{2}\rho q^2\, dA. \tag{11}$$

The potential energy of blood against gravity is ρgh per unit volume, where ρ is the density of the fluid, g is the gravitational acceleration, and h is the height of the fluid element. The total potential energy of the fluid particles that occupy the volume V instantaneously is

$$G = \int_V \rho gh\, dv, \tag{12}$$

and its rate of change is DG/Dt, and can be broken down into four integrals as in the case of the kinetic energy.

Finally, the change of internal energy is due to the generation of heat through viscosity. It can be shown that this is equal to the scalar product of the stress tensor σ_{ij} and strain rate tensor V_{ij},

$$V_{ij} = \frac{1}{2}\left(\frac{\partial u_i}{\partial x_j} + \frac{\partial u_j}{\partial x_i}\right).$$

Hence, the last term, the rate of dissipation of mechanical energy, is given by

$$\int_V \sigma_{ij} V_{ij} dv. \tag{13}$$

See Fung (1977, Sec. 10.8, pp. 255, 256) for a rigorous derivation.

Summarizing the above, we obtain the following energy equation:

$$\int_{A_1} pudA - \int_{A_2} pudA + \int_S \overset{v}{T}_i u_i dA + \text{heat input}$$

$$= \int_{A_2} \frac{1}{2}\rho q^2 udA - \int_{A_1} \frac{1}{2}\rho q^2 udA + \int_S \frac{1}{2}\rho q^2 u_i v_i dA$$

$$+ \int_V \frac{\partial}{\partial t}\left(\frac{1}{2}\rho q^2\right) dv + \frac{D}{Dt}\int_V \rho g h dv \tag{14}$$

$$+ \int_V \sigma_{ij} V_{ij} dv.$$

For the blood flow problem, usually some of the terms may be neglected. The heat input is often small. The deformation of the vessel wall may be so small that both the work done by the wall force and the kinetic energy crossing the vessel wall are negligible. Then the third and fourth terms on the left-hand side of the equation and the third term on the right can be omitted, and the gravitational potential term is simplified into $(\rho g h_2 - \rho g h_1)$ times the flow rate, h_1, h_2 being the height of stations 1 and 2, respectively.

The final equation is simplifed if we define a characteristic pressure $\hat{p}$ and a characteristic square of velocity $\hat{q^2}$ as follows:

$$\hat{p} = \frac{1}{Q}\int pudA, \qquad \hat{q^2} = \frac{1}{Q}\int q^2 udA, \tag{15}$$

where Q is the volume flow rate

$$Q = \int udA. \tag{16}$$

Then on dividing Eq. (14) by Q and writing $\mathscr{D}$ for the dissipation function

$$\mathscr{D} = \int \sigma_{ij} V_{ij} dv, \tag{17}$$

we have

$$\hat{p}_1 - \hat{p}_2 = \frac{1}{2}\rho\hat{q^2_2} - \frac{1}{2}\rho\hat{q^2_1} + \rho g h_2 - \rho g h_1 + \frac{\mathscr{D}}{Q} + \frac{1}{Q}\int \frac{\partial}{\partial t}\left(\frac{1}{2}\rho q^2\right) dv. \tag{18}$$

This final equation is most useful and important. If it is applied to a stream tube (a tube whose wall is composed of streamlines) of such a small cross section that the velocity and shear stress may be considered as uniform in it, then Eq. (3) of Sec. 1.6 results. If it is applied to tubes of finite cross section, then the definition of $\hat{p}$, $\hat{q^2}$, and $\mathscr{D}$ must be rigorously observed. For example, in Sec. 1.6 we speak of the pressure at the aortic valve. But the pressure varies from point to point at the aortic valve, and no single pressure can be assumed at the section. One might suggest to take the mean value, i.e., $(\int p\,dA)/A$, as "the" pressure, but that is not necessarily the p required by the energy equation. Similarly, the "square of velocity" would have to be $\hat{q^2}$. $\hat{p}$, $\hat{q^2}$ are "velocity-weighted" averages. If the pressure p is uniform over a cross section then $p = \hat{p}$. If the velocity u is uniform over the cross section, then $\hat{q^2} = u^2$. If the velocity profile is parabolic as in Poiseuille flow, then $\hat{u^2} = 2\bar{u}^2$, where $\bar{u}$ is the average value of u.

Equation (18) is a generalization of the Bernoulli's equation to viscous and nonstationary flows. It makes it possible for us to speak of "pressure drop" in terms of quantities that can be calculated from velocity measurements. It can be applied to the gas flow in the airway, and become the foundation on which the pulmonary ventilation theory is built.

Recapitulation

Although the energy principle is straightforward, the detailed statement above is long. Let us recapitulate it in another way. Recall a general formula for the material derivative for any integral of a function Φ over all the fluid particles in a volume V which is bounded by a surface S:

$$\frac{D}{Dt}\int_V \Phi\,dv = \int_V \frac{\partial \Phi}{\partial t}\,dv + \int_S \Phi v_j v_j\,dS, \tag{19}$$

where $\mathbf{v}$, with components v_1, v_2, v_3, is the velocity of the fluid, and $\mathbf{v}$, with components v_1, v_2, v_3, is the unit vector normal to the surface, and the summation convention is used: Repetition of an index means summation over the index. See Fung, (1977, Sec. 10.4, pp. 248–250). Applying this to the kinetic energy K, given by $\frac{1}{2}\rho q^2$ integrated over a volume V of the blood bounded by the wall S and cross sections A_1 and A_2 (Fig. 1.6:1), we obtain:

$$\frac{DK}{Dt} = \frac{D}{Dt}\int_V \frac{1}{2}\rho q^2\,dv = \int_V \frac{\partial}{\partial t}\left(\frac{1}{2}\rho q^2\right)dv$$
$$+ \int_{A_2} \frac{1}{2}\rho q^2 u_2\,dA_2 - \int_{A_1} \frac{1}{2}\rho q^2 u_1\,dA_1 + \int_S \frac{1}{2}\rho q^2 u_n\,dS, \tag{20}$$

where u_1, u_2, u_n are, respectively, velocity components normal to the cross sections A_1, A_2, and the vessel wall S. The right-hand side of Eq. (20) is the sum $(5) + (6) + (7) + (8)$ above.

Similar expressions are obtained for the gravitational energy G and the internal energy E:

$$G = \int_V \rho g h\,dv, \qquad E = \int_V \rho \mathscr{E}\,dv, \tag{21}$$

where $\mathscr{E}$ is the specific internal energy per unit mass of the fluid. The first law of thermodynamics states that

$$\frac{D}{Dt}(K + G + E) = \dot{W} + \dot{H}, \tag{22}$$

where $\dot{W}$ is the rate at which work is done on the fluid and $\dot{H}$ is the rate at which heat is transported into the fluid mass. $\dot{W}$ is the sum of the work done by the fluid pressure over the cross sections A_1, A_2, and the work done by shear and normal stresses over the vessel wall, Eqs. (1)', (2)', (3)' above, respectively. A similar expression can be written for $\dot{H}$.

The big equation given at the beginning of this section is a verbal statement of Eq. (22) or (14).

On substituting Eq. (20), etc., into (22) and making use of the equations of motion and continuity, we can show that the rate of change of internal energy is equal to the dissipation function $\sigma_{ij} V_{ij}$. This completes the derivation. The use of the final result is explained above and illustrated in Sec. 1.7.

Problems

1.1 Why is it that sometimes you can hear a turbulent flow, but you cannot hear a laminar flow?

1.2 To listen to a flow, you can use a stethoscope. Apply a stethoscope to an artery. In what range of the eddying frequencies can you hear?

1.3 Discuss the possible relationships between the eddy size, the velocity of mean flow, the velocity fluctuations, and the frequency of pressure fluctuations in a turbulent flow. To be concrete, think of listening to a stenosis in an artery.

1.4 Discuss the answer to the preceding question more rigorously in terms of the correlation functions of velocity components and the corresponding frequency spectrums.

1.5 In which way is venturi tube used in a hydrodynamics laboratory? Explain the function of a venturi tube on the basis that acceleration corresponds to negative pressure gradient and deceleration corresponds to positive pressure gradient, or in terms of the Bernoulli equation, Eq. (3) of Sec. 1.6.

1.6 Why is a red blood cell so deformable whereas a white blood cell is less so?

1.7 What is the evidence that the hemoglobin in the red blood cell is in a liquid state? When a hemoglobin solution is examined under X-ray, a definite diffraction pattern can be found. Why does the existence of such a crystalline pattern not in conflict with the idea that the solution is in liquid state?

1.8 What is the source of bending rigidity of a red-cell membrane?

1.9 What is the evidence that the bending rigidity of a red-cell membrane exists and in which way is it important?

1.10 What is the evidence that the hydrostatic pressure in the red blood cell is about the same as that outside the cell?

1.11 What are the factors that determine the volume of a red blood cell?

1.12 How can a red blood cell deform without changing its surface area and volume? Can a sphere do it?

1.13 In catheterization, the pressure reading varies with the position of the catheter as the catheter is advanced. Why?

1.14 Explain why the flow resistance depends on the Reynolds number as indicated in Eq. (13) of Sec. 1.7.

1.15 Consult a book on anatomy, describe the structure of the vascular system of an organ (such as a hand, an arm, or a lung, heart, kidney or brain). Can you estimate the total peripheral vascular resistance for the organ? What data are needed? Where can they be found?

1.16 Referring to Fig. 1.4:1, explain why the resistence to flow is higher in the case of turbulent flow as compared with laminar flow.

1.17 Design an artificial heart valve to replace a diseased one. Discuss the pros and cons of your design.

1.18 When you measure your blood pressure by inflating a cuff over your brachial artery and then listen to the sound in the brachial artery below the cuff with a stethoscope, what do you hear? What is the meaning of various sounds? How is the sound correlated with the physical phenomena happening in the artery? How are systolic and diastolic pressures defined and decided?

References

Most topics considered in this chapter will be discussed in greater detail in the rest of this book. See the Index to locate references. Fundamental equations of fluid and solid mechanics are given in the Appendix at the end of this book. Basic concepts and equations for the description of finite deformation are presented in the Appendix of the companion volume *Biodynamics: Flow, Motion, and Stress* (Fung, 1984). References mentioned in the text are the following:

Fåhraeus, R. (1975). Empty Arteries, Lecture delivered at the 15th International Congress of the History of Medicine, Madrid.

Fung, Y. C. (1977). *A First Course in Continuum Mechanics*, Prentice-Hall, Englewood Cliffs, N.J.

Harris, C. R. S. (1980). The arteries in Greco-Roman medicine. In *Structure and Function of the Circulation* (Schwartz, C. T., Werthessen, N. T., and Wolf, S., eds.)., Plenum Press, New York.

CHAPTER 2

The Heart

2.1 Introduction

The heart is the prime mover of blood. By periodic stimulation of its muscles it contracts periodically and pumps blood throughout the body. How the pump works is the subject of this chapter.

In each cycle the left and right ventricles are first filled with blood from the left and right atria, respectively, in the diastolic phase of the cycle. Then by the deceleration of the blood stream a pressure field is generated, which closes the valves between the atria and the ventricles. The contraction of the heart muscle begins and the pressures in the ventricles rise. When the pressure in the left ventricle exceeds that in the aorta, and the pressure in the right ventricle exceeds that in the pulmonary artery, the aortic valve in the left and the pulmonary valve in the right are pushed open, and blood is ejected into the aorta and the lung. This is the systolic phase. The ejection continues until the deceleration of the jets of blood creates pressure fields to close the valves. Then the muscle relaxes, the pressures decrease, and the diastolic phase begins.

Thus, in the left ventricle, the blood pressure fluctuates from a low of nearly zero (i.e., atmospheric) to a high of 120 mm Hg or so. But in the aorta, the pressure fluctuation is much less. How does the aorta do it? How is the large fluctuation of blood pressure in the heart converted to the pressure wave in the aorta, with a high mean value and a smaller fluctuation? The answer was given by Stephen Hales (1733), who credited the feat to the elasticity of the aorta. An analogy was drawn between the heart–and–artery system and the old-fashioned hand-pumped fire engine. In the case of the fire engine, the fireman pumps water into a high-pressure air chamber by periodic injections at higher pressure. Water is then drained from the air

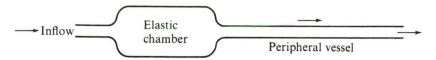

Figure 2.1:1 The "Windkessel" model of the aorta and peripheral circulation.

chamber, which has a high mean pressure that drives water out in a steady jet. This analogy was used by Otto Frank (1899) in his theory of the cardio-vascular system, and is known as the *Windkessel* (German: air vessel) theory. In this theory, the aorta is represented by an elastic chamber and the periph-eral blood vessels are replaced by a rigid tube of constant resistance. See Fig. 2.1:1. Let $\dot{Q}$ be the inflow (cm^3/sec) into this system from the left ven-tricle. Part of this inflow is sent to the peripheral vessels and part of it is used to distend the elastic chamber. If p is the blood pressure in the elastic chamber (aorta), then the flow in the peripheral vessel is assumed to be equal to p/R, where R is a constant called peripheral resistance. For the elastic chamber, its change of volume is assumed to be proportional to the pressure. The rate of change of the volume of the elastic chamber with respect to time, t, is therefore proportional to dp/dt. Let the constant of proportionality be written as K. Then, on equating the inflow to the sum of the rate of change of volume of the elastic chamber and the outflow p/R, the differential equation govern-ing the pressure p is

$$\dot{Q} = K(dp/dt) + p/R. \tag{1}$$

The solution of this differential equation is

$$p(t) = \frac{1}{K} e^{-t/(RK)} \int_0^t \dot{Q}(\tau) e^{\tau/(RK)} d\tau + p_0 e^{-t/(RK)}, \tag{2}$$

where p_0 is the value of p at time $t = 0$. This gives the pressure in the aorta as a function of the left ventricle ejection history $\dot{Q}(t)$. Equation (2) works remarkably well in correlating experimental data on the total blood flow $\dot{Q}$ with the blood pressure p, particularly during diastole. (See McDonald 1974, pp. 11, 310, 423; and Wetterer and Kenner, 1968.) Hence, in spite of the severity of the underlying assumptions it is quite useful.

Turning now to the question of stress in the heart itself, there is another very simple analysis that is quite good. Assume that the left ventricle can be approximated by a thick-walled hemispherical shell (Fig. 2.1:2), with inner radius a and outer radius b. Let the pressure acting on the inside be p_i (blood pressure) and that acting on the outside be p_o (pressure from pericardium), both assumed to be uniform. Consider the equilibrium of forces in the vertical direction. The force acting downward is equal to p_i times the projected area πa^2. The forces acting upward are $p_o \pi b^2$ and the product of the average wall stress $\langle \sigma_\theta \rangle$ and the area on which it acts, $\pi(b^2 - a^2)$. At equilibrium, these forces are balanced:

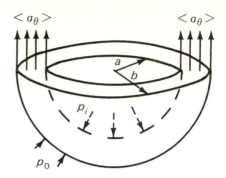

Figure 2.1:2 Balance of pressure forces acting on a thick-walled spherical shell.

$$\langle\sigma_\theta\rangle(b^2 - a^2) = p_i a^2 - p_o b^2. \tag{3}$$

Hence the average circumferential wall stress in the heart is

$$\langle\sigma_\theta\rangle = \frac{p_i a^2 - p_o b^2}{b^2 - a^2}. \tag{4}$$

The highest stress is obtained when p_i is equal to the maximum systolic pressure. The outer pressure p_o is normally close to the pleural pressure, which is subatmospheric (negative), but may become positive in disease states such as cardiac tamponade (large accumulation of pericardial fluid). The material of the heart wall is incompressible, so that the volume of the heart wall, $(\frac{2}{3})\pi(b^3 - a^3)$, remains a constant. Hence b is a function of a, and we see from Eq. (4) that the maximum stress acting in the heart wall is essentially proportional to $p_i a^2$: the higher the systolic pressure, and the larger the heart (radius a), the larger is the stress. From this we can make two deductions:

(1) Abnormal enlargement of the heart and increase in pressure will increase the wall stress and may lead to hypertrophy of the heart. The radius a is principally controlled by the diastolic pressure of the heart.
(2) The systolic pressure p_i is determined by the wall stress $\langle\sigma_\theta\rangle$, which is due to muscle contraction. The maximum tensile stress that can be generated in an isometric contraction of a cardiac muscle varies with the length of the sarcomere. See the length–tension curve in Fig. 2.1:3, and the explanation in Fung (1981, chapter 10). If a heart normally operates at a sarcomere length marked by the point A in the figure, then when the sarcomere is lengthened the maximum muscle tension will increase, and as a consequence the systolic pressure p_i will increase. Now the number of sarcomeres in a heart muscle is fixed, hence the sarcomere length is proportional to the heart radius a. Thus, if the radius of the heart a is increased, the muscle tension will increase, and so will be the systolic blood pressure. This is known as *Starling's law of the heart*.

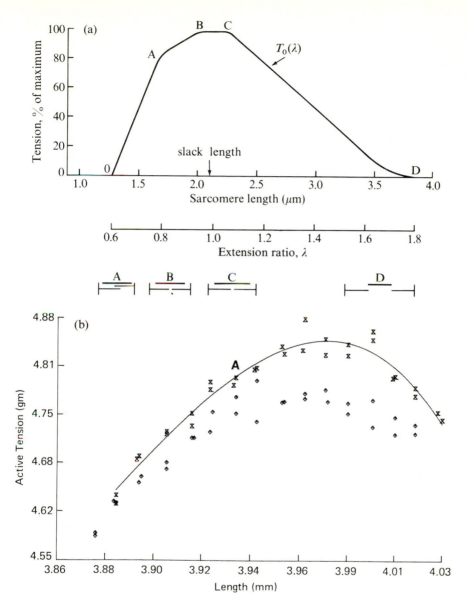

Figure 2.1:3 (a) The "length–tension" curve of a skeletal muscle. The sarcomere length is plotted on the abscissa. The maximum tension achieved in isometric contraction at the length specified is plotted on the ordinate. (b) The maximum active tension in single isometric twitches of the papillary muscle of the rabbit obtained by Paul Patitucci in the author's lab. Note that the maximum tension is not a unique function of the muscle length: its value depends on whether in successive experiments the length is increased (symbol **X**) or decreased (symbol ◇). Thus, there is hysteresis in active tension. The solid curve represents a fitted Fourier series.

Starling's law of the heart works as long as the operating point A lies on the upward-sloping leg of the curve shown in Fig. 2.1:3. It ceases to be valid when A moves off this leg.

As mentioned before, the size of the left ventricle in the isovolumetric phase is determined by how well the left ventricle is filled at the end diastolic condition. This, in turn, is determined by the balance between p_i, the diastolic pressure, p_o, the pericardial pressure, and $\langle \sigma_\theta \rangle$, the elastic stress in the ventricular wall when it is relaxed while the muscle is in the refractive period between successive stimulations. The same formula (3) applies. The major determinants are the diastolic pressure and the elasticity of the heart muscle in the resting state. By controlling the diastolic pressure, i.e., the filling of the heart, the size of the left ventricle, and hence the length of the sarcomeres in the isovolumetric phase, can be controlled. Thus, by controlling the diastolic pressure, the location of the point A on the upward leg of Fig. 2.1:3 can be controlled. In this way a physician or surgeon can make use of Starling's law to deal with some clinical problems.

This brief discussion shows the critical role played by biorheology in understanding the function of the organs. Biorheology is described in *Biomechanics: Mechanical Properties of Living Tissues* (Fung, 1981), which will be referred to frequently in the present work.

To know more about the heart we must know its geometry, its materials of construction and their mechanical properties, and the electric, chemical, and nervous events in each cycle of contraction, as well as the way heart is coupled with the vascular system. On the foundation of this information we should be able to predict the function of the heart by the method of continuum mechanics.

2.2 The Geometry and Materials of the Heart

The adult human heart has four chambers: two thin-walled atria separated from each other by an interatrial septum, and two thick-walled ventricles separated by an interventricular septum. As it is shown schematically in Fig. 2.2:1, the venous blood flows into the right atrium, through the tricuspid valve into the right ventricle, and then is pumped into the pulmonary artery and the lung, where the blood is oxygenated. The oxygenated blood then flows from the pulmonary veins into the left atrium, and through the mitral valve into the left ventricle, whose contraction pumps the blood into the aorta, and then to the arteries, arterioles, capillaries, venules, veins, and back to the right atrium.

The four valves are seated in a plane, as shown in Fig. 2.2:1. The mitral and tricuspid valves, which are opened in order to fill the ventricles with blood when the blood pressure is low and velocity is small, are relatively large in area. The aortic and pulmonary valves, used in ventricular systole to pump blood out of the ventricles at high velocity, are smaller. The mitral and

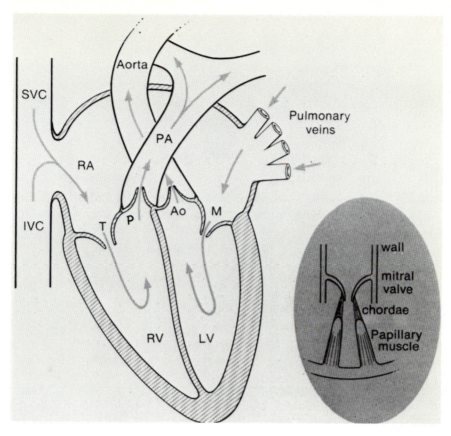

Figure 2.2:1 Blood flow through the heart. The arrows show the direction of blood flow. The symbols are: SVC, superior vena cava; IVC, inferior vena cava; RA, right atrium; RV, right ventricle; PA, pulmonary artery; LV, left ventricle. The valves are T, tricuspid, P, pulmonary, AO, aortic, M, mitral. From Folkow and Neil (1971) *Circulation*, Oxford Univ. Press, New York, p. 153, by permission.

triscuspid valves are attached to papillary muscles, which contract in systole, pull down the valves to generate systolic pressure rapidly, and prevent the valves from any danger of inversion into the atrium. The aortic and pulmonary valves have no strings attached. The closing and opening of all valves are operated by blood itself through hydrodynamic forces.

The heart is a muscle. The muscles of the atria and the ventricles are joined to a skeleton of fibrous tissue on which the rings of the four valves are seated. The *bundle of His* constitutes the only *muscle* connection between the atria and ventricles. The electric pacemaking activity of the right atrium can pass to the ventricles only via the bundle of His.

The muscle fibers in the heart are systematically oriented. Figure 2.2:2 shows the fiber orientation in the left ventricular wall of the dog. On the

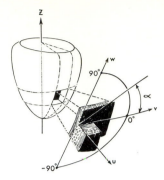

Figure 2.2:2 The orientation of muscle fibers in the left ventricular wall of the dog. From Streeter et al. (1969), by permission.

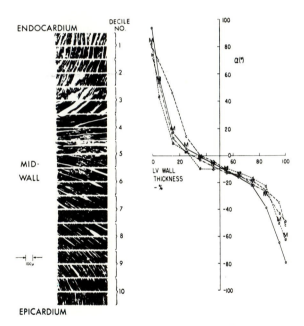

Figure 2.2:3 Variation of the inclination of the muscle fibers in the left ventricular wall of the dog from the apex-to-base (longitudinal) direction. From Streeter et al. (1969), by permission.

epicardium, the muscle fibers are oriented from the apex to the base, or, if we borrow the language used in geography in describing features on the globe, we say that the fibers are arranged in the direction of the longitudes. Away from the epicardium the muscle fiber orientation changes continuously. At the midwall the fibers are oriented parallel to the base, i.e., in the direction of the latitudes. The rotation continues until the fibers become longitudinal again in the endocardium. If the angle between a muscle fiber and a parallel circle is denoted by α, then the relationship between α and the depth through the ventricular wall is as shown in Fig. 2.2:3.

The valves are collagen membranes. They are thin and flexible. A membranous structure of similar flexibility is the pericardium, which encloses the entire heart. The pericardium is attached to arterial trunks above and the central tendon the diaphragm below. It is a sac containing a small amount of pericardial fluid that serves as a lubricant. It is lined with mesothelium. It limits the excursions of the heart.

The reader should enjoy looking over the beautifully illustrated book by Frank Netter, *The Heart* (1969). Details of the anatomy of the heart can be found in the *Handbook of Physiology* (Berne et al., 1979).

2.3 The Electric System

Since every contraction of the heart muscle needs an electric stimulation, the heart must have a center which generates a periodic electric signal which is conducted to every muscle cell. The main electric generating station of the heart lies in the *sinoatrial node*, (the S–A node). See Fig. 2.3:1. The S–A node is a pale, narrow structure. For man it is approximately 25 mm long, 3 to 4 mm wide, and 2 mm thick. It contains two types of cells: (1) the small, round *P cells*, which have few organelles and myofibrils, and (2) the slender, elongated *transitional cells*, which are intermediate in appearance between the *P* and the ordinary myocardial cells. The *P* cells are the dominant pacemaker cells of the heart. They exhibit rhythmicity very early in fetal life. (In human fetus rhythmic contraction of the heart tube begins on the 19th or 20th day.) Electrophysiological data show that the S–A node is the first region of the heart to display electric activity during each cardiac cycle.

From the S–A node, the cardiac electric signal spreads radially throughout the right atrium along ordinary myocardial fibers at a conduction velocity of approximately 1 m/sec. In the meantime, a special bundle of fibers carries the signal directly from the S–A node to the left atrium, and three other bundles conduct the signal directly from the S–A to the A–V node. These bundles consist of a mixture of ordinary myocardial cells and specialized conducting fibers similar to those that exist in the ventricles.

The *atrioventricular* (or A–V) *node*, is a substation of the signal transmission. See its location in Fig. 2.3:1. This node has dimensions $3 \times 10 \times 22$ mm in man. It contains the same two types of cells as the S–A node, but the *P*

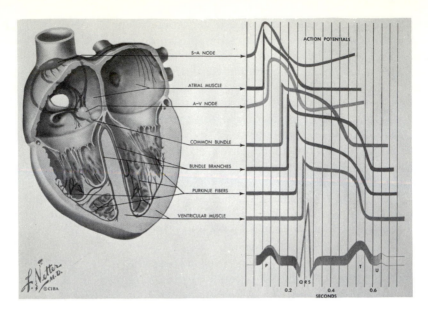

Figure 2.3:1 The electric system of the heart and the action potentials at various locations in the heart. From Frank Netter (1969). © Copyright 1969, CIBA Pharmaceutical Company, Division of CIBA-GEIGY Corporation. Reprinted with permission from THE CIBA COLLECTION OF MEDICAL ILLUSTRATIONS illustrated by Frank H. Netter, M.D. All rights reserved.

cells are more sparse and the transitional cells preponderate. When the signal from S–A node reaches the A–V node, it is delayed for a certain period of time, and then is passed to the ventricles via the *atrioventricular bundle*, or *bundle of His*. It is the only muscular tissue connecting the atria to the ventricles. In man it is about 12 mm long before it branches.

The delay of the electric signal transmission at the A–V node allows optimal ventricular filling during atrial contraction. It is this delay that is responsible for the interval between the *P wave* and the *QRS complex* in the electrocardiogram. Detailed studies attribute the delay to the small fibers in the junctional region between the atrial myocardium and the A–V node. It is known that the conduction velocity is directly related to fiber diameter, and in these small fibers the velocity is 0.05 m/sec as compared with 1m/sec in the main body of the A–V node. The cells in the A–V node have been found to be significantly less excitable than other cardiac cells, and the relative refraction period persists for an appreciable period of time after repolarization.

If the A–V delay were prolonged or if some or all of the atrial excitations were prevented from reaching the ventricles, then the conduction is said to be *blocked*. Pathological blocks may be provoked by nervous, inflammatory, circulatory, or drug factors, such as acute rheumatic fever or digitalis.

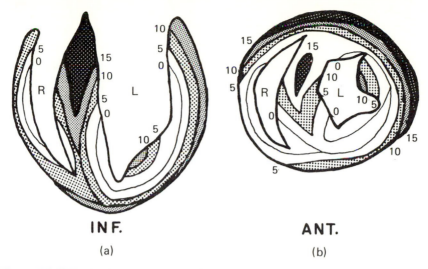

INF.   ANT.

(a)   (b)

Figure 2.3:2 Excitation sequence of the myocardium as determined by miniature electrodes. (a) Meridional section. (b) Latitudinal section. The numbers indicate the intervals in millseconds after the earliest excitation. The shading increases in darkness with increasing length of intervals. From W. G. Guntheroth, (1965) *Pediatric Electrocardiography*, W. B. Saunders Co., Philadelphia, on the basis of data in Scher and Young (1956). Reproduced by permission.

The bundle of His passes down the right side of the interventricular septum and then divides into the right and left *bundle branches*. From these further branches called *Purkinje fibers* spread over both ventricles. See Fig. 2.3:1. Electric signal propagates fast in the Purkinje fibers at a speed of 1 to 4 m/sec.

The last stage of electric transmission is done by the cardiac muscle itself, transmitting from one cell to the next. There is a semblance of *syncytium* between cardiac muscle cells, which make such excitation possible. The speed of signal transmission in the myocardium is 0.3 to 0.4 m/sec.

Figure 2.3:2 shows an example of the sequence of initiation of excitation spreading in the ventricles of man. Different parts of the heart are excited in a definite sequence of time. Such a map is important not only for the interpretation of the electrocardiogram, but also for the dynamics of the movement of the heart.

So far we have outlined the layout of the electric system and the sequence of spreading of electric signal in normal condition. However, apparently some cells in the walls of all four cardiac chambers are capable of initiating beats. Regions of the heart, other than the S–A node, that initiate beats under special circumstances are called *ectopic foci* or *ectopic pacemakers*. The special circumstances include block of conduction pathways, enhancement of rhythmicity of the ectopic foci, or depression of the rhythmicity of the S–A node.

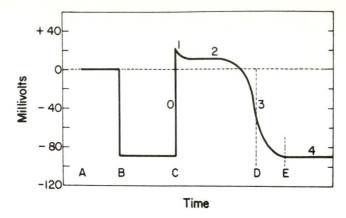

Figure 2.3:3 Changes in electric potential recorded by an intracellular microelectrode. From time A to B the electrode was outside the cell. At B the cell was impaled by the electrode. At C an action potential begins in the impaled cell. Time C–D represents the absolute refractory period. Time D–E is the relative refractory period, while E–F is the supernormal period. From Berne, R. M., and Levy, M. N. (1972) *Cardiovascular Physiology*, 2nd edn. C. V. Mosby Co., Saint Louis, p. 6, by permission.

The electric activity of the heart is of great clinical significance, particularly because it is revealed in the electrocardiogram (ECG). The ECG thus becomes a powerful clinical tool. The reader should consult articles in *Handbook of Physiology* (edited by Berne et al, 1979), especially Scher and Spach (1979), to learn something about the electrophysiology of the heart.

From the point of view of mechanics, it is probably sufficient to know the layout of the electric system and to know that the *action potential* of myocardial cells in different parts of the heart have somewhat different courses in time. The action potential of a cardiac muscle cell is recorded by inserting microelectrodes into the interior of the cell. A typical example of a record of potential changes occurring in a ventricular cell is shown in Fig. 2.3:3. When two electrodes are put next to a quiescent cell in an electrolyte solution there is no potential difference between the two electrodes (in the period of time from point *A* to point *B* in the figure.) At time *B* one of the microelectrodes is inserted into the cell. Immediately the galvanometer records a potential difference across the cell membrane, indicating that the potential of the interior of the cell is about 90 mV lower than that of the surrounding medium. At point *C* a propagated action potential is transmitted to the cell impaled with the microelectrode (assuming that the cell lies in a strip of ventricular muscle in which action potential is propagated). Very rapidly the cell membrane becomes depolarized and the potential difference reversed, so that the potential of the interior of the cell exceeds that of the exterior by about 20 mV. Immediately following the upstroke there is a brief rapid change of potential in the direction of repolarization. Repolarization then decelerates (phase 2),

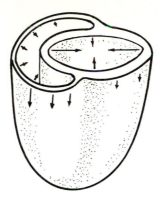

Figure 2.4:1 Patterns of ventricular contraction. (a) Right ventricular ejection is accomplished primarily by compression of the right ventricular cavity, but also by downward displacement of the tricuspid valve ring (shortening of the free wall). (b) Left ventricular ejection is accomplished primarily by constriction of the left ventricular chamber with only a minor contribution of shortening of the long axis. From Rushmer R., (1976) *Cardiovascular Dynamics*, W. B. Saunders, Philadelphia, p. 92, by permission.

and again accelerates (phase 3), until finally it decelerates asymptotically to the resting potential (phase 4).

Figure 2.3:1 shows that the time course of action potential at different parts of the heart is somewhat different.

Of mechanical significance is the difference in the duration of action potentials in the subendocardial cells from that in the subepicardial cells. As a result, although the wave of depolarization in the ventricles proceeds from endocardium to epicardium, the wave of repolarization travels in the opposite direction. It has been postulated that the compressive strain in the ventricular muscle during systole retards the repolarization process more in the subendocardial than in the subepicardial region.

2.4 Mechanical Events in a Cardiac Cycle

The electric events described in Sec. 2.3 determine the sequence in which the cardiac muscle cells contract. This contraction, operating in coordination with a set of valves, circulates the blood.

Figure 2.4:1 shows the ejection pattern of the two ventricles. The left ventricle, which pumps blood at a pressure much higher than that in the right ventricle, remains nearly ellipsoidal in shape. Since the net pressure load on the interventricular septum points toward the right ventricle, the septum has to assume the shape sketched in Fig. 2.4:1. The right ventricle then appears as a bellows, which is a geometry ideally suited to the ejection of a large volume of fluid at a low pressure. In both ventricles there is also

TABLE 2.4:1 Pressures and Volumes in the Normal Human Heart*

Left atrial pressure, mean ≤12 mm Hg
Left ventricular pressure
  Peak systolic, 100–150 mm Hg in adults
  End-diastolic, ≤12 mm Hg
Aortic pressure
  Systolic, 100–150 mm Hg in adults
  Diastolic, 60–100 mm Hg in adults
Right atrial pressure, mean ≤6 mm Hg
Right ventricular pressure
  Peak systolic, 15–30 mm Hg
  End-diastolic, ≤6 mm Hg
Pulmonary arterial pressure
  Systolic, 15–30 mm Hg
  Diastolic, 4–12 mm Hg
Left ventricular end-diastolic volume, at rest, 70–100 ml/m^2 body surface area
Left ventricular end-systolic volume, at rest, 25–35 ml/m^2 body surface area
Stroke volume, at rest, 40–70 ml/m^2 body surface area
Ejection fraction at rest, (stroke volume divided by end-diastolic volume), 0.55–0.80
Cardiac index, 2.8–4.2 liter/m^2/min.
Systemic vascular resistance, 770–1500 dyn sec cm^{-5}
Pulmonary vascular resistance, 20–120 dyn sec cm^{-5}

* Grossman, W. (ed.) (1974) *Cardiac Catherization and Augiography*. Lea & Febiger, Philadelphia: and Grossman, Brodie, Mann, and McLaurin (1977) Effects of sodium nitroprusside on left ventricular diastolic pressure–volume relations. *J. Chin. Inves.* **59**: 59–68. Body surface area is given approximately by (weight in kg + height in cm − 60)/100 m^2.

some shortening of the longitudinal axis, with the direction of motion as indicated in Fig. 2.4:1.

The pressures acting on the pericardium and in the ventricles are unsteady with respect to time and nonuniform with respect to space. These pressures, together with the inertial forces due to acceleration, and the elastic, viscoelastic, and active contraction stresses in the muscle, determine the dynamics of the heart. On the other hand, the pressure in the fluid in these cavities is determined by the movement of the walls. Thus, there is a hydroelastic feedback mechanism in operation.

Typical values of pressures and volumes of the chambers in the normal human heart are listed in Table 2.4:1. Volume changes and wall motion of the heart are affected significantly by posture (supine or erect), anesthetization, and surgery (open-chested or not, pericardium open or not). Measurement of shape and volume in an intact heart remains a challenging problem. Some experiments have shown that the strain is nonuniform in the left ventricle during systole: the shortening is greater in the neighborhood of the apex than that at the base. Opening of the pericardium has an important effect on the shape and size of the heart. All this is quite expected from the

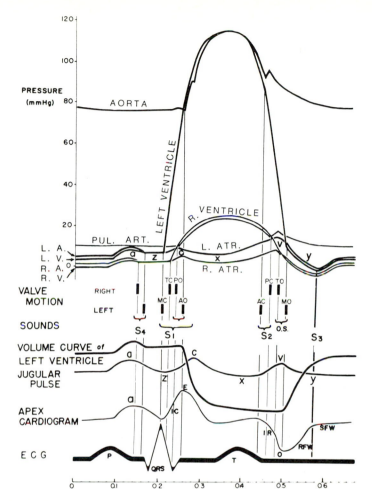

Figure 2.4:2 Correlation of various hemodynamic measurements in a single cardiac cycle. The time scale reference at the bottom is in tenths of a second. From Hurst, J. W., and Logue R. B. (1970) *The Heart*, 2nd edn., McGraw–Hill, New York, p. 76, by permission.

mechanical point of view, because any change in boundary conditions changes the stresses and strains in the heart.

Correlation with Electric Events

Figure 2.4:2 shows the relationship between the mechanical and electric events in the heart. The electrocardiogram, or ECG, is shown at the bottom. It shows the characteristic P wave of atrial electric activity, the QRS complex representing ventricular depolarization, and the T wave representing ventricular repolarization.

The valve motion is indicated in the middle of the figure. The opening O and closing C of each of the valves (A = aortic, T = tricuspid, P = pulmonic, M = mitral) are marked in the figure. Thus, TC means tricuspid valve closing, etc.

The curve above the ECG represents the displacement of the apex of the heart, which can usually be felt through the chest wall when a person lies horizontally on the left side. Starting from the left, the a wave coincides with the atrial contraction at the end of filling of the left ventricle. IC represents isovolumic contraction, ending at E the most outward position. The apex then moves away from the chest wall during the period of ejection of blood after E. In isovolume relaxation (IR) the apex moves further inward. At O the mitral valve opens. Then a rapid filling wave (RFW) follows due to the initial rush of blood into the left ventricle. This is followed by a slow-filling wave (SFW) during mid-diastole, up to the a wave contraction at end-diastole.

The jugular vein pulse shows a similar a wave due to right atrial contraction at end-diastole. The c wave reflects bulging backward of the tricuspid valve into the right atrium during right ventricular systole. The x wave is due to downward displacement of the base of the ventricles during systole and continued atrial relaxation. The xv wave is due to filling of the right atrium. The vy wave follows the opening of the tricuspid valve.

The right atrial pressure wave (R.A.) is essentially the same as the juglar vein pulse.

The volume curve of the left ventricle shows an a wave due to the contraction of the left atrium, followed by an isovolumic period of ventricular contraction. As the aortic valve opens, blood is ejected into the aorta and the left ventricular volume is rapidly decreased. This continues until end-systole. The blood volume remains constant during the isovolumic relaxation phase until the mitral valve opens to admit fresh blood.

The pressure curve of the left ventricle (L.V.) is shown in the uppermost part of the figure. When the ventricular pressure exceeds the pressure in the aorta the aortic valve opens and blood is ejected into the aorta. Later, when the ventricular pressure becomes smaller than that in the aorta the ejecting jet decelerates. At the instant marked as AC the aortic valve closes.

The aortic pressure curve reflects the closure of the aortic valve with a *dicrotic notch*.

The right ventricular pressure curve (R.V.) is similar to that of the left ventricle, but at a lower level. The pulmonary artery pressure curve is similar to that of the aorta but also at a lower level.

Certain sound is associated with these events. The timing of the four heart sounds, S_1, S_2, S_3, S_4, is indicated in the figure. They are associated with the movement of the valves and the acceleration and deceleration of blood, and the movement and vibration of the heart muscle, and their trans-

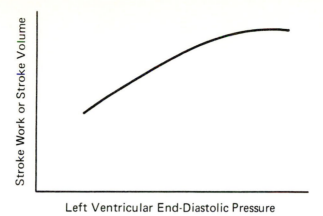

Figure 2.4:3 Schematic diagram of a left ventricular function curve. Some measure of ventricular performance, such as stroke work or stroke volume, is plotted on the ordinate as a function of some measure of preload, such as left ventricular end-diastolic pressure (LVEDP), on the abscissa.

mission through the thorax. If fully understood, the heart sounds can become as useful a tool to the clinician as seismic waves are to geologists.

The Ventricular Function Curve

A ventricular function curve is one that relates certain measure of preload (which determines the length of the heart muscle fibers in a relaxed state before contraction), such as the end-diastolic pressure, with some measure of cardiac performance, such as stroke volume or stroke work. See Fig. 2.4:3. Depending on the choice of the "measures," many different ventricular function curves can be plotted. The choice is usually based on considerations of clinical relevance. For example, as the filling pressure of the ventricle decreases symptoms of dyspnea appear; and as the stroke work decreases signs of insufficient peripheral perfusion occurs; hence a figure like Fig. 2.4:3 is useful. It tells a clinician a lot about a patient, especially with respect to therapeutic interventions which may shift the ventricular function curve up or down, left or right.

Pressure–Volume Loop

If we plot the pressure and volume of a ventricle throughout a cardiac cycle on a plane with respect to a set of coordinates as shown in Fig. 2.4:4, with volume as abscissa and pressure as ordinate, we see a clear representation of

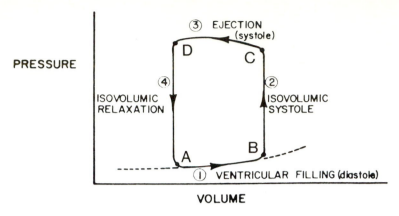

Figure 2.4:4 A plot of the pressure and volume in a ventricle during a cardiac cycle. Phase 1 represents ventricular filling during diastole. Phase 2 represents isovolumic pressure development. Phase 3 represents ejection of blood into the aorta. Phase 4 represents the isovolumic relaxation period.

the four phases of the cardiac cycle. The area within the loop describes the external work (stroke work) done by the left ventricle as it contracts.

The lower curve of the loop, phase 1, (the arc AB in Fig. 2.4:4), represents the ventricular filling. During this period the heart is in diastole and the muscle is resting. The curve AB, therefore, should be the same as the pressure–volume (P–V) curve of a resting heart. Some deviation of the arc AB from the P–V curve of a resting heart occurs at the corners A and B owing to the dynamic events in the heart.

The corner C in Fig. 2.4:4 represents the opening of the aortic valve, whereas the point D represents the closure of the aortic valve. The arc DA corresponds to isovolumic relaxation.

One may ask whether the point D in Fig. 2.4:4 corresponds to the maximum isometric tension in the heart muscle at the volume specified. To answer this question, Suga et al. (1973) made an experiment on dog's heart in which the aorta was transiently occluded at specified volumes of the heart and the heart muscle was allowed to go through cycles of contraction during which the heart could develop pressure but not eject blood. The maximum and minimum pressures developed in such cycles were noted, and plotted against the volume. Such a curve of the maximum pressure vs volume is called an *isovolumic pressure curve*, and was found to be approximately a straight line. When the isovolumic pressure line was plotted onto the P–V curves of Fig. 2.4:4, it was found that the corner D fell in the neighborhood of the isovolumic pressure line, as is shown in Fig. 2.4:5. Thus, the point D does seem to correspond to the maximum isometric tension of heart muscle at the volume specified. Of course, we should object to the use of the word "isometric," because isovolumic contraction does not guarantee constant

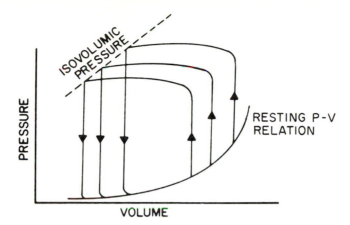

Figure 2.4:5 Relationship between the "isovolumic pressure line" and the cardiac cycle. The isovolumic pressure line represents the capacity of the ventricle to develop pressure at each initial end-diastolic volume if it were not allowed to eject blood. The three ejection cycles illustrated represent cardiac contractions at different initial end-diastolic volumes and aortic pressures.

length of the muscle fibers. Indeed, shape change of the ventricles in the isovolumic contraction period, as shown in Fig. 2.4:1, implies the lack of isometry in the muscle fibers. But roughly, isovolumic condition is an approximation to isometric condition.

The relationship plotted in Fig. 2.4:5 suggests that the upper left-hand corner of each loop approximates the isovolumic pressure line, independent of the initial end-diastolic volume and the aortic pressure against which the heart is working. The isovolumic pressure line, when extrapolated to the volume axis, intercepts that axis at approximately 5 ml (for the dog). If the contractility of the ventricle is increased by an inotropic drug such as epinephrine, the isovolumic pressure line is shifted upward and to the left, although the volume intercept remains approximately the same, as is shown in Fig. 2.4:6. Thus, under these circumstances, an increase in stroke volume can be produced at the same end-diastolic pressure and arterial pressure, since the end-systolic point of contraction will approximate the new iso-volumic pressure line. A reverse situation would occur during the process of heart failure, when the isovolumic pressure line would be shifted downward and to the right.

2.5 How Are the Heart Valves Operated?

The most interesting fluid-dynamical events in the heart are the filling and ejecting of blood in the ventricles, which are associated with the motion of the heart valves. The human heart has four valves: the tricuspid (T),

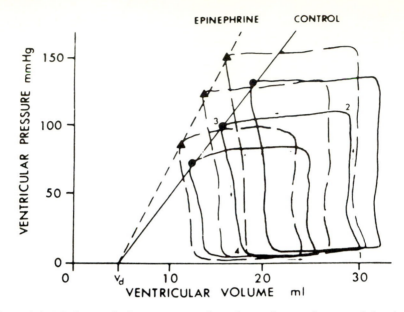

Figure 2.4:6 Left ventricular pressure–volume loops from a denervated dog heart. Mean aortic pressure was fixed at three different levels while cardiac output was kept constant during both the control (solid loops) and enhanced (2 µg/kg/min epinephrine infusion) (broken loops) contractile states. The upper left-hand corners of the pressure–volume loops form a line which intersects the volume axis at a point V_d of about 5 ml. From Suga et al. (1973), by permission.

pulmonic (P), aortic (AO), and mitral (M) (Fig. 2.2:1). They lie essentially in a plane.

The aortic valve consists of three thin, crescent-shaped cusps (whence the name semilunar), which in the open position are displaced outward toward the aorta. In the closed position the three cusps come together to seal the aortic orifice. Behind the cusps there are outpouchings of the aortic root, called the *sinuses of Valsalva*, which play a role in the closure of the valve. The pulmonic valve has a similar structure.

The mitral valve consists of two thin membranous cusps of roughly trape-zoidal shape which originate from the slightly elliptical mitral ring. In the open position these membranes form a scalloped, cone-like structure. The distal margins of the two cusps have an irregular appearance because they are pulled by the chordae tendinea which originate from the papillary muscle of the ventricular wall. The cusp adjacent to the aortic valve is called the anterior or aortic cusp, the other is called the posterior or mural cusp. In closed condition the free edges of the cusps are pressed together. The tricuspid valve structure is similar, except that it has three cusps.

The muscle bundles of the heart are organized into a unified whole, and one part cannot move without affecting other parts. The aortic and mitral

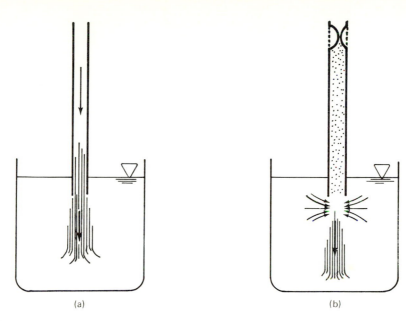

(a)   (b)

Figure 2.5:1 Schematic of Henderson and Johnson's first experiment drawn by Parmley and Talbot (1979).

valves, covering the base of the left ventricle, are an integral unit. The opening of the mitral valve occurs when the pressure above the aortic valve is low, so an enlargement of the mitral valve orifice coincides with a reduction of the orifice of the aortic valve. On the other hand, during systole, when the aortic valve is opened and its orifice is distended, the mitral valve is closed, and reduced in area.

The principle of opening and closing of the valves has been discussed in Sec. 1.5 of the preceding chapter. We shall now study the mechanism in greater details.

One of the earliest descriptions of fluid motion in a heart valve is Leonardo da Vinci's sketch of the vortices in the sinuses of Valsalva during ventricular systole. But the first correct fluid mechanical interpretation of the mechanism of closing of the heart valves was probably that of Henderson and Johnson (1912). They performed several experiments. In the first experiment they used a tube which was connected to the bottom of a reservoir of dye and dipped into a tank of water. When a valve was opened a distinct jet was produced (Fig. 2.5:1(a)). Then they pinched the tube (or closed the valve) to stop the flow (Fig. 2.5:1(b)). As the flow was halted, the jet was seen to conserve its forward motion and hence break away from the fluid in the tube, while clear water was drawn suddenly into the wake of the jet in the vicinity of the tube opening. In the second experiment a section of curved tube was attached to the midportion of a straight tube to form a "D" configuration, as shown in

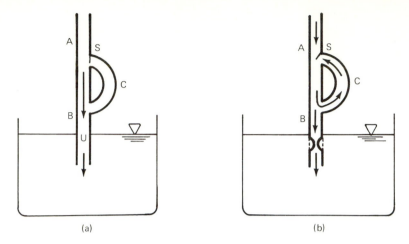

Figure 2.5:2 Henderson and Johnson's second experiment.

Fig. 2.5:2. An excised bovine heart valve membrane was installed across the entrance to the curved section, as indicated by the short line drawn at S. Fluid flow was directed down the straight tube into a water-filled tank and it was observed that little, if any, motion occurred in the curved part of the D as shown in Fig. 2.5:2(a). The straight-through flow was then halted by occluding the tube, thereupon the fluid began to circulate in the curved portion of D, as indicated in Fig. 3.5:2(b). The circulating fluid in the curved tube caused the valve to close against the forward flow coming from A.

In another of their experiments, a glass tube fitted with a flexible rubber sleeve was dipped into a tank of water (Fig. 2.5:3) and the column of water within the tube was raised to a level above that of the tank. Upon release of the column of fluid, it was observed that when the level in the tube fell below that of the tank, the fluid within the tank moved inward to collapse the sleeve and seal the tube.

Lee and Talbot (1979) explained Henderson and Johnson's experiment shown in Fig. 2.5:2 as follows: Consider the phenomenon described in Fig. 2.5:2. On assuming that the flow velocity U is uniform across the tube between A and B, and that there is initially little flow in the curved section C, and neglecting gravity and viscous effects, the equation of motion for the fluid contained in AB is

$$\frac{\partial U}{\partial t} + U\frac{\partial U}{\partial x} = -\frac{1}{\rho}\frac{\partial p}{\partial x}, \tag{1}$$

where U is the velocity in the x (flow) direction, ρ is the fluid density, p is the fluid pressure, and t is time. However, since the section AB is of constant area, there is no velocity gradient along the tube (according to the principle of conservation of mass), and the convective acceleration $U(\partial U/\partial x)$ vanishes. We are thus left with

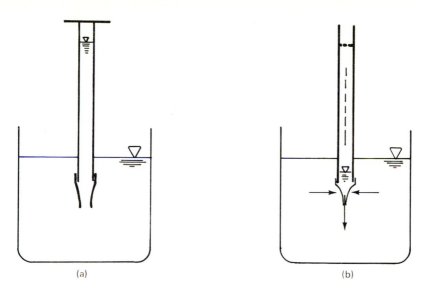

Figure 2.5:3 Henderson and Johnson's third experiment.

$$\frac{\partial U}{\partial t} = -\frac{1}{\rho}\frac{\partial p}{\partial x}. \tag{2}$$

Now, when the flow in AB is caused to decelerate, $\partial U/\partial t$ takes on a negative value. Accordingly, the pressure gradient $\partial p/\partial x$, must take on a positive value. Thus, the pressure at B becomes higher than that at A. This causes the fluid initially at rest in the curved section C to be set in motion, in the direction shown in Fig. 2.5:2. Other experiments sketched in Figs. 2.5:1 and 2.5:3 can be explained similarly.

The Operation of the Aortic Valve

An aortic valve with the sinus of Valsalva behind it is sketched in Fig. 2.5:4. According to model experiments by Bellhouse and Bellhouse (1969, 1972) and Bellhouse and Talbot (1969), the flow issuing from the ventricle immediately upon opening of the valve at the inception of systole is split into two streams at each valve cusp, as shown in the figure. Part of the flow is directed into the sinus behind the valve cusp, where it forms a vortical flow before re-emerging, out of the plane of the figure, to rejoin the main stream in the ascending aorta.

When the aortic pressure rises sufficiently so that deceleration of the flow occurs, an adverse pressure gradient is produced, p_2 at the valve cusp tip exceeds the pressure p_1 at a station upstream. The higher pressure p_2 causes a greater flow into the sinus which carries the cusp toward apposition.

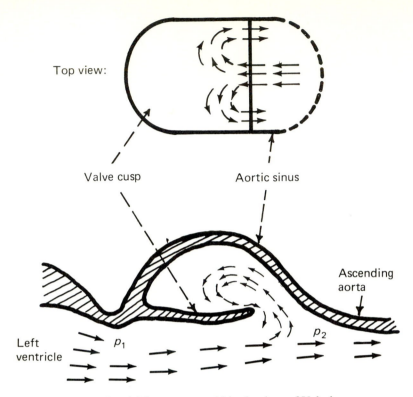

Figure 2.5:4 Flow pattern within the sinus of Valsalva.

The peak deceleration occurs just before the valve closure. The vortical motion established earlier upon the opening of the valve has the merit of preventing the valve cusp from bulging outward to contact the walls of the sinuses. The open sinus chamber thus can be supplied with fluid to fill the increasing volume behind the valve cusps as they move toward closure.

The Operation of the Mitral Valve

The flow through the mitral valve can be illustrated by the photographs of a model by Lee and Talbot (1979) shown in Fig. 2.5:5. The model consists of two freely hinged rigid cusps, with a simulated flexible ventricle and an atrium. In Fig. 2.5:5(a), at $t = 450$ msec after the onset of diastole, the valve has opened. The fluid motion in the ventricle is predominantly outward. At $t = 800$ msec, Fig. 2.5:5(b), a vortex motion can be seen behind the cusps. At $t = 1100$ msec and 1600 msec (Fig. 2.5:5(c) and (d)) the fully developed diastolic flow pattern is seen, which continues till the period of active diastole terminates at $t = 1650$ msec. It can be seen that the vortices behind the valve cusps have decayed in strength, and there is very little

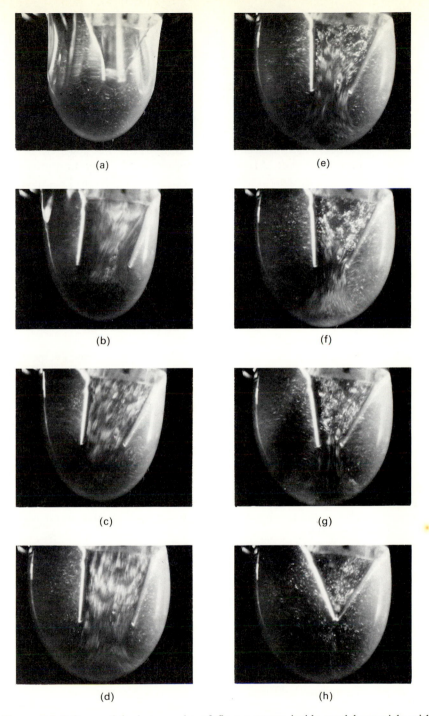

Figure 2.5:5 Sequential photographs of flow patterns inside model ventricle with mitral valve. (a) $t = 450$ msec, (b) $t = 800$ msec, (c) $t = 1100$ msec, (d) $t = 1600$ msec, (e) $t = 1800$ msec, (f) $t = 1850$ msec, (g) $t = 1900$ msec, (h) $t = 1950$ msec. Time t was measured with respect to onset of ventricular diastole. The flow pattern was made visible by hydrogen bubbles evolved from fine wires. From Lee and Talbot (1979), by permission.

motion in this region. In Fig. 2.5:5(e), at $t = 1800$ msec an early stage of valve closure is seen. A strong jet through the valve is still evident, although the fluid in the upper portion of the valve is moving much less rapidly. At $t = 1850$ msec (Fig. 2.5:5(f)) a stagnation point has formed in the flow within the valve, and the fluid in the upper portion of the valve has begun to move in the reverse direction. We see here the "breaking of the jet" mentioned earlier. Also, a circulating motion within the ventricle behind the valve cusps is evident. At $t = 1900$ msec (Fig. 2.5:5(g)) although the valve is nearly closed, there is still a narrow jet issuing from the valve, and the circulatory motion within the ventricles has become stronger. Closure is complete at $t = 1950$ msec, 50 msec before the onset of ventricle systole.

Lee and Talbot's model uses water as the circulating fluid, and the *Reynolds number* and *Strouhal number* of the heart are simulated. The Strouhal number is defined as $L/(U_m T)$, where L is the mitral valve cusp length, U_m is the maximum velocity of flow through the mitral valve, T is the time interval of one heartbeat. It is also called the *reduced frequency*. The Reynolds number and Strouhal number together define the dynamic similarity for model testing.

The flow patterns in Fig. 2.5:5 show that the deceleration of the jet and the associated adverse pressure gradient are the mechanism responsible for valve closure during diastole. The deceleration causes the pressure within the valve to fall below that of the surrounding fluid in the ventricle, and an inward motion of the ventricular fluid results which closes the valve.

Based on these observations, Lee and Talbot formulated a mathematical theory to calculate the valve cusp motion from a knowledge of the velocity–time history of the flow through the valve, under the assumptions that the valve cusps are massless and passive, and the velocity in the valve cross section is uniform. Using the theory in reverse, they showed also how to calculate the velocity of flow from known motion of the valve cusps. This theory is useful because valve cusp motion can be measured noninvasively by echocardiography.

What Are the Papillary Muscles For?

The operation of the mitral valves does not need the help of the papillary muscles, although these muscles do pull on the edge of the membranes (see Figs. 2.2:1 and 2.3:1). In the human heart the papillary muscles constitute about 10% of the total heart mass. What are they for?

To understand the function of the papillary muscles we should go back to the law of Laplace (see Fung, 1981, p. 17), which states that for a curved surface with principal curvatures $1/r_1$ and $1/r_2$, and principal membrane stress resultants T_1 and T_2, resisting an internal pressure p_i and an external pressure p_e, the equation of equilibrium is

$$p_i - p_0 = \frac{T_1}{r_1} + \frac{T_2}{r_2}. \tag{3}$$

Now, during isovolumic contraction the papillary muscles are not restrained in length, and they can shorten, pulling on the valve membrane, increasing its tension T_1, T_2, and decreasing its radii of curvature r_1, r_2, so that the ventricular pressure p_i is increased. Thus the papillary muscle may be regarded as the controller of the ventricular pressure when the mitral or tricuspid valve is closed.

2.6 Fluid Mechanics of the Heart

To analyze the motion of the heart and the coupling of the heart with the lung and aorta, we must deal with the fluid mechanics of the heart. As an introduction, let us consider a simplified mathematical model of flow in a pulsating bulb presented by R. T. Jones (1969). Consider flows with a velocity potential ϕ given by

$$\phi = \alpha x^2 + \beta y^2 + \gamma z^2, \tag{1}$$

where α, β, γ are functions of time with

$$\alpha(t) + \beta(t) + \gamma(t) = 0 \tag{2}$$

and x, y, z are Cartesian coordinates. The velocity components u, v, w in the directions of x, y, z are given by the derivatives of ϕ:

$$u = \frac{\partial \phi}{\partial x}, \qquad v = \frac{\partial \phi}{\partial y}, \qquad w = \frac{\partial \phi}{\partial z}. \tag{3}$$

They are functions of time and linear in x, y, z. Hence flows represented by Eq. (1) have the property that initially plane surfaces convected with the fluid remain plane. Successive changes in the shape of a bulb are thus related to an (arbitrary) initial shape by affine transformation. If x, y, z are the initial coordinates of a particle of fluid (or of the boundary) we have

$$\zeta = 2x \int \alpha dt, \qquad \eta = 2y \int \beta dt, \qquad \xi = 2z \int \gamma dt, \tag{4}$$

for the Lagrangian coordinates. This is an affine transformation between (x, y, z) and (ξ, η, ζ).

If the time dependence in Eq. (1) is represented by a single function, as in

$$\phi = f(t)[ax^2 + by^2 + cz^2], \tag{5}$$

where a, b, c are constants with

$$a + b + c = 0, \tag{6}$$

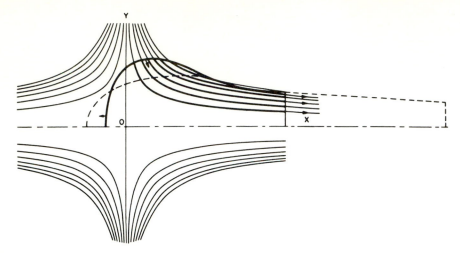

Figure 2.6:1 Streamlines for a collapsing bulb. From Jones (1972), by permission.

then the streamlines are stationary though the flow is time dependent. The streamlines for a flow of this type, with $a = 2$, $b = -1$, $c = -1$, is shown in Fig. 2.6:1. In this case the flow is axially symmetric with a stagnation point at the origin. Starting with a bulb of arbitrary shape, successive shapes are obtained by a simple stretching transformation. Figure 2.6:1 illustrates this process. Here a bulb is drawn in heavy line; its mouth opens to the right. At a later moment the bulb's shape is changed into the one outlined by the dotted curve.

With the effect of viscosity omitted, the pressure at points within the bulb is given by the generalized Bernoulli's equation (cf. Sec. 1.11)

$$p = p_o(t) - \frac{\rho}{2}(u^2 + v^2 + w^2) - \rho\frac{d\phi}{dt}, \tag{7}$$

where ρ is the density of the fluid. Equation (7) contains an arbitrary function, $p_o(t)$, which must be determined by the impedance into which the bulb works.

For flows with stationary streamlines the isobaric surfaces given by $u^2 + v^2 + w^2$ and ϕ in Eq. (5) are also stationary. Figure 2.6:2 shows these isobaric surfaces for flows with axial symmetry. Jones called the component associated with ϕ the "acceleration pressure," while $(\rho/2)(u^2 + v^2 + w^2)$ is called the "Bernoulli pressure." In an oscillatory flow the latter component will oscillate at twice the frequency of the former.

Figure 2.6:3 shows pressures computed by the above formula for the initial instant of contraction of the bulb shown. Here $u^2 + v^2 + w^2 = 0$ and the pressures are entirely due to acceleration of the flow ($p = p_o - \rho d\phi/dt$). For an ejection curve of the type shown in Fig. 2.4:4, the pressure variation within the bulb amounts to 3 to 5 mm Hg, and the pressures due

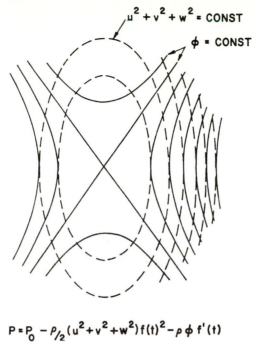

$$P = P_0 - \rho/_2 \, (u^2 + v^2 + w^2) f(t)^2 - \rho \, \phi \, f'(t)$$

Figure 2.6:2 Isobaric surfaces of Jones's solution. From Jones (1972), by permission.

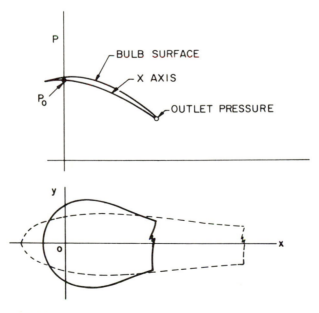

Figure 2.6:3 Initial distribution of pressure within a collapsing bulb. From Jones (1972). Reproduced by permission.

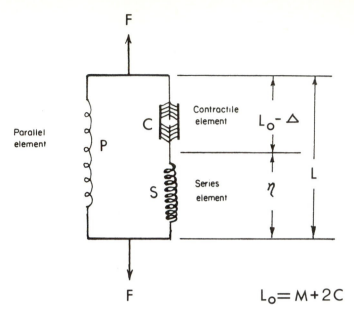

Figure 2.7:1 A schematic diagram of the action of the parallel, series, and contractile elements in a heart muscle.

to the acceleration of flow within the heart are of the same order as the "Bernoulli pressures."

More complete analysis of fluid motion in the heart can be done with numerical methods. See, for example, Peskin (1977).

2.7 The Heart Muscle

The structure and the mechanical properties of the heart muscle have been discussed in Chap. 10 of the first volume of this series: *Biomechanics: Mechanical Properties of Living Tissues* (Fung, 1981). For the purpose of analyzing the whole heart, we shall use the mathematical description of the mechanical properties of each muscle fiber, and assemble the fibers according to the structure exhibited in Figs. 2.2:2 and 2.2:3.

The most useful current model of the mechanical properties of the heart muscle considers each muscle fiber as composed of a parallel element and a contractile element (Fig. 2.7:1). It is assumed that when the muscle is resting the contractile element is completely relaxed, with zero tension, and free to extend or shorten. In the resting state the tissue behaves as an ordinary viscoelastic material with a nonlinear stress–strain relationship. When the muscle is stimulated the contractile element is activated, tension develops, and shortening occurs, if permitted. The tension and shortening is due to the activation of cross bridges between actin and myosin fibers in the sarcomere. The tension in the contractile element is revealed by the elastic extension of the actin and myosin fibers and cross bridges, denoted by the "series elastic" element, S, in Fig. 2.7:1. Thus the total force, F, acting in the fiber is

$$F = P + S, \tag{1}$$

where P and S represent the forces in the parallel and series elements, respectively. To discuss shortening and its relationship to P and S let us regard Fig. 2.7:1 as representing one sarcomere. P is a function of the length L (or the history of L if viscoelasticity is emphasized). Each sarcomere consists of one myosin fiber of length M and two actin fibers of length C each. Hence if the fibers were lined up end-to-end the length would be $M + 2C$. But they overlap by an amount Δ; so the length of an unstressed contractile element is $M + 2C - \Delta$. In the unstressed state the series element extension (i.e., the contractile element's elastic extension) is zero. When the tension is S the series elastic length becomes η. Hence in the stressed state the sarcomere length is

$$L = M + 2C - \Delta + \eta. \tag{2}$$

By differentiation, we have

$$\frac{dL}{dt} = -\frac{d\Delta}{dt} + \frac{d\eta}{dt}, \tag{3}$$

which is a basic kinematic relation connecting the rate of muscle length change with the rate at which the actin–myosin overlap changes, and the velocity of extension of the series element.

Experimental data on resting heart muscles show that (Pinto and Fung, 1973)

$$\frac{dP}{d\lambda} = \alpha(P + \beta) \tag{4}$$

or

$$P + \beta = ce^{\alpha\lambda}, \tag{5}$$

where λ is the stretch ratio of the muscle (measured from the state of zero tension in resting state), α, β are material constants. c is an integration constant. To determine c, let a point be chosen on the curve, so that $P = P^*$ when $\lambda = \lambda^*$; then

$$P = (P^* + \beta)e^{\alpha(\lambda - \lambda^*)} - \beta. \tag{6}$$

Experimental results on series element show that (Sonnenblick, 1964, Parmley and Sonnenblick, 1967, Edman and Nilsson, 1968)

$$\frac{dS}{d\eta} = \alpha'(S + \beta'), \tag{7}$$

where α', β' are also constants. Hence S is also an exponential function of the extension η:

$$S = (S^* + \beta')e^{\alpha'(\eta - \eta^*)} - \beta'. \tag{8}$$

The contractile element shortening velocity may be represented by the following modified Hill's equation (Fung, 1970)

$$\frac{d\Delta}{dt} = \frac{b[S_o f(t) - S]}{a + S}, \tag{9}$$

in which the constants a and b are functions of muscle length L, S_o is the peak tensile stress arrived in an isometric contraction at length L, t is the time after stimulus, and $f(t)$ is a function which may be represented as

$$f(t) = \sin\left[\frac{\pi}{2}\left(\frac{t + t_o}{t_{ip} + t_o}\right)\right]. \tag{10}$$

Here t_o is a phase shift related to the initiation of the active state at stimulation, and t_{ip} is the time to reach the peak isometric tension after the instant of stimulation. The constant a as a function of L is known empirically to be proportional to S_o which is also a function of L, and can be written as

$$a(L) = \gamma S_o(L). \tag{11}$$

The value of γ is of the order of 0.45. The relationship between S_o and L is shown in Fig. 2.1:3.

If active tension history $S(t)$ is known, then from Eq. (7) we can compute the series element velocity

$$\frac{d\eta}{dt} = \frac{1}{\alpha'(S + \beta')}\frac{dS}{dt}. \tag{12}$$

Using Eqs. (9), (11) and (3), we can obtain the velocity of muscle contraction dL/dt. If the length history $L(t)$ is known, then from Eqs. (3) and (9) we can compute $d\eta/dt$, and then by an integration to obtain η. Then Eq. (8) yields S, Eq. (6) yields P, and Eq. (1) yields the tension in the muscle. In some important problems, however, one would have to find both $S(t)$ and $L(t)$ from specified boundary conditions.

The above is a condensation of a huge amount of experimental data into one set of mathematical expressions. It represents one approach. The data base is, however, somewhat controversial. The curve fitting is sometimes doubtful. Many other approaches have been proposed. See *Biomechanics* (Fung, 1981) for details. Some physiologists (see Brady, 1979) doubt whether one has any right to hope for such a simple set of formulas to represent the mechanical properties of the heart muscle. Others have advanced theories of actin–myosin interaction on the basis of chemical reaction rates, electromagnetic fields, or optimum design principles. These elegant approaches are either too crude to yield realistic relations required in the analysis of the

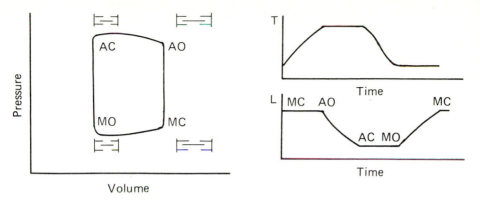

Figure 2.7:2 Sarcomere lengths at different stages of contraction of the heart.

heart, or are many, many times more complex than the formulas presented above, or contain a large number of unknown constants.

A rational analysis of the heart must use Eqs. (1)–(12) together with the fluid mechanical equations for the blood and solid mechanical equations for the wall. Fluid, solid, and muscle mechanics are coupled together. The coupling is indicated in Fig. 2.7:2 in which mitral valve opening (MO), mitral valve closing (MC), aortic valve opening (AO), aortic valve closing (AC), tension (T), sarcomere length (L), and cross bridge configuration (≡≡) are noted as functions of time and cardiac contraction cycle (≡≡ is pronounced as *ken*, one of the ancient Chinese words, meaning water). The solution of these equations is difficult, but valuable. To solve these equations, we have essentially all the basic information we need, except one: the residual stress in the heart wall, which will be discussed in the sections to follow.

2.8 Stresses in the Heart Wall

We need to know stresses and strains in the heart wall in order to know *how* the muscle contracts (Sec. 2.7), *where* on the length–tension curve (Sec. 2.1, Fig. 2.1:3) the points MC, AC of Fig. 2.7:2 correspond to, *how* the blood vessels in the heart wall are deformed and so affect the coronary circulation and health of the heart muscle (Chaps. 3, 4, 5). A rational analysis of systolic and diastolic pressures and stroke volume requires information on the stresses and strains in the heart muscle. We can anticipate that the task of stress analysis will not be simple because of the nonlinear time-dependent stress–strain relationship of the heart muscle. Many papers (Mirsky, 1973, Mirsky, Ghista, and Sandler, 1979, Janz et al, 1973, 1974, Wong and Rautaharju, 1968 etc.) have been published which show terrifying complexity even under strong simplifying assumptions. A major feature of the results in these papers is the great nonuniformity of stress distribution in the heart wall. The inner wall is shown to be the site of large stress concentration.

The general feature may be illustrated by a simple model: Consider a spherical shell of inner radius a and outer radius b, subjected to a uniform internal pressure p_i and external pressure p_o; see Fig. 2.1:2. Assume that the material obeys Hooke's law, and that when p_i and p_o are zero the shell is stress free, i.e., all stresses are zero everywhere. Under these hypotheses, the stress distribution was found by Lamé (1852) a long time ago, (see Fung, *Foundations of Solid Mechanics*, 1965, p. 191).

The classical solution gives the radial stress σ_r:

$$\sigma_r = \frac{p_o b^3 (r^3 - a^3)}{r^3 (a^3 - b^3)} + \frac{p_i a^3 (b^3 - r^3)}{r^3 (a^3 - b^3)} \tag{1}$$

and the circumferential stress σ_θ:

$$\sigma_\theta = \frac{p_o b^3 (2r^3 + a^3)}{2r^3 (a^3 - b^3)} - \frac{p_i a^3 (2r^3 + b^3)}{2r^3 (a^3 - b^3)}. \tag{2}$$

If $p_o = 0$, the greatest circumferential stress is at the inner surface, at which

$$(\sigma_\theta)_{\text{max}} = \frac{p_i}{2} \frac{2a^3 + b^3}{b^3 - a^3}. \tag{3}$$

If $a = 1$, $b = 2$, then $(\sigma_\theta)_{\text{max}} = (5/7)p_i$, which is 2.14 times the mean circumferential stress (see the Laplace formula Eq. (4) in Sec. 2.1), and 3.33 times the circumferential stress at the outer wall.

It is remarkable that in this case the solution is independent of the material constants. If the stress–strain relationship is nonlinear, or the shell is not spherical, or if the load and deformation are not spherically symmetric, the solution would depend on the material constants and the analysis would be harder. That is why the analyses given in the papers named above are so difficult.

I feel that such a large stress and strain concentration in a diastolic heart is unreasonable. I will state my case in the following section.

2.9 The Need for a New Hypothesis for Residual Stress Distribution

The Question of Residual Stress

Biological material is not static. It responds to stress by growth or resorption. If tensile stress in a connective tissue is increased beyond the normal value new collagen and elastin grows to increase the load-bearing material, and the stress will be reduced afterward. (See examples of lungs and arteries in Chap. 7 of *Biodynamics: Flow, Motion, and Stress* (Fung, 1984). If compressive stress in bone is increased beyond the normal value, the bone material may either grow or resorb (again, see examples in Chap. 7, *loc cit*). Depending on the circumstances, either growth or resorption may reduce the stress: Growth may be efficient when the stress distribution is quite uniform. Resorption may be more economical to reduce stress concentration. These mechanisms are unique to the living tissues, they are not available to engineers dealing with inanimate structures.

It is well known that in a *statically indeterminate* structure* the stress distribution depends on the "residual" (or "initial") stresses in its members, i.e., the stresses that remain when all of the external load is removed. To discover the initial stresses in a steel truss, the engineer cuts open a sufficient number of bars to make the truss statically determinate and measures the gaps that are opened up by the cuts. Then he uses the theory of elasticity to calculate the initial stresses that are necessary to close these gaps. In another example, an engineer uses shrink fit to fasten a ring onto a shaft, (by heating the ring, slipping it on the shaft, then letting the system cool down). This creates initial compression in the shaft and initial tension in the ring. To discover how large the initial stresses are, he may cut the ring open and measure the gap that appears. Unfortunately, this kind of method generally cannot be used for living organs. It is extremely difficult to discover the initial stresses in biological tissues.

Need for a New Hypothesis

In practically all publications, the assumption is made that the body is stress free when all external loads are removed. This is a good strategy for a linear system, because in such a system one can compute the stresses induced by the external loads and then superpose them on the initial stresses, if any. However, for a nonlinear system the principle of superposition does not apply, and the effect of such an assumption would be far reaching and difficult to evaluate.

For example, Fig. 2.9:1 shows the stresses in the wall of an artery (the thoracic aorta of the rabbit) subjected to an internal pressure of 120 mm Hg ($\sim$ 16 kPa), and an external pressure of zero, computed on the basis of the measured nonlinear stress–strain relationship of the wall material, and the assumption that the wall is stress free when the internal pressure is zero. The concentration of the circumferential stress σ_θ at the inner wall is seen to be very large (being 6.5 times larger than the average value across the

---

* A structure is *statically determinate* (such as a simple truss) if the stresses in all its members can be determined by equations of static equilibrium alone. The stresses in a statically determinate structure do not depend on the elastic deformation of the structure. All other structures are *statically indeterminate*.

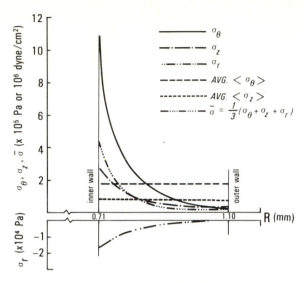

Figure 2.9:1 Distribution of stresses in the wall of the thoracic aorta of the rabbit computed under the assumptions that the wall is stress-free when all the external loads are removed and the internal pressure is 120 mm Hg, the external pressure is zero, and the longitudinal stretch ratio λ_z is 1.691. σ_θ, σ_z, σ_r are the circumferential, longitudinal, and radial stresses, respectively, defined in the sense of Cauchy. $\langle \sigma_\theta \rangle$, $\langle \sigma_z \rangle$ are the values of σ_θ, σ_z averaged thoroughout the wall. $\bar{\sigma} = (\sigma_\theta + \sigma_z + \sigma_r)/3$ is the mean stress (negative of pressure) in the vessel wall. From Chuong and Fung (1983), by permission.

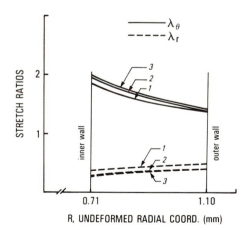

Figure 2.9:2 The distribution of the circumferential stretch ratio λ_θ and the radial stretch ratio λ_r in the thoracic aorta of the rabbit computed as in Fig. 2.9:1. Curve (1) is for $p_i = 60$ mm Hg, $\lambda_z = 1.542$. Curve (2) is for $p_i = 120$ mm Hg, $\lambda_z = 1.691$. Curve (3) is for $p_i = 160$ mm Hg, $\lambda_z = 1.696$. From Chuong and Fung (1983), by permission.

wall). This large stress concentration is a consequence of the large deformation of the artery. For this rabbit artery the inner–radius–to wall-thickness ratio was 1.8 when the blood pressure was zero, but it became 9.5 when the blood pressure was increased to 120 mm Hg, while the longitudinal stretch was maintained at an approximately physiological value. The deformation of the artery between the states of zero blood pressure and normal blood pressure is shown to be very large. The circumferential strain, computed according to Green's definition, is much larger at the inner surface of the vessel wall than that at the outer surface (see Fig. 2.9:2). The stress–strain relationship is exponential as exhibited in Fig. 2.9:3. The large stress concentration at the inner wall is obviously the consequence of the large difference in circumferential strains at the inner and outer walls.

Of all the assumptions leading to this result, the most doubtful is the assumption that the vessel wall is stress free when all external loads are removed. Otherwise the calculations leading to Figs. 2.9:1 and 2.9:2 are quite rigorous, and they are based on the experimentally determined stress–strain law and rigorous equations of continuum mechanics. The zero initial stress assumption, however, has no experimental verification.

In normal life, the blood pressure in the thoracic aorta is never zero. It varies from the systolic pressure to the diastolic pressure, say, from 120 mm Hg to 80 mm Hg. There seems to be no reason for the cells of the blood vessel ever to "remember" a state of zero blood pressure. In the course of development in the embryo there might have been a time when such a condition did prevail, but the cells have gone through many, many generations of new birth and the "memory" cannot be expected to be that good, because new cells must grow in their new environment (new stress field). We can visualize many ways in which the high stress concentration depicted in Fig. 2.9:1 can be attenuated. For example, let more cells be grown on the intima and inner layers of the media, and let more collagen or elastin material be laid down in these layers. The added material will reduce the circumferential strain $E_{\theta\theta}$, and hence the stress $\sigma_{\theta\theta}$, in the normal physiological condition. This growth, however, will introduce a residual compressive stress in the intimal region if the blood pressure were reduced to zero. I am not sure how the cell gets the message that it should divide, grow, or die in this manner, but it is very difficult to imagine a mechanism to regulate the cell growth according to the rule that the residual stress must be zero in a state of zero blood pressure at which the vessel never was.

The same situation applies to the heart, the lungs, and other organs. The hypothesis that the organ is stress free when all of the external load is removed is not so natural. There is a need for a new hypothesis.

There is much experimental evidence of the existence of residual stresses when the external loads are removed. Let us show a few.

Arteries. Fig. 2.9:4 shows the cross section of a thoracic artery of the rabbit freshly taken from a live animal: (a) when it is unloaded, internal and

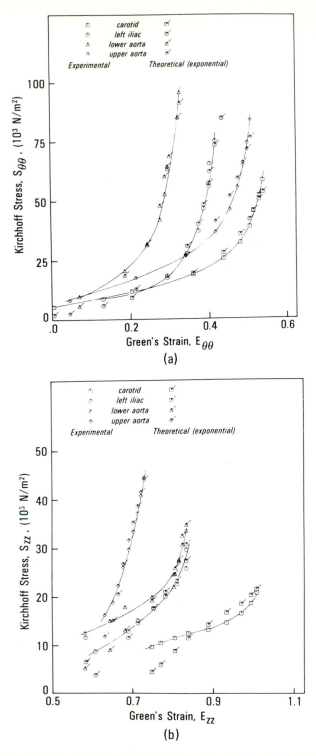

Figure 2.9:3 The stress–strain relationship of the thoracic aorta of the rabbit. From Fung, Fronek, and Patitucci (1979), by permission.

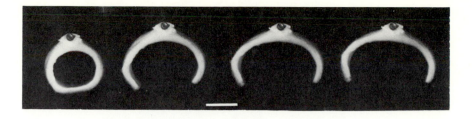

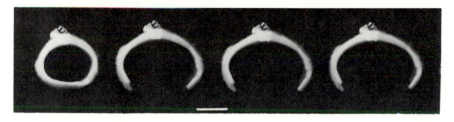

Figure 2.9:4 The cross sectional shape of the thoracic aorta of the cat. *Upper row:* vessel soaked in normal saline. *Left to right:* (1) before cut, (2) 15 sec after cut, (3)15 min after cut, (4) 30 min after cut. *Lower row:* Normal saline + 2 mg. papaverine/cc. *Left to right:* same time sequence, before cut, 15 sec, 15 min, 30 min after cut. Photograph by courtesy of Paul Patitucci. Bar length: 2 mm. The artery segment was glued to a small pin to support it vertically for photography.

external pressures = 0, longitudinal tension = 0; (b) Immediately after the unloaded specimen is cut open longitudinally. The spring back in (b) is evidence that the intimal region in (a) is in compression and the adventitial region in (a) is in tension. By cutting, these stresses are eliminated and the change of strain is made evident by the change of curvature of the wall, and the opening of the gap. Continued change after cutting is evidence of tissue viscoelasticity.

Left Ventricle. Fig. 2.9:5(a) shows an unloaded left ventricle of a rabbit, freshly taken from a live animal, with the right ventricle removed, and the left ventricle cut open longitudinally from apex to base along a line in the middle of the interventricular septa. The ventricle is seen opened up, revealing the residual compressive stress in the inner wall when the pressure load was reduced to zero. The left ventricle was then cut laterally into several slices. Further deformation took place as a result of relieving of residual stress in the longitudinal direction (see Fig. 2.9:5(b)).

Since living tissues are very soft in the stress-free condition, photographs shown in Figs. 2.9:4 and 2.9:5 were taken with the tissues floating in saline, thus avoiding gravitational and frictional disturbances. The pH was controlled at 7.4, and the left ventricle continued to beat and responded to stimulations long after it was excised.

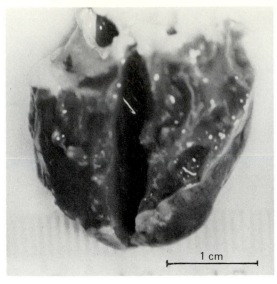

(a)

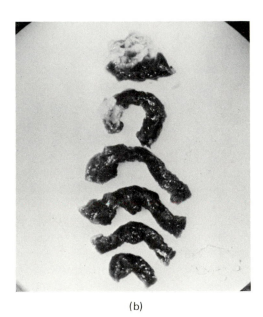

(b)

Figure 2.9:5 The change of shape of the left ventricle of the rabbit when it was cut open. (a) The appearance of the left ventricle after a longitudinal cut was made through the interventricular septum. (The right ventricle was removed.) (b) The cut left ventricle was further sliced into 6 strips. Further large deformation was seen, revealing large residual stresses. Photograph by courtesy of Paul Patitucci.

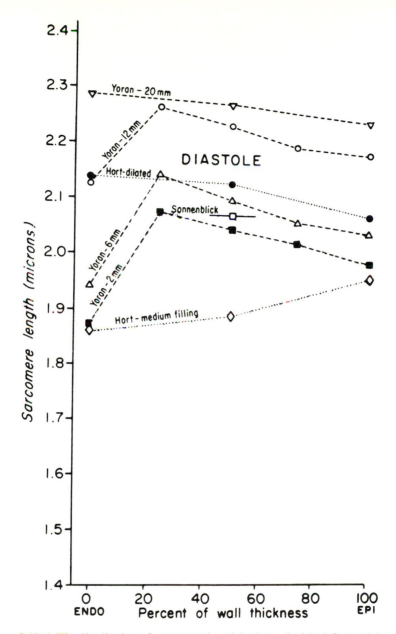

Figure 2.10:1 The distribution of sarcomere length in the wall of the left ventricle of the dog in diastolic condition as given by Hort (1960), Yoran et al. (1973), and Sonnenblick et al. (1967).

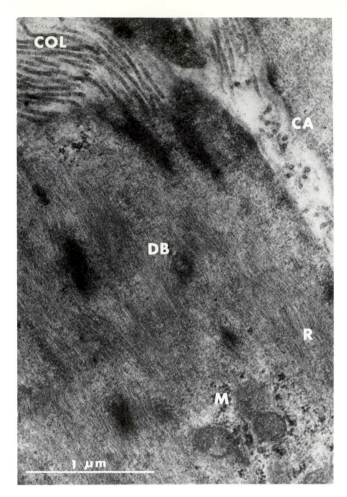

Figure 2.10:2 *Left panel:* Vascular smooth muscle in a small artery of the mesentery of the rabbit, at a magnification of 53,185, showing the dense bodies (DB), collagen (COL) caveoli (CA), ribosomes (R), mitochondria (M). Electron micrograph by John Hardy in Los Angeles County-USC Cardiovascular Research Lab., Sid Sobin, Director.

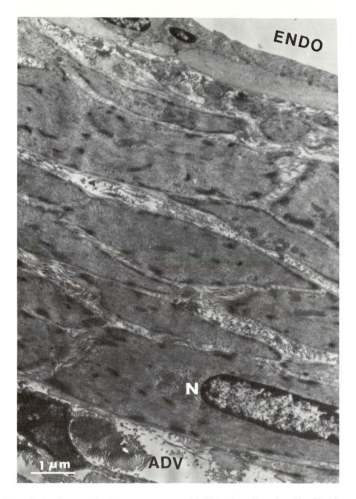

Figure 2.10:2 *Right panel:* Same artery, × 10,725, showing the distribution of dense bodies in the muscle layers, and endothelium (ENDO), nucleus (N), adventitia (ADV). Blood pressure = 100 mm Hg. Inner diameter of blood vessel = 320 μm.

2.10 The Principle of Optimal Operation

I will put forward the following hypothesis: Each organ operates in a manner to achieve optimal performance in some sense. In particular, the residual stress in the tissue distributes itself in a way to assure such a performance. The optimal condition may vary from organ to organ; but, in general, it is not the same as zero residual stress when all of the external loads are removed.

For example, the heart is a pump. When the left ventricle is filled and systolic contraction begins, all muscle cells will contract in approximately isometric condition until the aortic valve is opened. Let us assume that the optimal condition be that every muscle cell of the heart contributes equally to the contraction in this period. Since the maximum tensile stress in an isometric contraction varies with the length of the sarcomere, and the velocity of contraction varies with the tensile stress, we see that a requirement of uniform performance of every muscle cell is equivalent to requiring all the sarcomeres to have the same length throughout the heart in this period. But at the end-diastolic condition the sarcomere length is determined by the preload on the muscle cells. Hence, in order to achieve a uniform sarcomere length throughout the heart, the stress (in the direction of the muscle fibers) must be uniform everywhere. Now, the stress in a relaxed muscle is a unique function of the stretch ratio. Hence, the stretch ratio of every muscle fiber should be the same at the end-diastolic condition. From this the residual stress when the ventricles are unloaded can be computed.

Is there evidence for this? In a crude way, yes. Figure 2.10:1 shows some existing data on the distribution of sarcomere length in the wall of the left ventricle of the dog. The data are taken from the papers of Hort (1960), Yoran et al. (1973), and Sonnenblick et al. (1967). While none of them shows exactly uniform distribution of the sarcomere length at end-diastole (at some finite ventricular pressure), they are all far different from what one would have predicted from the hypothesis that the sarcomere length is uniform when the left ventricle is load free (with zero transmural pressure). If the last-mentioned hypothesis were true, then at the end-diastolic condition (when the ventricular transmural pressure is finite) the sarcomere length would be longest at the endocardium and shortest in the epicardium, similar to λ_θ the case shown in Fig. 2.9:2. This is obviously not the case.

It is fortunate that the sarcomeres can serve as natural grid lines to measure the change of strains in a muscle. For arteries and veins, the dense bodies of the smooth-muscle cells (see *Biomechanics*, Fung, 1981, p. 358) can serve as markers also, although they are not as evenly spaced as the Z-lines of the sarcomeres of the heart muscle. The dense bodies are smooth muscle's equivalent of the Z-lines of the skeletal and heart muscles. Fig. 2.10:2 shows the distribution of dense bodies in the mesenteric artery of the rabbit. It can be seen that the dense bodies are either attached to the cell membranes or are free-floating. By measuring the number of the dense bodies per unit length of the cell membrane as seen in these electronmicrographs, we can obtain a measure of the spacing of the dense bodies. Our results are

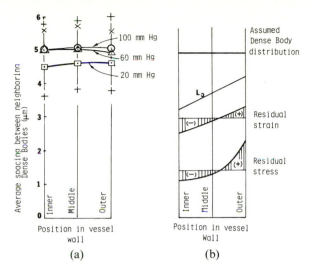

Figure 2.10:3 (a) The distribution of dense bodies on the cell membranes of the smooth muscles in the small mesenteric arteries of the rabbit (inner diameter 300–425 μm). Spacing between neighboring dense bodies averaged over inner, middle, and outer one-third of the vessel wall, in μm. Mean $\pm$ S.D. (+ for 20 and 100 mm Hg, $\times$ for 60 mm Hg). (b) Probable distribution of residual circumferential stress and strain in arterial wall calculated under the assumption that the circumferential stress and strain are distributed uniformly in the wall at 60 mm Hg blood pressure. See text.

shown in Fig. 2.10:3. (a) shows the spacing between neighboring dense bodies attached to the cell membranes in longitudinal cross sections of the smooth muscle. It is seen that the spacing is statistically uniform throughout the vessel wall when the blood pressure is 20 mm Hg and above. (b) shows some results calculated under the assumption that the stress is uniformly distributed at a blood pressure of 60 mm Hg. L_0 is the reference length of wall material at zero stress. The residual circumferential strain and stress in the vessel wall when the blood pressure is reduced to zero are calculated on the basis of a nonlinear stress–strain relationship (Eq. (1), p. 66). At zero pressure the inner wall is compressed and the outer wall is in tension. If the wall is cut longitudinally, the relief of the circumferential stress will cause the artery to spring open, in agreement with the result shown in Fig. 2.9:4.

2.11 Consequences of Our New Hypothesis

It remains to discover what the optimal condition is for each organ. Once the optimal condition is found, one can then proceed to analyze the stress and strain in the organ. For example, in the case of the left ventricle, if we can assume that the optimal condition is the uniformity of sarcomere length at the end diastolic condition, which corresponds to a uniform stretch ratio λ throughout the ventricle wall, then we can calculate, step by step, the shape of the left ventricle when the transmural pressure vanishes, and the contraction process of the heart. The dynamics of the left ventricle, the fluid mechanics of blood in the heart, the ejection process, the coupling of the heart with the aorta and pulmonary artery, and the coupling of the cardiac fluid dynamics with the pulmonary and peripheral circulations, are all affected by the initial hypothesis.

Problems

2.1 Consider a blood vessel, Fig. P2.1. Let us make the following assumptions: (1) When the internal and external pressures are both zero and the length is fixed, it is a uniform long circular cylindrical tube with inner radius R_i and outer radius R_o. (2) In this state the circumferential stress is zero everywhere. (3) The vessel wall material is incompressible. (4) The relationship between the circumferential stress T and the circumferential stretch ratio λ is given by Eq. (5) on p. 269 of *Biomechanics* (Fung, 1981):

$$T = (T^* + \beta)e^{\alpha(\lambda - \lambda^*)} - \beta, \tag{1}$$

where α, β are material constants and (T^*, λ^*) represent a point on the curve, $T = T^*$ when $\lambda = \lambda^*$. The values of α and $E_0 = \alpha\beta$ are given in Fig. 8.3:2, p. 270 of that book.

Now let the vessel be subjected to an internal pressure p and an external pressure of zero. The inner radius then becomes r_i. Under assumption (3) (incompressibility), how large would the outer radius r_o be? and what would be the stress distribution in the wall? Express r_o in terms of r_i, R_i, and R_o. Do the same for every point r in the wall, which has an original radius of R. Then compute λ as a function of R or r, and finally the stress T as a function of R or r.

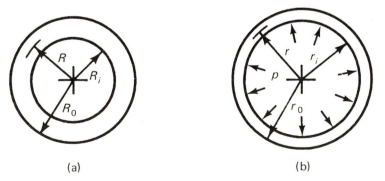

(a)   (b)

Figure P2.1 Cross section of a blood vessel when it is (a) unloaded, and (b), loaded.

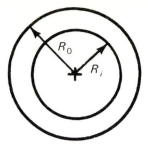
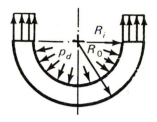

Diastolic condition

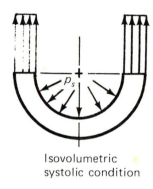
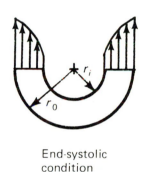

Isovolumetric
systolic condition

End-systolic
condition

Figure P2.3 Simplified ventricular analysis.

2.2 In the problem above, change the second hypothesis to: (2′) At an internal pressure
of p, outer pressure of zero, and an inner radius of r_i, the circumferential stress T
is uniform throughout the vessel wall. λ is, therefore, a constant. Now, let the
internal pressure be reduced to zero. The blood vessel diameter will be reduced.
Calculate the new stress distribution. What assumptions must be made in order to
get an answer? Is the solution unique?

2.3 Consider an approximate theory of the heart, Fig. P2.3. Let the left ventricle be
approximated by a spherical shell of uniform wall thickness. In the *end diastolic*
condition the internal pressure is p_d, the active tension in the muscle is zero, the
inner and outer radii are R_i and R_o, respectively. Let us *assume that in the end
diastolic condition the circumferential stress in the wall is uniformly distributed in the
wall*. Now let the valves be closed and the muscle be stimulated and the left ventricle
*contracted isometrically. Assume that the active muscle tension is also uniformly
distributed throughout the wall in this isometric condition*. When the systolic pressure
becomes p_s, what would the active tensile stress be?

You may analyze the problem with algebraic symbols. When you have finished,
try the following numerical values and find the values of the passive and active
tensile stresses:

$$R_i = 3 \text{ cm}, \qquad R_o = 3.6 \text{ cm},$$

$$p_d = 11 \text{ cm H}_2\text{O} \doteq 11 \times 10^3 \text{ dyn/cm}^2,$$

$$p_s = 150 \text{ cm H}_2\text{O} \doteq 150 \times 10^3 \text{ dyn/cm}^2.$$

Assume that the active tension corresponds to the point A on the curve of length–tension diagram shown in Fig. 2.1:3. What is the sarcomere length of this heart in the end diastolic condition?

In the second stage of systolic contraction, the aortic valve is open and blood is ejected. At the end of systole the inner and outer radii become r_i, r_o respectively and the aortic valve is closed again.

Assume that the wall material is uniform and incompressible, that the passive property of the muscle obeys the stress–strain relationship given by Eq. (1) of Problem **2.1**, and that the total stress is the sum of the passive stress and the active stress as in Hill's model. In this contracted condition, what is the strain (or stretch ratio) in the ventricular wall? What is the passive stress distribution in the wall? What is the active stress distribution in the wall? What assumptions must be made in order to get a reasonable approximate answer?

2.12 Embedding Muscle Fibers in a Continuum

A mathematical formalism of embedding muscle fibers into a continuum (such as the heart) was developed by the author (Fung, 1971a) and used by him (Fung, 1971b) in an analysis of ureteral peristalsis. Since large deformation is concerned, we must use the method of finite strain (see, for example, Fung, 1965, Ch. 16; or Fung, 1984, Appendix). Let a rectangular Cartesian frame of reference x_i ($i = 1, 2, 3$) be chosen. Let e_{ij} and E_{ij} be the Eulerian and Lagrangian strain tensors, respectively, which describe the deformation of the heart from a reference state, (e.g., the end diastolic state). If da_i is a differential element in the reference state, and dx_i is the corresponding element after deformation, and if ds_0 and ds represent the lengths of the elements da_i and dx_i respectively, then, by definition (see Fung (1977), p. 126),

$$ds^2 - ds_0^2 = 2E_{ij}da_i da_j = 2e_{ij}dx_i dx_j. \tag{1}$$

Hence the stretch ratio

$$\lambda = ds/ds_0, \tag{2}$$

is related to the direction cosines

$$n_i = da_i/ds_0, \qquad v_i = dx_i/ds, \tag{3}$$

by the equations

$$\lambda^2 - 1 = 2E_{ij}n_i n_j, \qquad 1 - \frac{1}{\lambda^2} = 2e_{ij}v_i v_j. \tag{4}$$

Now, if da_i is an element, say a sarcomere of a muscle fiber so that ds_0 represents the sarcomere length in the reference state, then dx_i is the deformed element and ds represents the instantaneous sarcomere length, which can be identified with the length L in Eq. (2.7:2). In Sec. 2.7 we distinguish the muscle length L from the "insertion," $-\Delta$, (the overlap of the actin and myosin fibers in a sarcomere), and the series elastic element extension η. Similarly, we *decompose the strain tensor* e_{ij} *into an insertion tensor* $-\Delta_{ij}$ *and a series elastic strain tensor* η_{ij}. Thus,

$$e_{ij} = -\Delta_{ij} + \eta_{ij}. \tag{5}$$

The strain e_{ij} is defined for the continuum. The insertion, Δ_{ij}, is supposed to occur in individual sarcomeres. Equation (5) imposes constraints on Δ_{ij} and η_{ij} so that together they must fit into a continuum.

Corresponding to the strains there are stresses. The stress tensor τ_{ij} will be decomposed into a "series element" due to the actin–myosin contractile machinery and a "parallel element" due to connective tissues, $\tau_{ij}^{(s)}$ and $\tau_{ij}^{(p)}$, respectively,

$$\tau_{ij} = \tau_{ij}^{(s)} + \tau_{ij}^{(p)}. \tag{6}$$

In Sec. 2.7 we have summarized results on the series and parallel tensions in uniaxial loading experiments on papillary muscles. We shall assume that in a three-dimensional continuum the contractile mechanism in each sarcomere remains the same as that in the papillary muscle. Modifications of the papillary muscle properties to those of the heart will be done by modifying and generalizing P and η to the tensors $\tau_{ij}^{(P)}$ and η_{ij}. $\tau_{ij}^{(P)}$ is related to the strain e_{ij} by a constitutive equation of the type discussed in *Biomechanics* (Fung, 1981, chaps. 7, 9). $\tau_{ij}^{(s)}$ is related to η_{ij} as discussed below.

Let a set of local cartesian coordinates y_1, y_2, y_3 be chosen so that y_1 lies in the direction of the muscle fiber. Then both the actin–myosin insertion Δ and the series elastic tension, S, generated by the contractile mechanism, act in the direction of y_1. If we denote the insertion and series elasticity tensors referred to the muscle axes y_1, y_2, y_3 by $\bar{\Delta}_{ij}$ and $\bar{\tau}_{ij}^{(s)}$, respectively, then their components are

$$(\bar{\Delta}_{ij}) = \begin{pmatrix} \Delta & 0 & 0 \\ 0 & 0 & 0 \\ 0 & 0 & 0 \end{pmatrix}, \qquad \bar{\tau}_{ij}^{(s)} = \begin{pmatrix} S & 0 & 0 \\ 0 & 0 & 0 \\ 0 & 0 & 0 \end{pmatrix}. \tag{7}$$

Only the first elements are nonvanishing. If the axes x_1, x_2, x_3 are related to y_1, y_2, y_3 by the equations

$$x_i = \beta_{ij} y_j, \tag{8}$$

then, according to the usual tensor transformation law,

$$\Delta_{ij} = \bar{\Delta}_{kl} \beta_{ik} \beta_{jl}, \qquad \tau_{ij}^{(s)} = \bar{\tau}_{kl}^{(s)} \beta_{ik} \beta_{jl}. \tag{9}$$

Note that if, as in Eq. (3), the direction cosines of a muscle fiber are v_1, v_2, v_3, then, since the axis y_1 lies in the direction of the muscle,

$$\beta_{11} = v_1, \qquad \beta_{21} = v_2, \qquad \beta_{31} = v_3, \tag{10}$$

we have

$$\varDelta_{ij} = v_i v_j \varDelta, \qquad \tau_{ij}^{(s)} = v_i v_j S. \tag{11}$$

The properties of $\varDelta$ and S will be assumed to be the same as those described in Sec. 2.7. The stress tensor τ_{ij} is fully determined when the history of stimulation and constraints are prescribed. The structural details of the heart are prescribed by the vector v_i or tensor β_{ij}. The equation of motion is, as usual,

$$\rho \frac{DV_i}{Dt} = \frac{\partial \tau_{ij}}{\partial x_j} + \rho X_i, \tag{12}$$

where V_i is the velocity vector, DV_i/Dt is the acceleration, X_i is the body force per unit mass, and ρ is the density. In most problems X_i is zero and the inertia force is negligible. Then the equation of equilibrium is

$$\frac{\partial \tau_{ij}}{\partial x_j} = 0. \tag{13}$$

Together with the equation of continuity (conservation of mass), the system of field equations is now complete.

The Fluid–Fiber Model

Chadwick (1981) proposed a "fluid–fiber" model, and Skalak (1982) used it to develop some approximate formulas. Neither of them considered active contraction specifically. In their model, the stress tensor is assumed to be of the form

$$\tau_{ij} = -p\delta_{ij} + Tv_i v_j. \tag{14}$$

This is interpreted as saying that the fiber, in the direction of v_i, has a tensile stress T in the direction of the fiber. The continuum is assumed to be incompressible, so an arbitrary parameter, p, the "pressure," is added. The last term is identical in form with the contractile stress given in Eq. (11). Actually, as a model of contraction, this is reasonable; but as a model of a resting myocardium, this is quite doubtful. There is no evidence that a resting muscle is so orthotropic that tension can develop only along the length of the fibers. The fibers are so well embedded in connective tissues that they can respond normally to any kind of loading: tension, compression, or shear, in any direction. Experiments on the diaphragm, a skeletal muscle, show that at the resting state its mechanical behavior is anisotropic, but not much more directionally dependent than the abdominal skin. The diaphragm can sustain tension very well in the direction perpendicular to the muscle fibers. For this reason we believe that Eq. (14) is not a good model of the resting myocardium.

Skalak's Approximations

Skalak (1981) derived an interesting formula based on the following assumptions: (a) The tension T is constant along the fiber, so that $\partial T/\partial x_j$ vanishes. (b) $\partial v_j/\partial x_j = 0$, i.e., that the fibers are "parallel curves." Then the equation of equilibrium, Eq. (13), becomes

$$\frac{\partial p}{\partial x_i} = T\frac{\partial v_i}{\partial x_j}v_j = T\frac{\partial v_i}{\partial s} = T\frac{1}{R_f}n_i, \tag{15}$$

where s is the distance measured along the fiber, R_f is the radius of curvature of the fiber, and n_i is the ith component of the principal normal vector of the space curve that the fiber follows. This equation may be regarded as a form of the "Laplace law," in which the gradient of p, $\partial p/\partial x_i$, represents the pressure difference per unit normal distance and the tension T acts only along the fiber so that only one term, T/R_f, appears in Eq. (15).

Now, if one makes a third assumption (c) that there is a direction s parallel to the normal $\mathbf{n}$ at every point so that a sequence of normals going from the outside of the ventricle to the inside surface allows a straight line to be drawn normal to the inner and outer surfaces of the ventricular wall and being parallel to the fiber normal $\mathbf{n}$ at every point; then Eq. (15) is reduced to

$$\frac{\partial p}{\partial s} = \frac{T}{R_f}. \tag{16}$$

Further simplification can be obtained by more restrictive assumptions. For example, if we assume $T/R_f = \text{const.}$, then Eq. (16) yields

$$p_1 - p_2 = \frac{Th}{R_f}, \tag{17}$$

where p_1, p_2 are the pressures on the inner and outer surfaces of the ventricle, respectively, and h is the ventricular wall thickness. If we assume $T = \text{const.}$ for all fibers, then by integrating Eq. (16) from the inner wall to the outer surface, one obtains

$$p_1 - p_2 = T\int_0^h \frac{1}{R_f}ds = \frac{Th}{\bar{R}_f}, \tag{18}$$

where $\bar{R}_f$ is the mean fiber radius of curvature along the integration path.

Problems

2.4 Formulate a mathematical analysis of the blood flow in the opening process of the aortic and mitral valves. According to experimental results, it is allowable to assume velocity of flow as uniform across the cross section of the valve at any time. Use of this assumption will simplify the analysis.

An example can be found in Lee and Talbot (1978).

2.5 Stenotic heart valves have increased resistance to flow. Use dimensional analysis (by comparing the physical dimensions of various terms, e.g., pressure,
$[ML^{-1}T^{-2}]$, where M, L, T, stand for mass, length, and time; velocity $[LT^{-2}]$);
and the so-called Π-theorem), find the relationship between the pressure drop
across a heart valve, the average velocity of flow through the valve, the cross
sectional area of the valve, and the density of the fluid. An empirical constant will
be involved, which can be determined by experiments. Find a formula for the
determination of the cross sectional area of the valve.

    Note: For dimensional analysis, see *Biomechanics*, (Fung, 1981, p. 143). For
experiments on stenotic heart valves, see Gorlin and Gorlin (1951).

2.6 Write down a full set of basic equations and boundary conditions governing the
flow of blood in the left ventricle.

    Cf. Peskin (1977).

2.7 Write down a full set of field equations and boundary conditions governing the
deformation of the myocardium.

2.8 Write down a full set of equations governing blood flow through the heart valves
in the process of closing.

2.9 The flow through heart valves was analyzed by Lee and Talbot (1978) using a cone
with straight walls to simulate the aortic valve and a pair of rigid flaps (see Fig.
2.5:5) to simulate the mitral valve. As a result of this simplifying simulation, a
singularity exists at the instant of valve closing: the velocity becomes infinitely
large and the valves cannot close without regurgitation (backward flow). To
remove this difficulty, the valve leaflets should be assumed flexible, with a curved
wall. Formulate an improved theory.

2.10 At the end of the diastolic state, the left ventricular wall may be considered as a
layered orthotropic pseudoelastic material. One of the material axes of symmetry
must coincide with the direction of muscle fibers. Since fiber direction changes
systematically throughout the ventricular wall the directions of the material axes
of symmetry change in different layers. Assume a pseudo strain energy function
for the temporarily resting myocardium in a form similar to those presented in
Chapters 7 and 8 of *Biomechanics* (Fung, 1981, Sec. 7.9, and pp. 249, 252, 277).
Use it to specialize the general equations obtained in Prob. 2.7.

2.11 In many publications on stress analysis of the myocardium, the mechanical
property of the material is assumed to be isotropic. Discuss qualitatively the effect
of this hypothesis on the stress distribution in the myocardium. (Mirsky (1979).)

2.12 Consider the question of stress concentration in a thick-walled spherical shell
subjected to internal pressure. Under the hypotheses that (1), the initial stress is
zero when the shell is unloaded and (2), the material obeys Hooke's law, we have
the classical solution by Lamé, Eqs. (1) and (2) of Sec. 2.8. Now, retain the assumption (1) but replace the assumption (2) by a more realistic exponentially stiffening
stress-strain law, e.g., by one of incompressible material with a pseudo-strain-
energy function

$$\rho_0 W = C \exp\left[a_1 E_{\theta\theta}^2 + a_2 E_{\phi\phi}^2 + a_4 E_{\theta\theta} E_{\phi\phi}\right]$$

where $E_{\theta\theta}$, $E_{\phi\phi}$ are strains in the circumferential (θ) and longitudinal (ϕ) directions, respectively, and C, a_1, a_2, a_4 are constants. Will the stress concentration be increased or decreased? Give an estimate.

Note: The pseudo-strain-energy function given above is discussed in detail in *Biomechanics* (Fung, 1981, Ch. 7 and 8).

2.13 The finite-element method should be suitable for the analysis of the stress distribution in the myocardium. For an analysis of myocardium at the end diastolic state considered in Prob. 2.7, how can a finite element be formulated?

2.14 The finite-element method should be useful also for the analysis of the contraction process of the heart. In formulating a finite element of the heart muscle in active contraction, what basic information is needed? For the whole heart, what additional information is needed? How can the coupling of the circulation in the heart to that in the lung and aorta be described mathematically? (The last question is discussed in Waldman (1983)).

References

Bellhouse, B. J. (1972). The fluid mechanics of heart valves. In *Cardiovascular Fluid Dynamics* (D. H. Bergel ed.), Vol. 1, Academic Press, New York, Ch. 8, pp. 261–285.

Bellhouse, B. J. and Bellhouse, F. H. (1969). Fluid mechanics of model normal and stenosed aortic valves. *Circulation Research*, **25**: 693–704.

Bellhouse, B. J. and Bellhouse, F. H. (1972). Fluid mechanics of a model mitral valve and left ventricle. *Cardiovascular Research* **6**: 199–210.

Berne, R. M., Sperelakis, N. (ed.) (1979). *Handbook of Physiology*. Sec. 2. *The Cardiovascular System*, Vol. 1. *The Heart*. American Physiological Society, Bethesda, Md.

Bohr, D. F., Somlyo, A. P., and Spark, H. V., Jr. (eds.) (1980). *Handbook of Physiology*. Sec. 2. *The Cardiovascular System*. Vol. 2. *Vascular Smooth Muscle*. American Physiological Society, Bethesda, Md.

Brady, A. J. (1979). Mechanical properties of cardiac fibers. In *Handbook of Physiology*, Sec. 2, Vol. 1. *The Heart*. (Berne, R. M. and Sperelakis, N. eds.), American Physiological Society, Bethesda, Md, pp. 461–474.

Chadwick, R. S. (1981). The myocardium as a fluid-fiber continuum: passive equilibrium configurations. In *1981 Advances in Bioengineering* (Viano, D. C. ed.), American Society of Mechanical Engineers, New York, pp. 135–138.

Chuong, C. J. and Fung, Y. C. (1983). Three-dimensional stress distribution in arteries. *J. Biomechanical Engineering*. **105**: 268–274.

Danielson, D. A. (1977). Mechanics of muscular organs. *Journal of Biomechanics* **10**: 355–356.

Durrer, D., and van der Tweel, L. H. (1957). Excitation of the left ventricular wall of the dog and goat. *Ann. New York Academy of Science*, **65**: 779–802.

Edman, K. A. P. and Nilsson, E. (1972). Relationship between force and velocity of shortening in rabbit papillary muscle. *Acta Physiol. Scand.* **85**: 488–500.

Frank, O. (1899). Die grundform des arteriellen pulses. Erste Abhandlung, Mathematische Analyse. *Z. Biol.* **37**: 483–526.

Fung Y. C. (1965). *Foundations of Solid Mechanics*. Prentice-Hall, Englewood Cliffs, N. J.

Fung, Y. C. (1970). Mathematical representation of the mechanical properties of the heart muscle. *J. of Biomechanics*. **3**: 381–404.

Fung, Y. C. (1971a). Muscle controlled flow. In *Development in Mechanics, Proc. of 12th Midwest Mechanics Conf*. Vol. 6, Univ. of Notre Dame, Ind, art. 3, pp. 33–62.

Fung, Y. C. (1971b). Peristaltic pumping: A bioengineering model. In *Urodynamics: Hydrodynamics of the Ureter and Renal Pelvis*. (Boyarsky, S., Gottschalk, C. W., Tanago, E. A. and Zimskind, P. D., eds.) Academic Press, New York.

Fung, Y. C. (1977). *A First Course in Continuum Mechanics*. 2nd edn. Prentice-Hall, Englewood Cliffs, N.J.

Fung, Y. C. (1981). *Biomechanics: Mechanical Properties of Biological Materials*. Springer-Verlag, New York.

Fung, Y. C. (1984). *Biodynamics: Flow, Motion, and Stress*. Springer-Verlag, New York. In press.

Gay, W. A. and Johnson, E. A. (1967). Anatomical evaluation of the myocardial length-tension diagram. *Circulation Research* **21**: 33–43.

Gorlin, R. and Gorlin, S. G. (1951). Hydraulic formula for calculation of the area of the stenotic mitral valve, other cardiac valves, and central circulatory shunts. *Am. Heart J*. **41**: 1–29.

Hales, S. (1733). *Statical Essays. II. Haemostaticks*. Innays and Manby, London, Reprinted by Hafner, New York.

Henderson, Y. and Johnson, F. E. (1912). Two modes of closure of the heart valves. *Heart*. **4**: 69–82.

Hill, A. V. (1939). The heat of shortening and the dynamic constants of muscle. *Proc. Roy. Soc. London (Biol.) B*. **126**: 136–195.

Hort, W. (1960). Makroskopische und mikrometrische untersuchungen am Myokard verschieden stark gefullter linker kammern. *Virchows Arch Path. Anat*. **333**: 523–564.

Iwazumi, T. (1970). A new field theory of muscle contraction. Ph. D. Thesis, University of Pennsylvania, Pa.

Janz, R. F. and Grimm, A. F. (1973). Deformation of the diastolic left ventricle. I. Nonlinear elastic effects. *Biophys. J*. **13**: 689–704.

Janz, R. F., Grimm, A. F., Kubert, B. R., and Moriarty, T. F. (1974). Deformation of the diastolic left ventricle. II. Nonlinear geometric effects. *J. of Biomechanics* **7**: 509–516.

Janz, R. F. and Waldron, R. J. (1976). Some implications of a constant fiber stress hypothesis in the diastolic left ventricle. *Bull. Math. Biol*. **38**: 401–413.

Jones, R. T. (1969). Blood flow. In *Annual Review of Fluid Mechanics* (W. R. Sears and M. van Dyke, eds.) Annual Reviews, Palo Alto, Ca.

Jones, R. T. (1972). Fluid dynamics of heart assist devices. In *Biomechanics: Its Foundations and Objectives*. (ed. by Y. C. Fung, N. Perrone, and M. Anliker), Prentice-Hall, Englewood Cliffs, N.J., Chapter 21, pp. 549–565.

Lamé, E. (1852). *Lecons sur la theorie de l'elasticite*. Paris.

Lee, C. S. F. and Talbot, L. (1979). A fluid mechanical study on the closure of heart valves. *J. Fluid Mechanics* **91**(1): 41–63.

McDonald, D. A. (1974). *Blood Flow in Arteries*. Williams & Wilkins, Baltimore, Md.

Milnor, W. R. (1975). Arterial impedance as ventricular afterload. *Circulation Res.* **36**: 565–570.

Mirsky, I. (1973). Ventricular and arterial wall stresses based on large deformation analysis. *Biophysical J.* **13**: 1141–1159.

Mirsky, I., Ghista, D. N., and Sandler, H. (eds.) (1974). *Cardiac Mechanics: Physiological, Clinical, and Mathematical Considerations.* John Wiley & Sons Inc., New York.

Mirsky, I. (1979). Elastic properties of the myocardium: a quantitative approach with physiological and clinical applications. In *Handbook of Physiology, Sec. 2, Vol. 1. The Heart.* (Berne, R. M. and Sperelakis, N. eds.), American Physiological Society, Bethesda, Md., pp. 497–531.

Netter, F. (1969). *The Ciba Collection of Medical Illustrations*, Vol. 5, *Heart*, CIBA Publications Dept., Summit, N.J.

Parmley, W. W. and Sonnenblick, E. H. (1967). Series elasticity of heart muscle: Its relation to contractile element velocity and proposed muscle models, *Circulation Res.* **20**: 112–123.

Parmley, W. W., Brutsaert, D. L. and Sonnenblick, E. H. (1969). The effects of altered loading on contractile events in isolated cat papillary muscle. *Circulation Res.* **24**: 521–532.

Parmley, W. and Talbot, L. (1979). Heart as a pump. In *Handbook of Physiology. Sec. 2. The Cardiovascular System, Vol. 1, The Heart.* (Berne, R. M. and Sperelakis, N. eds.), American Physiological Society, Bethesda, Md., pp. 429–460.

Peskin, C. S. (1977). Numerical analysis of blood flow in the heart. *J. Comput. Phys.* **25**: 220–252.

Peskin, C. S. and Wolfe, A. W. (1978). The aortic sinus vortex. *Federation Proc.* **37**: 2784–2792.

Pinto, J. G. and Fung, Y. C. (1973a). Mechanical properties of the heart muscle in the passive state. *J. Biomechanics* **6**: 597–616.

Pinto, J. G. and Fung, Y. C. (1973b). Mechanical properties of stimulated papillary muscle in quick-release experiments. *J. Biomechanics* **6**: 617–630.

Scher, A. M. and Spach, M. S. (1979). Cardiac depolarization and repolarization and the electrocardiogram. In *Handbook of Physiology, Sec. 2, Vol. 1, The Heart.* (Berne, R. M. and Sperelakis, N., eds.), American Physiological Society, Bethesda, Md., pp. 357–392.

Skalak, R. (1982). Approximate formulas for myocardial fiber stresses. *J. Biomechanical Engineering.* **104**: 162–163.

Sonnenblick, E. H. (1962). Implications of muscle mechanics in the heart. *Federation Proc.* **21**: 975–990.

Sonnenblick, E. H. (1964). Series elastic and contractile elements in heart muscle: changes in muscle length. *Am. J. Physiol.* **207**: 1330–1338.

Sonnenblick, E. H., Braunwald, E., Covell, J. W., and Ross, Jr., J. (1966). Alterations in resting length-tension relations of cardiac muscle induced by changes in contractile force. *Circulation Res.* **19**: 980–988.

Sonnenblick, E. H., Spotnitz, H. and Spiro, D. (1964). The relation of sarcomere structure to the pressure-volume curve of the intact dog ventricle. *Supp.* III to *Circulation*, Vol. **29–30**, p. 111–163.

Sonnenblick, E. H., Ross, Jr., Jr, Covell, J. W., Spotnitz, H. M. and Spiro, D. (1967). Ultrastructure of the heart in systole and diastole: changes in sarcomere length. *Circulation Res.* **21**: 423–431.

Streeter, D. Jr. (1979). Gross morphology and fiber geometry of the heart. In *Handbook of Physiology, Sec. 2, Cardiovascular System. Vol. 1. The Heart* (Berne, R. M. and Sperelakis, N. eds.), American Physiology Society, Bethesda, Md., pp. 61–112.

Streeter, D., Jr., Spotnitz, H. M., Patel, D. J., Ross, J. Jr., and Sonnenblick, E. H. (1969). Fiber orientation in the canine left ventricle during diastole and systole. *Circulation Res.* **24**: 339–347.

Streeter, D., Jr., and Hanna, W. T. (1973). Engineering mechanics for successive states in canine left ventricular myocardium. I. Cavity and Wall Geometry. II. Fiber angle and sarcomere length. *Circulation Res.* **33**: 639–655(I), 656–664(II).

Suga, H., Sagawa, K. and Shoukas, A. A. (1973). Load independence of the instantaneous pressure-volume ratio of the canine left ventricle and effects of epinephrine and heart rate on the ratio. *Circulation* **32**: 314–322.

Waldman, L. K. (1983). On the mechanical coupling of the Heart to the Circulation. Ph.D. thesis. University of California, San Diego.

Wetterer, E. and Kenner, T. (1968). *Die Dynamik des Arterien-pulses.* Springer-Verlag, New York & Berlin.

Wong, A. Y. K. and Rautaharju, P. M. (1968). Stress distribution within the left ventricular wall approximated as a thick ellipsoidal shell. *Am. Heart J.* **75**: 649–662.

Yoran, C., Covell, J. W., and Ross, J., Jr. (1973). Structural basis for the ascending limb of left ventricular function. *Circulation Res.* **32**: 297–303.

CHAPTER 3

Blood Flow in Arteries

3.1 Introduction

The larger systemic arteries, shown in Fig. 3.1:1, conduct the blood from
the heart to the peripheral organs. Their dimensions are given in Table
3.1:1. In man, the aorta originates in the left ventricle at the aortic valve,
and almost immediately curves about 180°, branching off to the head and
upper limbs. It then pursues a fairly straight course down through the
diaphragm to the abdomen and legs. The aortic arch is tapered, curved,
and twisted (i.e., it does not lie in a plane). The other arteries have a constant
diameter between branches, but every time a daughter branch forks off the
main trunk the diameter of the aorta is reduced. Overall, the aorta may be
described as tapered. In the dog, the change of area fits the exponential
equation:

$$A = A_0 e^{(-Bx/R_0)},$$

where A is the area of the aorta, A_0 and R_0 are, respectively, the area and
radius at the upstream site, x is the distance from that upstream site, and
B is a "taper factor," which has been found to lie between 0.02 and 0.05.
Figure 3.1:2 shows a sketch of the dog's aorta.

At a given blood pressure the stress in the arterial wall depends on the
radius and wall thickness of the vessel. These quantities change considerably
with age (see, for example, Fig. 3.1:3). Associated with these geometric
changes are changes in elastic properties. In the thoracic aorta, at a physiological pressure of 1.33×10^4 Nm^{-2} (100 mm Hg), the incremental Young's
modulus E increases steadily with age; but in more peripheral vessels there
is either no change or a fall (see Fig. 3.1:4(a) and (b)). The explanation for
this appears to be that the diameter of the thoracic aorta increases with age,

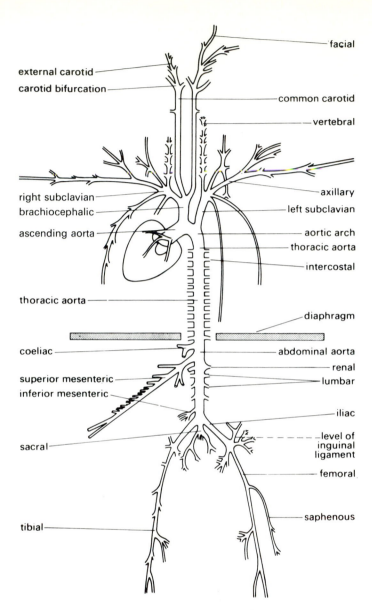

Figure 3.1:1 Major branches of the canine arterial tree. From McDonald (1974), by permission.

TABLE 3.1:1 Normal Values for Canine Cardiovascular Parameters. An Approximate Average Value, and Then the Range, Is Given Where Possible. From Caro, Pedley, and Seed (1974). Reproduced by permission.

Site		Ascending aorta	Descending aorta	Abdominal aorta	Femoral artery	Carotid artery	Arteriole	Capillary	Venule	Inferior vena cava	Main pulmonary artery
Internal diameter d_i	cm	1.5 1.0–2.4	1.3 0.8–1.8	0.9 0.5–1.2	0.4 0.2–0.8	0.5 0.2–0.8	0.005 0.001–0.008	0.0006 0.0004–0.0008	0.004 0.001–0.0075	1.0 0.6–1.5	1.7 1.0–2.0
Wall thickness h	cm	0.065 0.05–0.08		0.05 0.04–0.06	0.04 0.02–0.06	0.03 0.02–0.04	0.002	0.0001	0.0002	0.015 0.01–0.02	0.02 0.01–0.03
h/d_i		0.07 0.055–0.084		0.06 0.04–0.09	0.07 0.055–0.11	0.08 0.053–0.095	0.4	0.17	0.05	0.015	0.01
Length	cm	5	20	15	10	15 10–20	0.15 0.1–0.2	0.06 0.02–0.1	0.15 0.1–0.2	30 20–40	3.5 3–4
Approximate cross-sectional area	cm²	2	1.3	0.6	0.2	0.2	2×10^{-5}	3×10^{-7}	2×10^{-5}	0.8	2.3
Total vascular cross-sectional area at each level	cm²	2	2	2	3	3	125	600	570	3.0	2.3
Peak blood velocity	cm s⁻¹	120 40–290	105 25–250	55 50–60	100 100–120		0.75 0.5–1.0	0.07 0.02–0.17	0.35 0.2–0.5	25 15–40	70
Mean blood velocity	cm s⁻¹	20 10–40	20 10–40	15 8–20	10 10–15						15 6–28
Reynolds number (peak)		4500	3400	1250	1000		0.09	0.001	0.035	700	3000
α (heart rate 2 Hz)		13.2	11.5	8	3.5	4.4	0.04	0.005	0.035	8.8	15
Calculated wave-speed c_0	cm s⁻¹	580		770	840	850				100	350
Measured wave-speed c	cm s⁻¹	500 400–600		700 600–750	900 800–1030	800 600–1100				400 100–700	250 200–330
Young's modulus E	Nm⁻² × 10⁵	4.8 3–6		10 9–11	10 9–12	9 7–11				0.7 0.4–1.0	6 2–10

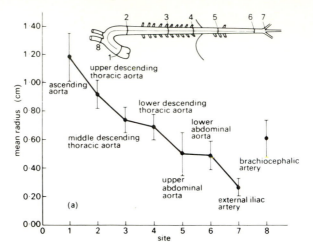

Figure 3.1:2 A sketch of the dog's aorta from data measured at physiological pressure in 10 large dogs. From Fry, Griggs, Jr., and Greenfield, Jr. (1963) In vivo studies of pulsatile blood flow. In *Pulsatile Blood Flow*, Attinger, (ed.). McGraw–Hill, New York, p. 110, by permission.

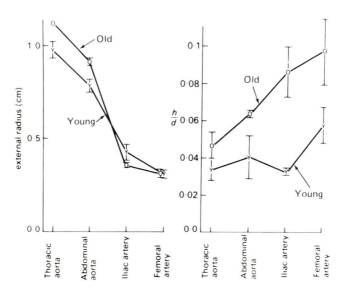

Figure 3.1:3 The radius and wall thickness of human arteries for young (*Y*) and old (*O*) persons. From Learoyd and Taylor, (1966) Alterations with age in the viscoelastic properties of human arterial walls. *Circ. Res.* **18**: 278–292, by permission of the American Heart Association.

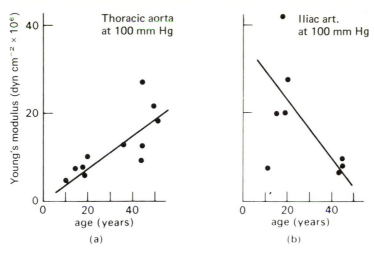

Figure 3.1:4 Incremental modulus of elasticity of arteries of normal young and old persons at a pressure of 100 mm Hg. (a) Thoracia aorta. (b) Iliac artery. From Learoyd and Taylor, (1966) *Circulation Res.* **18**: 278–292, by permission of the American Heart Association.

whereas that of the iliac and femeral arteries either decreases or changes little with age (see Fig. 3.1:3); thus at the same transmural pressure the stress in the thoracic aorta of the old is greater than that of the young, whereas the reverse is true for the iliac or femeral arteries. A glance at the nonlinear stress–strain relationship, as shown in Fig. 7.5:1 of *Biomechanics*, (Fung, 1981, p. 220), or Fig. 2.9:3 of the preceding chapter, tells us that at higher stress the incremental Young's modulus is larger.

A detailed discussion of the mechanical properties of arteries is given in Chap. 8 of *Biomechanics* (Fung, 1981). In the present chapter we shall consider the flow of blood in these elastic vessels. The basic equations of hemodynamics are presented in the Appendix at the end of this book. A serious reader should read the Appendix before proceeding to the rest of the book.

We shall proceed from the simple to the complex. First, we give a solution to the problem of steady flow in a uniform rigid pipe. It is interesting to see that this simple solution has important applications. We shall see also that even this simple case has some very difficult aspects, e.g., the questions of stability and turbulence. We then proceed to study aspects of flow in elastic tubes, first steady flow, and then wave propagation. Reflection and transmission of waves in branching vessels is a subject of major interest. This brings us to the subject of real pulsatile flow in the arteries. To explain the real features of the pulse waves observed *in vivo*, a number of simplifying assumptions used in earlier sections must be removed. The mathematical problem then becomes more difficult, and we will offer some physical explanations based on model experiments.

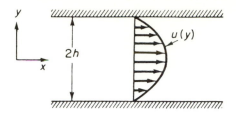

Figure 3.2:1 Laminar flow in a channel.

3.2 Laminar Flow in a Channel or Tube

Consider first a steady flow of an incompressible Newtonian fluid in a rigid, horizontal channel of width $2h$ between two parallel planes, as shown in Fig. 3.2:1. The channel is assumed horizontal so that the gravitational effect (a body force) may be ignored. The walls are assumed to be so rigid that their geometry is uninfluenced by the flow.

We search for a flow,

$$u = u(y), \qquad v = 0, \qquad w = 0, \tag{1}$$

that satisfies the Navier–Stokes equations, the equation of continuity, and the no-slip conditions on the boundaries $y = \pm h$:

$$u(h) = 0, \qquad u(-h) = 0. \tag{2}$$

These equations are discussed in the Appendix at the end of this book. Obviously Eqs. (1) satisfy the equation of continuity (Eq. (A.3:3)), p. 373, exactly; whereas the equations of motion (Eq. (A.3:6)), p. 373, become, with the body force ignored,

$$0 = -\frac{\partial p}{\partial x} + \mu \frac{d^2 u}{dy^2}, \tag{3}$$

$$0 = \frac{\partial p}{\partial y}, \tag{4}$$

$$0 = \frac{\partial p}{\partial z}. \tag{5}$$

Equations (4) and (5) show that p is a function of x only. If we differentiate Eq. (3) with respect to x and use Eq. (1), we obtain $\partial^2 p/\partial x^2 = 0$. *Hence $\partial p/\partial x$ must be a constant.* Equation (3) then becomes

$$\frac{d^2 u}{dy^2} = \frac{1}{\mu} \frac{dp}{dx}, \tag{6}$$

which has a solution

$$u = A + By + \frac{1}{\mu} \frac{y^2}{2} \frac{dp}{dx}. \tag{7}$$

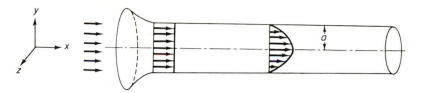

Figure 3.2:2 Laminar flow in a circular cylindrical tube.

The two constants A and B can be determined by the boundary conditions (2) to yield the final solution

$$u = -\frac{1}{2\mu}(h^2 - y^2)\frac{dp}{dx}. \tag{8}$$

Thus, the velocity profile is a parabola.

A corresponding problem is the flow through a horizontal circular cylindrical tube of radius a (see Fig. 3.2:2). We search for a solution

$$u = u(y, z), \qquad v = 0, \qquad w = 0.$$

In analogy with Eq. (6), the Navier–Stokes equation becomes

$$\frac{\partial^2 u}{\partial y^2} + \frac{\partial^2 u}{\partial z^2} = \frac{1}{\mu}\frac{dp}{dx}, \tag{9}$$

where dp/dx is a constant. For convenience we will use cylindrical polar coordinates x, r, θ, with $r^2 = y^2 + z^2$, instead of the cartesian coordinates x, y, x. Then Eq. (9) becomes

$$\frac{\partial^2 u}{\partial y^2} + \frac{\partial^2 u}{\partial z^2} = \frac{1}{r}\frac{\partial}{\partial r}\left(r\frac{\partial u}{\partial r}\right) + \frac{1}{r^2}\frac{\partial^2 u}{\partial \theta^2} = \frac{1}{\mu}\frac{dp}{dx}. \tag{10}$$

Let us assume that the flow is symmetric so that u is a function of r only; then $\partial^2 u/\partial \theta^2 = 0$, and the equation

$$\frac{1}{r}\frac{d}{dr}\left(r\frac{du}{dr}\right) = \frac{1}{\mu}\frac{dp}{dx} \tag{11}$$

can be integrated immediately to yield

$$u = \frac{1}{\mu}\frac{r^2}{4}\frac{dp}{dx} + A \log r + B. \tag{12}$$

The constants A and B are determined by the conditions of no-slip at $r = a$ and symmetry on the center line, $r = 0$:

$$u = 0 \qquad \text{at } r = a, \tag{13}$$

$$\frac{du}{dr} = 0 \qquad \text{at } r = 0. \tag{14}$$

The final solution is

$$u = -\frac{1}{4\mu}(a^2 - r^2)\frac{dp}{dx}. \tag{15}$$

This is the famous parabolic velocity profile of the *Hagen–Poiseuille flow*; the theoretical solution was worked out by Stokes. The profile is sketched in Fig. 3.2:2.

From the solution (15) we can obtain the *rate of flow* through the tube by an integrations:

$$\dot{Q} = 2\pi \int_0^a u r \, dr. \tag{16}$$

This leads to

$$\dot{Q} = -\frac{\pi a^4}{8\mu}\frac{dp}{dx}. \tag{17}$$

Dividing the rate of flow by the cross-sectional area of the tube yields the *mean velocity of flow*

$$u_m = -\frac{a^2}{8\mu}\frac{dp}{dx}. \tag{18}$$

Finally, the shear stress at the tube wall is given by $-\mu(\partial u/\partial r)$ at $r = a$. If we divide the shear stress by the mean dynamic pressure $\frac{1}{2}\rho u_m^2$ the ratio is called the *skin friction coefficient*. Denoting the skin friction coefficient by C_f, we obtain

$$C_f = \frac{\text{shear stress}}{\text{mean dynamic pressure}} = \frac{-\mu(\partial u/\partial r)_{r=a}}{\frac{1}{2}\rho u_m^2} = \frac{16}{N_R}, \tag{19}$$

where

$$N_R = 2a u_m / \nu. \tag{20}$$

The formula for shear stress on the wall is then

$$\text{shear stress} = C_f \tfrac{1}{2}\rho u_m^2. \tag{21}$$

This classical solution by Hagen and Poiseuille has been subjected to innumerable experimental observations. It is not valid near the entrance to a tube. It is satisfactory at a sufficiently large distance from the entrance but is again invalid if the tube is too large or if the velocity is too high. The difficulty at the entry region is due to the transitional nature of the flow in that region, so that our assumption $v = 0$, $w = 0$ is not valid. The difficulty with too large a Reynolds number, however, is of a different kind: the flow becomes turbulent! Osborne Reynolds demonstrated the transition to turbulent flow in a classical experiment in which he examined an outlet from a large water tank

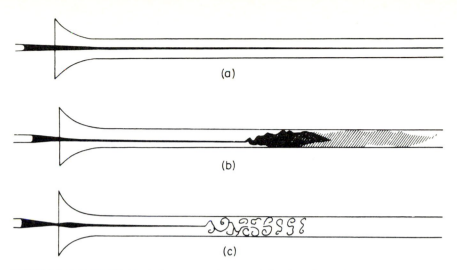

Figure 3.2:3 Reynolds' turbulence experiment: (a) laminar flow; (b) and (c) transition from laminar to turbulent flow. After Reynolds, O. (1883): An experimental investigation of the circumstances which determine whether the motion of water shall be direct or sinuous, and of the law of resistance in parallel channels. *Phil. Trans., Roy. Soc.* **174**: 935–982.

through a small tube. At the end of the tube there was a stopcock used to vary the speed of water through the tube. The junction of the tube with the tank was nicely rounded, and a filament of colored fluid was introduced at the mouth. When the speed of water was slow, the filament remained distinct through the entire length of the tube. When the speed was increased, the filament broke up at a given point and diffused throughout the cross section (see Fig. 3.2:3). Reynolds identified the governing parameter $u_m d/v$—the Reynolds number—where u_m is the mean velocity, d is the diameter, and v is the kinematic viscosity. The point at which the color diffuses throughout the tube is the transition point from laminar to turbulent flow in the tube. Reynolds found that transition occurred at Reynolds numbers between 2000 and 13,000, depending on the smoothness of the entry conditions. When extreme care is taken, the transition can be delayed to Reynolds numbers as high as 40,000. On the other hand, a value of 2000 appears to be about the lowest value obtainable on a rough entrance.

Turbulence is one of the most important and difficult problems in fluid mechanics.

The Hagen–Poiseuille solution can be modified to account for the non-Newtonian rheological properties of blood, which have been discussed in Secs. 3.1 and 3.2 in *Biomechanics* (Fung, 1981). Steady flow of blood in circular cylindrical tubes is discussed in Sec. 3.3 of that book. It is shown that the effect of nonlinear blood rheology on the resistance of blood flow in arteries is relatively minor but its effect on flow separation can be great.

3.3 Applications of Poiseuille's Formula:
Optimum Design of Blood Vessel Bifurcation

Poiseuille's formula has many uses. It tells us that the most effective factor controlling blood flow is the radius of the blood vessel. For a given pressure drop, a 1% change in vessel radius will cause a 4% change in blood flow. Conversely, if an organ needs a certain amount of blood flow to function, then the pressure difference needed to send this flow through depends on the vessel radius. For a fixed flow a 1% decrease in vessel diameter will cause a 4% increase in the required pressure difference. This is seen from Eq. (3.2:17):

(a) If Δp, μ, and L are constant, then by taking logarithm on both sides of the equation and differentiating, we obtain

$$\frac{\delta \dot{Q}}{\dot{Q}} = 4\frac{\delta a}{a}. \tag{1}$$

(b) If $\dot{Q}$, μ, and L are constant, then a logarithmic differentiation yields

$$\frac{\delta(\Delta p)}{\Delta p} = -4\frac{\delta a}{a}. \tag{2}$$

Hence an effective way of controlling blood pressure is to change the vessel radius. Hypertension (high blood pressure) is caused by narrowing of blood vessels, and can be reduced by relaxing the smooth muscle tension that controls the blood vessel radius.

Reducing blood viscosity is another way of reducing the resistance to blood flow, and hemodilution is sometimes used in surgery.

Now let us consider a different application. We know that arteries bifurcate many times before they become capillaries. Can we guess at a design principle of the blood vessel bifurcation?

To be more concrete, let us consider three vessels, AB, BC, and BD, connecting three points, A, C, and D, in space (Fig. 3.3:1). There is a flow $\dot{Q}_0$ coming through A into AB. The flow is divided into $\dot{Q}_1$ in BC and $\dot{Q}_2$ in BD. Let the points A, C, D be fixed, but the location of B and the vessel radii are left for the designer to choose. Is there an optimal position for the point B?

By asking such a question we are seeking a principle of optimum design. Some *cost function* is assumed, and the design parameters are chosen so that the cost function is minimized. Some of the great theories of physics and chemistry are based on such principles. One may recall the principle of minimum potential energy in elasticity, the principle of minimum entropy production in irreversible thermodynamics, the Fermat principle of least time of travel in optics, Maupertius' principle of least action, Hamilton's principle in physics, and so on. The potential energy, entropy production, travel time, action, and the Hamiltonian are the cost functions in these cases.

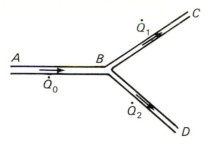

Figure 3.3:1 Bifurcation of a blood vessel AB into two branches BC and BD, supplying blood at a rate of $\dot{Q}_0$(cm³/sec) from point A to points C and D, with outflow of $\dot{Q}_1$. at C and $\dot{Q}_2$ at D.

For blood vessels, Murray (1926) proposed a cost function which is the sum of the rate at which work is done on the blood and the metabolic rate of the vessel. The former is the product of $\dot{Q}\Delta p$. The latter is assumed to be proportional to the volume of the vessel $\pi a^2 L$, with a proportional constant K. Hence

$$\text{Cost function for blood vessels} = \dot{Q}\Delta p + K\pi a^2 L. \qquad (3)$$

With Eqs. (3.2:17) we can write

$$\text{Cost function} = \frac{8\mu L}{\pi a^4}\dot{Q}^2 + K\pi a^2 L. \qquad (4)$$

The cost function of the entire system of blood vessels is the sum of the cost functions of individual vessel segments. Hence, each vessel must be optimal and the system must be put together optimally. For a given vessel of length L and flow $\dot{Q}$, there is an optimal radius a, which can be calculated by minimizing the cost function with respect to a. At the optimal condition, the following derivative must vanish:

$$\frac{\partial}{\partial a}(\text{cost function}) = -\frac{32\mu L}{\pi}\dot{Q}^2 a^{-5} + 2K\pi La = 0. \qquad (5)$$

This yields the solution

$$a = \left(\frac{16\mu}{\pi^2 K}\right)^{1/6}\dot{Q}^{1/3}. \qquad (6)$$

Hence, the optimal radius of a blood vessel is proportional to $\dot{Q}$ to the 1/3 power. On substituting (6) into (4), we obtain the minimum value of the cost function:

$$\text{Min. cost function} = \frac{3\pi}{2}KLa^2. \qquad (7)$$

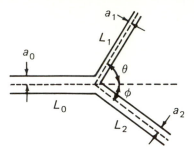

Figure 3.3:2 Geometric parameters of the branching pattern. Theory shows that B should lie in the plane of ACD.

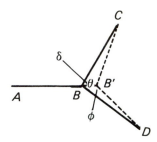

Figure 3.3:3 A particular variation of δL_0, δL_1, δL_2 by a small displacement of B in the direction of AB.

Bifurcation Pattern

Now consider the bifurcation problem. Since the cost functions of all vessels are additive, we see at once that the vessels connecting A, C, and D in Fig. 3.3:1 should be straight and lie in a plane (because this minimizes the length, L, when other things are fixed.) To find out the details let the geometric parameters be specified as shown in Fig. 3.3:2. The three branches will be denoted by subscripts 0, 1, 2. The total cost function will be denoted by P:

$$P = \frac{3\pi K}{2}(a_0^2 L_0 + a_1^2 L_1 + a_2^2 L_2). \tag{8}$$

The lengths L_0, L_1, L_2 are affected by the location of the point B, the radii a_0, a_1, a_2 are related to the flows $\dot{Q}_0$, $\dot{Q}_1$, $\dot{Q}_2$ through Eq. (6). Let us now minimize P by properly choosing location of the bifurcation point B.

Since a small movement of B changes P by

$$\delta P = \frac{3\pi K}{2}(a_0^2 \delta L_0 + a_1^2 \delta L_1 + a_2^2 \delta L_2), \tag{9}$$

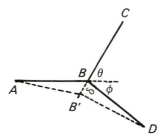

Figure 3.3:4 Another particular variation of δL_0, δL_1, δL_2 by a displacement of B to B' along BC.

an optimal location of B would make $\delta P = 0$ for arbitrary small movement of B. Let us consider three special movements of B. First, let B move to B' in the direction of AB as shown in Fig. 3.3:3. In this case

$$\delta L_0 = \delta, \qquad \delta L_1 = -\delta \cos \theta, \qquad \delta L_2 = -\delta \cos \phi,$$

$$\delta P = \frac{3\pi K}{2} \delta(a_0^2 - a_1^2 \cos \theta - a_2^2 \cos \phi). \tag{10}$$

The optimum is obtained when

$$a_0^2 = a_1^2 \cos \theta - a_2^2 \cos \phi = 0. \tag{11}$$

Next, let B move to B' in the direction of CB, as shown in Fig. 3.3:4. Then

$$\delta L_0 = -\delta \cos \theta, \qquad \delta L_1 = \delta, \qquad \delta L_2 = \delta \cos (\theta + \phi),$$

$$\delta P = \frac{3\pi K \delta}{2} [-a_0^2 \cos \theta + a_1^2 + a_2^2 \cos (\theta + \phi)], \tag{12}$$

and the optimal condition is

$$-a_0^2 \cos \theta + a_1^2 + a_1^2 \cos (\theta + \phi). \tag{13}$$

Finally, let B move a short distance δ in the direction of DB (Fig. 3.3:5). Then the optimal condition is obviously,

$$-a_0^2 \cos \phi + a_1^2 \cos (\theta + \phi) + a_2^2 = 0. \tag{14}$$

Solving (11), (13), (14) for $\cos \theta$, $\cos \phi$, and $\cos (\theta + \phi)$, we obtain

$$\cos \theta = \frac{a_0^4 + a_1^4 - a_2^4}{2a_0^2 a_1^2},$$

$$\cos \phi = \frac{a_0^4 - a_1^4 + a_2^4}{2a_0^2 a_2^2}, \tag{15}$$

$$\cos (\theta + \phi) = \frac{a_0^4 - a_1^4 - a_2^4}{2a_1^2 a_2^2}.$$

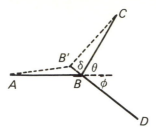

Figure 3.3:5 A third variation caused by a displacement of B to B' along BD.

These equations can be simplified by the fact that $Q_0 = Q_1 + Q_2$, and hence, by (6), $a_0^3 = a_1^3 + a_2^3$. Thus Eq. (15) can be reduced to

$$\cos \theta = \frac{a_0^4 + a_1^4 - (a_0^3 - a_1^3)^{4/3}}{2a_0^2 a_1^2}, \qquad \text{etc.} \qquad (16)$$

Applications of these formulas are illustrated in the following Problems.

Problems

3.1 Show that, if $a_1 = a_2$, then $\theta = \phi$. Thus, if the radii of the daughter branches are equal, the bifurcating angles are equal.

3.2 Show that, if $a_2 > a_1$, then $\theta > \phi$.

3.3 Show that, if $a_2 \gg a_1$, then $a_2 \doteq a_0$ and $\theta \doteq \pi/2$.

3.4 When $a_1 = a_2$, show that $a_1/a_0 = 2^{-1/3} = 0.794$, and $\cos \theta = 2^{\tau+1/3} = 0.794$. Thus $\theta \doteq 37.5°$.

These results are in reasonable agreement with empirical observations, suggesting that Rosen's cost function and minimization principles are probably correct.

The result of Problem 3.4 is especially interesting. Let a_0 denote the radius of the aorta, and assume equal bifurcation in all generations. Then the radius of the first generation is $0.794 \, a_0$, that of the second generation is $(0.794)^2 a_0$, and, generally, that of the nth generation is

$$a_n = (0.794)^n a_0. \qquad (17)$$

If a capillary blood vessel has a radius of 5×10^{-4} cm and the radius of the aorta is $a_0 = 1.5$ cm, then Eq. (17) yields $n \doteq 30$. Thus 30 generations of equal bifurcation are needed to reduce that aorta to the capillary dimension. Since each generation multiplies the number of vessels by 2, the total number of blood vessels is $2^{30} \doteq 10^9$. But these estimates cannot be taken too seriously, because arteries rarely bifurcate symmetrically (as required by the hypothesis $a_1 = a_2$). Of the arteries of man there is one symmetric bifurcation; of the dog there are none.

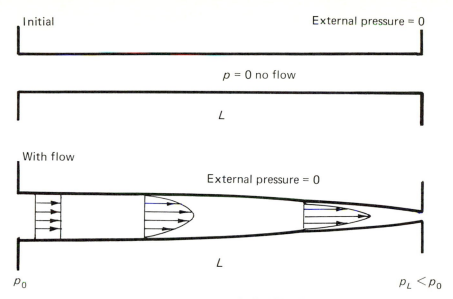

Figure 3.4:1 Flow in an elastic tube of length L.

Problem

3.5 The cost function specified in Eq. (4) is somewhat arbitrary. Develop some other
cost functions and deduce the consequences, such as

(a) Minimum total surface area of the blood vessels,
(b) Minimum total volume of the blood vessels,
(c) Minimum power for the blood flow,
(d) Minimum total shear force on the vessel wall.

See Zamir (1976), Murray (1926), and Kamiya and Togawa (1972).

3.4 Steady Laminar Flow in an Elastic Tube

As another application of Poiseuille's formula, let us consider the flow in a
circular cylindrical elastic tube (Fig. 3.4:1). The flow is maintained by a
pressure gradient. The pressure in the tube is, therefore, nonuniform—
higher at the entry end and lower at the exit end. Because the tube is elastic,
the high-pressure end distends more than the low-pressure end. The diameter
of the tube is, therefore, nonuniform (if it were uniform originally) and the
degree of nonuniformity depends on the flow rate.

  If we wish to determine the pressure–flow relationship for such a system,
we may break down the problem into two familiar components. This is
illustrated in Fig. 3.4:2. In the lower block, we regard the vessel as a rigid
conduit with a specified wall shape. For a given flow, we compute the pressure

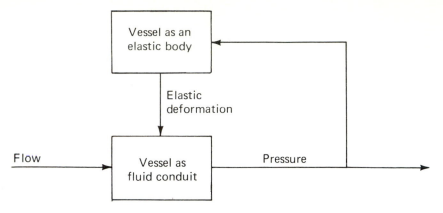

Figure 3.4:2 A hemoelastic system analyzed as a feedback system of two functional units: an elastic body, and a fluid mechanism.

distribution. This pressure distribution is then applied as loading on the elastic tube, represented by the upper block. We then analyze the deformation of the elastic tube in the usual manner of the theory of elasticity. The result of the calculation is then used to determine the boundary shape of the hydrodynamic problem of the lower block. When a consistent solution is obtained, the pressure distribution corresponding to a given flow is determined.

Let us put this in a mathematical form. Assume that the tube is long and slender, that the flow is laminar and steady, that the disturbances due to entry and exit are negligible, and that the deformed tube remains smooth and slender. These assumptions permit us to consider the solution given in Sec. 3.2 as valid (a good approximation) everywhere in the tube. Assuming a Newtonian fluid, we have (Eq. (17) of Sec. 3.2)

$$\frac{dp}{dx} = -\frac{8\mu}{\pi a^4}\dot{Q}. \tag{1}$$

Here $\dot{Q}$ is the volume–flow rate. In a stationary, nonpermeable tube $\dot{Q}$ is a constant throughout the length of the tube. The tube radius is a, which is a function of x because of the elastic deformation. An integration of Eq. (1) yields

$$p(x) = p(0) - \frac{8\mu}{\pi}\dot{Q}\int_0^x \frac{1}{[a(x)]^4}dx. \tag{2}$$

The integration constant is $p(0)$, the pressure at $x = 0$. The exit pressure is given by Eq. (2) with $x = L$. L is the length of the tube.

Now let us turn our attention to the calculation of the radius $a(x)$. Let the tube be initially straight and uniform, with a radius a_0. Assume that the tube is thin walled, and that the external pressure is zero (Fig. 3.4:3). (If the

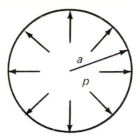

Figure 3.4:3 Distension of an elastic tube due to internal pressure.

external pressure is not zero, we should replace p, below, by the difference of internal and external pressures.) Then a simple analysis yields the average circumferential stress in the wall:

$$\sigma_{\theta\theta} = \frac{p(x)a(x)}{h}, \tag{3}$$

where h is the wall thickness. (See *First Course in Continuum Mechanics* (Fung, 1977), p. 22.) Let the axial tension be zero, and assume that the material obeys Hooke's law. Then the circumferential strain is

$$e_{\theta\theta} = \frac{\sigma_{\theta\theta}}{E}, \tag{4}$$

where E is the Young's modulus of the wall material. (Strictly, the right-hand side of Eq. (4) should be

$$\frac{1}{E}(\sigma_{\theta\theta} - v\sigma_{xx} - v\sigma_{rr}),$$

where v is the Poisson's ratio. But σ_{xx} is assumed to be zero and σ_{rr} is, in general, much smaller than $\sigma_{\theta\theta}$ for thin-walled tubes.) The strain $e_{\theta\theta}$ is equal to the change of radius divided by the original radius, a_0:

$$e_{\theta\theta} = \frac{a(x) - a_0}{a_0} = \frac{a(x)}{a_0} - 1. \tag{5}$$

Combining (5), (4), and (3), we obtain:

$$a(x) = a_0 \left[1 - \frac{a_0}{Eh} p(x) \right]^{-1}. \tag{6}$$

Substituting (6) into (1), we may write the result as

$$\left(1 - \frac{a_0}{Eh} p \right)^{-4} dp = -\frac{8\mu}{\pi a_0^4} \dot{Q} dx. \tag{7}$$

Recognizing the boundary conditions $p = p(0)$ when $x = 0$ and $p = p(L)$ when $x = L$, and integrating Eq. (7) from $p(0)$ to $p(L)$ on the left and 0 to L on the right, we obtain the pressure–flow relationship:

$$\frac{Eh}{3a_0}\left\{\left[1-\frac{a_0}{Eh}p(L)\right]^{-3}-\left[1-\frac{a_0}{Eh}p(0)\right]^{-3}\right\}=-\frac{8\mu}{\pi a_0^4}L\dot{Q}, \tag{8}$$

which shows that the flow is not a linear function of pressure drop $p(0) - p(L)$.

Another Solution

The solution obtained above is based on the assumption that the tube-wall material obeys Hooke's law; blood vessel walls do not. Hence the solution is not valid for blood vessels except possibly as an approximation.

A simpler result can be obtained if we assume the pressure–radius relationship to be linear:

$$a = a_0 + \alpha p/2. \tag{9}$$

Here a_0 is the tube radius when the transmural pressure is zero. α is a compliance constant. Equation (9) is a good representation of the pulmonary blood vessels. See Sec. 4.9, Fig. 4.9:2, and Sec. 6.4, Figures 6.4:1, 6.4:2.

Using Eq. (9), we have

$$\frac{dp}{dx} = \frac{dp}{da}\frac{da}{dx} = \frac{2}{\alpha}\frac{da}{dx}. \tag{10}$$

On substituting Eq. (10) into Eq. (1) and rearranging terms, we obtain

$$a^4\frac{da}{dx} = \frac{1}{5}\frac{da^5}{dx} = -\frac{4\mu\alpha}{\pi}\dot{Q}. \tag{11}$$

Since the right-hand side term is a constant independent of x, we obtain at once the integrated result

$$[a(x)]^5 = -\frac{20\mu\alpha}{\pi}\dot{Q}x + \text{const.} \tag{12}$$

The integration constant can be determined by the boundary condition that when $x = 0$, $a(x) = a(0)$. Hence the constant $= [a(0)]^5$. Then, by putting $x = L$, we obtain from Eq. (12) the elegant result

$$\frac{20\mu\alpha L}{\pi}\dot{Q} = [a(0)]^5 - [a(L)]^5. \tag{13}$$

The pressure–flow relationship is obtained by substituting Eq. (9) into Eq. (13). Thus the flow varies with the difference of the fifth power of the tube radius at the entry section ($x = 0$) minus that at the exit section ($x = L$). If the ratio $a(L)/a(0)$ is 1/2, then $[a(L)]^5$ is only about 3% of $[a(0)]^5$, and is negligible by comparison. Hence when $a(L)$ is one-half of $a(0)$ or smaller, the flow varies directly with the fifth power of the tube radius at the entry, whereas the radius (and the pressure) at the exit section has little effect on the flow.

Problems

3.6 If the elastic deformation is small,

$$\frac{a_0 p(0)}{Eh} \ll 1, \qquad \frac{a_0 p(L)}{Eh} \ll 1,$$

show that the pressure–flow relationship Eq. (8) or (13) then becomes linear.

3.7 Plot curves to show the flow–pressure relationship given by Eqs. (8) and (13) and discuss the results.

3.8 The actual relationship between the pressure and radius in peripheral blood vessel is nonlinear. See Chapter 8 of *Biomechanics* (Fung, 1981). Outline a theory which will take into account the nonlinear pseudo elastic stress–strain relationship in deriving the pressure–flow relationship of the blood vessel.

3.9 Outline further a theory that will take into account the viscoelastic behavior of the blood vessel in deriving the pressure–flow relationship of the blood vessel.

3.5 Turbulent Flow in a Tube

In Sec. 3.2 we mentioned that when the Reynolds number exceeds a certain critical value the flow becomes turbulent. Turbulence is marked by random fluctuations. With turbulence the velocity field can no longer be predicted with absolute precision, but its statistical features (mean velocity, root mean square velocity, mean pressure gradient, etc.) are perfectly well defined. If a steady flow in a straight, long pipe changes from laminar to turbulent, two important changes will occur: (a) the profile of the mean velocity will become much more blunt at the center of the pipe, and (b) the shear gradient will become much greater at the wall. This is shown in Chap. 1, Fig. 1.4:1. As a consequence of this change of velocity profile, the resistance to flow is greatly increased.

The best way to express the resistance change is via the *friction coefficient*, C_f, defined in Eq. (3.2:21):

$$\text{Shear stress on pipe wall} = C_f(\tfrac{1}{2}\rho U_m^2). \qquad (1)$$

Here ρ is the fluid density, U_m is the mean velocity over the cross section of the tube, capitalized here to show that this velocity is not only averaged over space, but also over a sufficiently long period of time so that the random fluctuations of turbulence are averaged out. C_f is a function of the Reynolds number (based on tube radius and the mean velocity of flow, U_m) and the roughness of the tube surface. Roughness influences the position of transition from the laminar to the turbulent boundary layer, and it affects the skin-friction drag on that portion of the surface over which the layer is turbulent.

The experimental results of Nikuradse are shown in Fig. 3.5:1. The surface of the tube was sprinkled with sand of various grain sizes, which are

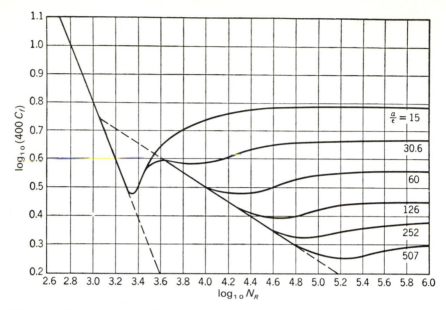

Figure 3.5:1 Resistance coefficient for fully developed flow through a tube of radius
a with various sizes of roughness elements on the wall. ε is roughly the diameter of sand
grain sprinkled on the wall. The solid curves represent the average experimental results
by Nikuradse. The dashed line on the left represents a theoretical result for laminar
flow. The dashed line on the right is Blasius empirical formula for turbulent flow in a
smooth tube. Based on Nikuradse, J. (1933) *Strömungsgesetze in Rauhen Rohren*,
Forschungsheft 361, Ver. deutsch. Ing.

expressed in the ratio a/ε in the figure, where a is the radius of the tube and
ε is the mesh size of the screen through which the sand will just pass. The
dotted straight line on the left refers to a fully developed laminar flow
(Eq. (3.2:19)):

$$C_f = 16 \left(\frac{2aU_m}{v} \right)^{-1} = \frac{16}{N_R}, \tag{2}$$

where N_R is the Reynolds number based on tube diameter and mean speed
of flow. The dotted line on the right is an empirical formula given by Blasius
for turbulent flow in smooth pipes:

$$C_f = 0.0655 \left(\frac{U_m a}{v} \right)^{-1/4} = \frac{0.0779}{(N_R)^{1/4}}. \tag{3}$$

The solid curves represent the mean experimental results. It is clear that at
large Reynolds numbers the friction coefficient of turbulent flow is much
greater than that of laminar flow. For example, at a Reynolds number of
4000, (i.e., $\log_{10} N_R \doteq 3.6$), a rough pipe with $a/\varepsilon = 30$ will have a skin friction about the same as that in a smooth pipe if the flow is turbulent, but it

would be 2.51 times larger than that of a laminar flow if laminar flow were possible. At $N_R = 10^5$ the skin friction of a smooth pipe with turbulent flow would be 27 times larger than that given by Eq. (2), and for a rough pipe with $a/\varepsilon = 30$ the skin friction would be increased again 2.77-fold.

It seems natural to expect that natural selection in the animal world would favor laminar flow in the blood vessels so that energy is not wasted in turbulence. Furthermore, a high shear stress on the wall of the arteries is implicated in atherogenesis. To avoid turbulent flow in aorta, the Reynolds number should be kept below a certain critical value. Let the cardiac output (volume flow per unit time) be $\dot{Q}$, and the radius of the aorta be R_a. Then the cross-sectional area of the aorta is πR_a^2, and the mean velocity of flow is

$$U_m = \frac{\dot{Q}}{\pi R_a^2}. \tag{4}$$

The Reynolds number is

$$N_R = \frac{2U_m R_a}{v} = \frac{2\dot{Q}}{\pi v R_a}. \tag{5}$$

Rosen (1967) plotted the radius of the aorta of animals versus the cardiac output, and obtained a regression line

$$R_a = 0.013\dot{Q}. \tag{6}$$

On substituting R_a from Eq. (6) into Eq. (5), we obtain a Reynolds number $2/(0.013\pi v)$, which is 1224 if $v = 0.04$, 1632 if $v = 0.03$. These values are fairly close to but somewhat lower than the transition Reynolds number in steady flow, which seems to mean that animal aortas are designed for laminar flow, but are fairly close to the borderline of transition to turbulence.

So far our discussion of turbulence is based on steady mean flow. Pulsatile flow makes the phenomenon of laminar–turbulence transition much more complex, as will be shown presently.

3.6 Turbulence in Pulsatile Blood Flow

Reynolds' experiment (Fig. 3.2:3) shows that in pipe flow the entry region remains laminar even though turbulence develops downstream when the Reynolds number exceeds the critical value. This shows that turbulence must develop gradually in a laminar flow. It takes time for some unstable modes of motion in a flow to grow into turbulence. We may apply this concept to the pulsatile blood flow in the arteries. The flow velocity changes with time. The Reynolds number, $2aU/v$, based on the instantaneous velocity of flow averaged over the cross section, varies with time. Figure 3.6:1 shows a record of velocity of flow versus time. In a period of rising velocity the Reynolds number increases slowly until it reaches a level marked by the dotted line ($N_R = 2300$), at which the flow could be expected to become

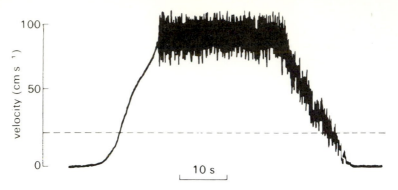

3.6:1 A turbulent flow velocity-vs-time record made with a hot-film probe in a pipe in which the flow-rate was slowly increased until turbulence occurred, and later stopped. Peak Reynolds number was 9500. The dotted line corresponds to Reynolds number 2300. From Nerem, R., and Seed, W. A. (1972) An in vivo study of aortic flow disturbances, *Cardiovasc. Res.* **6**: 1–14, by permission.

turbulent if it were steady. But an accelerating flow is more stable than a steady flow, because turbulence cannot develop instantaneously. So, when the turbulence finally sets in, the velocity and N_R are much higher than the dotted line level. On the other hand, in a period of decreasing velocity the disappearance of turbulence occurs at a level considerably below the dotted line. This is partly because decelerating flow is inherently less stable than steady flow, and partly because existing eddies take a finite time to decay. Thus, the *critical Reynolds number* of laminar–turbulent transition depends on the rate of change of velocity, as well as on the eddies upstream and roughness of the pipe wall.

The experiment corresponding to Fig. 3.6:1 was designed to show the transition from laminar to turbulent flow and vice versa. Figure 3.6:2 shows a record of velocity waves from the upper descending aorta of an anesthetized dog. Turbulence is seen during the deceleration of systolic flow. Hot-film anemometry was used to obtain such records.

Quantitative studies of the laminar–turbulent transition may seek to express the critical Reynolds number as a function of the frequency parameter (see the next Sec. 3.7) of the pulsatile flow. With the frequency expressed in terms of the dimensionless *Womersley number*, (see p. 101)

$$N_W = a \cdot \sqrt{\frac{\omega}{\nu}},$$

where a is the radius, ω is the circular frequency of heartbeat, and ν is the kinematic viscosity, experimental results can be plotted as shown in Fig. 3.6:3. The ordinate is the peak Reynolds number. The stippled area indicates the conditions under which the flow is stable and laminar.

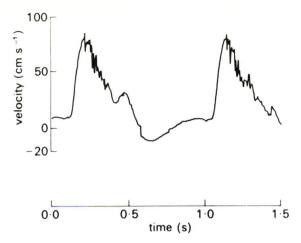

Figure 3.6:2 A record of velocity-*vs*-time of blood flow in the upper descending aorta of a dog, showing turbulence during the deceleration of systolic flow. From Seed, W. A., and Wood, N. B. (1971) Velocity patterns in the aorta. *Cardiovasc. Res.*, **5**: 319–333, by permission.

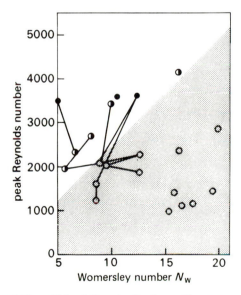

Figure 3.6:3 The stability of blood flow in the descending aorta of anesthetized dogs as influenced by the peak Reynolds number and the Womersley number. Points joined by the lines refer to the same animal. Open circles: laminar flow; filled circles: turbulent flow; half-filled circles; transiently turbulent flow. From Nerem, R. M., and Seed, W. A. (1972) An in vivo study of aortic flow disturbances. *Cardiovasc. Res.* **6**: 1–14, by permission.

In the experiments whose results are shown in Fig. 3.6:3, the wide variations of velocity and heart rate were obtained with drugs and nervous stimuli
in anesthetized dogs. In normal, conscious, free-ranging dogs the peak
Reynolds number usually lies in an area high above the stippled area of
Fig. 3.6:3. This suggests that some turbulence is generally tolerated in
deceleration of systolic flow in the dog.

Turbulence in blood flow implies fluctuating pressure acting on the
arterial wall, and fluctuating, increased shear stress. These stresses are
implicated in murmurs, poststenotic dilatation, and atherogenesis. On the
absolute scale the intensity of turbulence may be minor and the effects on
the arterial wall may be small, but the cumulative effect over a long period
of time may still be significant. The borderline between continued health
and slow, degenerative effects (aging, atherosclerosis, etc.) is tenuous, and
research in this area is needed.

Problems

3.10 The total volume rate of flow in all generations of blood vessels is the same. In
man and dog, in which vessel is the Reynolds number largest?

3.11 If the diameter of the aorta of a person is unusually small, would the blood flow
be more likely to be laminar or turbulent? If cardiac output is the same but the
heart rate is increased, would the blood flow be more likely to become turbulent?

3.12 Estimate the difference between the peak Reynolds number and the mean Reynolds
number of blood flow in the aorta of the dog.

3.7 The Frequency Parameter of Pulsatile Flow

The rest of this chapter will be concerned with pulsatile blood flow as
generated in the arteries by the pumping action of the heart. We shall begin
with a general discussion of the significance of various terms in the Navier–
Stokes equation (see Sec. A.3, p. 373):

$$\rho\frac{\partial u_i}{\partial t} + \rho\left(u_1\frac{\partial u_i}{\partial x_1} + u_2\frac{\partial u_i}{\partial x_2} + u_3\frac{\partial u_i}{\partial x_3}\right)$$

$$= X_i - \frac{\partial p}{\partial x_i} + \mu\left(\frac{\partial^2}{\partial x_1^2} + \frac{\partial^2}{\partial x_2^2} + \frac{\partial^2}{\partial x_3^2}\right)u_i. \tag{1}$$

This equation represents the balance of four kinds of forces. Term by term,
they are

| transient inertia | + | convective inertia | = | body force | + | pressure force | + | viscous force |

Not all the forces are important all the time. In a steady flow the transient inertial force vanishes. In an ideal fluid the viscous force vanishes. In hydrostatic equilibrium all but the body and pressure forces vanish. Simplifications are recognized for these cases.

In some problems the recognition of the relative importance of various terms in the Navier–Stokes equation is not as easy as in the cases cited above, and it is then useful to estimate the order of magnitude of individual terms systematically. In Sec. A.6 in the Appendix at the end of the book, we compared the order of magnitude of the convective inertia with that of the viscous force, and we obtained the Reynolds number. When the Reynolds number is high the convective inertia force is more important than the viscous forces. When the Reynolds number is low the opposite is true.

In pulsatile blood flow the transient inertial force term may become important when compared with the viscous force term. To make an estimate, let U be a characteristic velocity, ω a characteristic frequency, and L a characteristic length. Then the first term in Eq. (1) is of the order of magnitude $\rho \omega U$ and the last term is of the order of magnitude $\mu U L^{-2}$. The ratio is:

$$\frac{\text{transient inertia force}}{\text{viscous force}} = \frac{\rho \omega U}{\mu U L^{-2}} = \frac{\rho \omega L^2}{\mu} = \frac{\omega L^2}{v}. \tag{2}$$

This is a dimensionless number. If it is large, the transient inertial force dominates. If it is small, the viscous force dominates.

The dimensionless number $\omega L^2 / v$ is a *frequency parameter*, and is called the *Stokes' number* because its significance was pointed out by George Stokes in 1840. It is better known by its square root,

$$N_{\mathrm{W}} = L \sqrt{\left(\frac{\omega}{v}\right)}, \tag{3}$$

which is called *Womersley number* in honor of J. R. Womersley, who made extensive calculations on pulsatile blood flow in 1950s. If L is taken to be the radius of the blood vessel, then Womersley's number is often written as α:

$$\alpha = N_{\mathrm{W}} = \frac{D}{2} \sqrt{\left(\frac{\omega}{v}\right)}, \tag{4}$$

D being the blood vessel diameter. In large arteries of all but the smallest mammals the value of α calculated from the frequency of the heartbeat is considerably larger than 1. For example, a typical value of α in the aorta of man is 20, in a dog it is 14, in a cat, 8, and in a rat, 3. Hence in these aortas the inertial force dominates in pulsatile flow.

Another way of looking at the Womersley number is the following. In a pulsatile flow in blood vessel the velocity of flow oscillates, but on the vessel wall the velocity is always zero because of the no-slip condition. In the central portion of the vessel the velocity reaches a value U periodically. The transition from 0 on the wall to U in the central portion is accomplished in a time period π/ω and within a distance δ adjacent to the vessel wall. In the layer next to the wall the viscous force dominates. Between δ and the center of the tube the inertial force dominates. At δ the two forces are equally important. This fact can be used to estimate the magnitude of δ. Since u changes from 0 to U in a distance δ, the last term of Eq. (1) is of the order of magnitude $\mu U/\delta^2$. The first term of Eq. (1) is of the order of magnitude $\rho\omega U$. At the place where these two forces are equal we have

$$\rho\omega U = \frac{\mu U}{\delta^2},$$

or

$$\delta = \sqrt{\frac{\mu}{\rho\omega}} = \sqrt{\frac{v}{\omega}}. \tag{5}$$

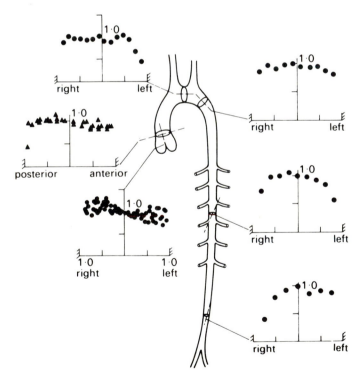

Figure 3.7:1 Normalized mean velocity profiles in dog's aorta. The mean velocity at each site is normalized by dividing through by the center-line mean velocity. From Schultz, D. L. (1972) Pressure and flow in large arteries. In *Cardiovascular Fluid Dynamics* Bergel, D. H. (ed.). vol. 1. Academic Press, New York, by permission.

The ratio of the radius of the tube to the wall layer thickness δ is

$$\frac{D}{2\delta} = \frac{D}{2}\sqrt{\frac{\omega}{\nu}} = \alpha, \tag{6}$$

which is exactly the Womersley number α.

Thus, if α is large, the effect of the viscosity of the fluid does not propogate very far from the wall. In the central portion of the tube (at a distance δ away from the wall) the transient flow is determined by the balance of the inertial forces and pressure forces (first and fourth terms in Eq. (1), and the elastic forces in the wall (through the boundary conditions), as if the fluid were nonviscous. We therefore expect that when the Womersley number is large the velocity profile in a pulsatile flow will be relatively blunt, in contrast to the parabolic profile of the Poiseuillean flow, which is determined by the balance of viscous and pressure forces. That this is indeed the case can be seen from Figs. 3.7:1 and 3.7:2. In Fig. 3.7:1 the velocity profiles constructed from time-mean measurements at several sites along the aorta of the dog are shown. They are seen to be quite blunt in the central portion of the aorta. Similar profiles constructed from instantaneous measurements show that this is true throughout the flow cycle.

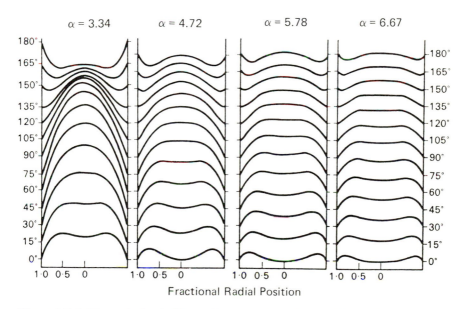

Figure 3.7:2 Theoretical velocity profiles of a sinusoidally oscillating flow in a pipe, with pressure gradient varying like $\cos \omega t$. α is the Womersley number. Profiles are plotted for phase angle steps of $\Delta \omega t = 15°$. For $\omega t > 180°$, the velocity profiles are of the same form but opposite in sign. From McDonald (1974), by permission.

Figure 3.7:2 shows the theoretical velocity profiles computed for a straight circular cylindrical tube in which a sinusoidally oscillating pressure gradient acts. As α increases from 3.34 to 6.67, the profiles are seen to become flatter and flatter in the central portion of the tube.

3.8 Wave Propagation in Blood Vessels

Before taking up the full complexity of pulse-wave propagation in arteries, let us consider some idealized cases and learn a few basic facts. Let us consider first an infinitely long, isolated, circular, cylindrical, elastic tube containing a homogenous, incompressible, and nonviscous liquid. When this tube is disturbed at one place, the disturbance will be propagated as waves along the tube at a finite speed. The problem is to determine this speed.

Let us impose some further simplifications.* Let the wave amplitude be small and the wave length be long compared with the tube radius, so that the slope of the deformed wall remains $\ll 1$ at all times. Under these conditions we can introduce an important hypothesis that the flow is essentially one-dimensional, with a longitudinal velocity component $u(x, t)$ which is a function of the axial coordinate x and time t. In comparison with u, other velocity components are negligibly small. Then the basic equations can be obtained from the general equations listed in the Appendix at the end of the book. They are the equation of continuity (or conservation of mass)

$$\frac{\partial A}{\partial t} + \frac{\partial}{\partial x}(uA) = 0, \tag{1}$$

and the equation of motion

$$\frac{\partial u}{\partial t} + u\frac{\partial u}{\partial x} + \frac{1}{\rho}\frac{\partial p_i}{\partial x} = 0. \tag{2}$$

Here $A(x, t)$ is the cross-sectional area of the tube and $p_i(x, t)$ is the pressure in the tube. The relationship between p_i and A may be quite complex. For simplicity we introduce another hypothesis, that A depends on the transmural pressure, $p_i - p_e$, alone:

$$p_i - p_e = P(A), \tag{3}$$

where p_e is the pressure acting on the outside of the tube. Equation (3) is a gross simplification. In the theory of elastic shells we know that the tube deformation is related to the applied load by a set of partial differential equations and that the external load includes the inertial force of the tube wall (see Eqs. (4) and (5) of Sec. 3.15 *infra*). Hence Eq. (3) implies that the

---

* In subsequent sections we shall relax these assumptions and evaluate their effects.

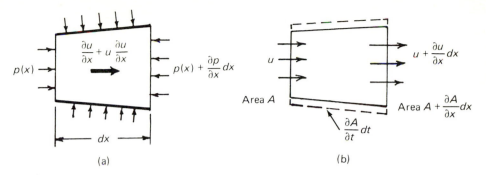

Figure 3.8:1 Free-body diagram of an arterial element, showing pressure, velocity, and wall displacement.

mass of the tube is ignored, and that the partial differential equations are replaced by an algebraic equation. By assuming Eq. (3) the dynamics of the tube is replaced by statics. The viscoelasticity of tube wall is ignored.

In the theoretical development, the derivative of the function $P(A)$ is very important, particularly in the combination

$$c = \sqrt{\frac{A}{\rho}\frac{dP}{dA}}. \qquad (4)$$

We shall see later that c is the velocity of propagation of progressive waves.

These equations are not difficult to solve since Georg Riemann (1826–1866) has shown the way. But before solving these equations we shall derive them once more from elementary considerations to make sure that we know them well.

Consider first the balance of forces acting in the axial direction on a fluid element of length dx and cross sectional area A. A free-body diagram is shown in Fig. 3.8:1(a). Since the fluid is nonviscous there is no shear stress acting on it. The force acting on the left end due to the pressure is pA toward the right, that acting on the right end is $[p + (\partial p/\partial x)dx][A + (\partial A/\partial x)dx]$ toward the left. The pressure acting on the lateral sides contributes an axial force $p(\partial A/\partial x)dx$ toward the right. Therefore, on neglecting the second-order term, the net pressure force is $A(\partial p/\partial x)dx$ acting toward the left. The mass is $\rho A dx$, ρ being the density of the blood. According to Newton's law the net force will cause an acceleration $\partial u/\partial t + u\partial u/\partial x$. On equating the force with mass times acceleration, we obtain Eq. (2).

Next, consider the conservation of mass in a segment of the tube of length dx as is illustrated in Fig. 3.8:1(b). In a unit time the mass influx at the left end is equal to $\rho u A$; the efflux at the right is $\rho\{uA + [\partial(uA)/\partial x]dx\}$. In the mean time the volume of the element is increased by $(\partial A/\partial t)dx$. The law of conservation of mass then leads to Eq. (1).

Next, consider the elasticity of the tube. If the tube behaves like a pulmonary artery or vein, then the situation is simple. The pulmonary arterial diameter $2a_i$ is linearly proportional to the blood pressure in the vessel p_i (see Sec. 6.4 and 6.11):

$$2a_i = 2a_{i0} + \alpha p_i, \tag{5}$$

where a_{i0} and α are constants which depend on the pleural pressure p_{PL} and airway pressure p_A, but are independent of blood pressure p_i. α is the compliance constant of the vessel, and a_{i0} is the radius when $p_i = 0$. A differentiation of Eq. (5) then yields the relationship

$$da_i = \frac{\alpha}{2} dp_i. \tag{6}$$

Equations (1), (2), and (6) govern the wave propagation phenomenon. Let us first solve a linearized version of these equations. Consider small disturbances in an initially stationary liquid-filled circular cylindrical tube. In this case u is small and the second term in Eq. (2) can be neglected. Hence

$$\frac{\partial u}{\partial t} + \frac{1}{\rho} \frac{\partial p_i}{\partial x} = 0. \tag{7}$$

The area A is equal to πa_i^2. Substituting πa_i^2 for A in Eq. (1), remembering the hypothesis that the wave amplitude is much smaller than the wave length, so that $\partial a_i/\partial x \ll 1$, then, on neglecting small quantities of the second order, we can reduce Eq. (1) to the form

$$\frac{\partial u}{\partial x} + \frac{2}{a_i} \frac{\partial a_i}{\partial t} = 0. \tag{8}$$

Combining Eqs. (8) and (6), we obtain

$$\frac{\partial u}{\partial x} + \frac{\alpha}{a_i} \frac{\partial p_i}{\partial t} = 0. \tag{9}$$

Differentiating Eq. (7) with respect to x and Eq. (9) with respect to t, subtracting the resulting equations, and neglecting the second order term (α/a_i^2) $(\partial a_i/\partial t)(\partial p_i/\partial t)$, we obtain

$$\frac{\partial^2 p_i}{\partial x^2} - \frac{1}{c^2} \frac{\partial^2 p_i}{\partial t^2} = 0, \tag{10}$$

where

$$c^2 = \frac{a_i}{\rho \alpha}. \tag{11}$$

Equation (10) is the famous *wave equation*. The quantity c is the *wave speed*:

$$c = \sqrt{\frac{a_i}{\rho \alpha}}. \tag{12}$$

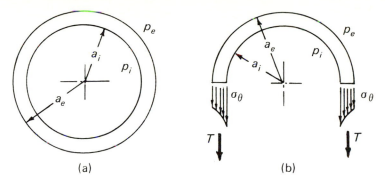

Figure 3.8:2 The balances of forces in an arterial wall.

Thin-Walled Elastic Tube

If the tube is thin-walled and the material obeys Hooke's law then for a small change in radius da_i the circumference is changed by $2\pi da_i$ and the circumferential strain is $2\pi da_i/2\pi a_i = da_i/a_i$. If E is the Young's modulus of the wall material the circumferential stress is changed by the amount Eda_i/a_i. If the wall thickness is h the tension in the wall is changed by $Ehda_i/a_i$. This increment of tension is balanced by the change of pressure dp_i. According to the condition of equilibrium of the forces acting on a free body shown in Fig. 3.8:2(b), we have

$$\frac{Ehda_i}{a_i} = a_i dp_i. \tag{13}$$

This equation is of the same form as Eq. (6) with

$$\frac{\alpha}{2} = \frac{a_i^2}{Eh}. \tag{14}$$

The wave speed in such a tube is, therefore,

$$c = \sqrt{\frac{Eh}{2\rho a_i}}. \tag{15}$$

This formula was first derived by Thomas Young in 1808 (see Table 3.15:1), and is known as the Moens–Korteweg formula.

Note that if the thin-wall assumption is not made the accuracy of the result can be improved by computing the strain on the mid wall of the tube: $da_i/(a_i + h/2)$. Then the wave speed is

$$c = \sqrt{\frac{Eh}{2\rho(a_i + h/2)}}. \tag{16}$$

Nonlinear Elasticity of Systemic Arteries

The radius to wall thickness ratio of systemic arteries is of the order of 2 or 3 when the transmural pressure is reduced to zero, or of the order of 10 when the blood pressure is high. These vessels cannot be regarded as thin-walled. The stress-strain relationship of the blood vessel wall is nonlinear (see *Biomechanics* (Fung, 1981), Sec. 8.5). Hence it is important to determine under what condition can Eq. (6) apply to systemic arteries.

Let the internal and external radii of the vessel be a_i and a_e, respectively, and the corresponding pressures be p_i and p_e; see Fig. 3.8:2(a). Let the radii be a_{i0} and a_{e0} when the pressures p_i and p_e are zero. The stress in the vessel wall is nonuniformly distributed, but the conditions of equilibrium of the forces acting on a free body shown in Fig. 3.8:2(b) yields the average circumferential stress

$$\langle \sigma_\theta \rangle = (p_i a_i - p_e a_e)/(a_i - a_e). \tag{17}$$

Let us define the stretch ratio λ_θ and strain $E_{\theta\theta}$ on the midwall by the formulas

$$\lambda_\theta = \frac{a_i + a_e}{a_{i0} + a_{e0}}, \qquad E_{\theta\theta} = \frac{1}{2}(\lambda_\theta^2 - 1). \tag{18}$$

Then, if $\rho_0 W^{(2)}$ denotes the strain energy function in the arterial wall expressed as a function of the strains $E_{\theta\theta}$ and E_{zz} (the longitudinal strain), we have (see *Biomechanics, loc. cit.*, p. 276)

$$\langle \sigma_\theta \rangle = \lambda_\theta^2 \frac{\partial(\rho_0 W^{(2)})}{\partial E_{\theta\theta}}. \tag{19}$$

Combining Eqs. (17) and (19) we have

$$p_i a_i - p_e a_e = (a_i - a_e)\lambda_\theta^2 \frac{\partial(\rho_0 W^{(2)})}{\partial E_{\theta\theta}}. \tag{20}$$

The function $\rho_0 W^{(2)}$ is given in *Biomechanics*, p. 277:

$$\rho_0 W^{(2)} = \frac{1}{2}C' \exp[a_1 E_{\theta\theta}^2 + a_2 E_{zz}^2 + 2a_4 E_{\theta\theta} E_{zz}], \tag{21}$$

where C', a_1, a_2, a_4 are constants. The radii a_i and a_e are related by the condition of incompressibility of the wall:

$$\pi(a_e^2 - a_i^2) = \pi(a_{e0}^2 - a_{i0}^2). \tag{22}$$

On computing $\partial a_e/\partial a_i$ from Eq. (22) and using it in an equation obtained by differentiating Eq. (20), we obtain

$$a_i dp_i + p_i da_i - p_e \frac{a_i}{a_e} da_i = \lambda_\theta^2 \frac{\partial(\rho_0 W^{(2)})}{\partial E_{\theta\theta}}\left(1 - \frac{a_i}{a_e}\right) da_i$$

$$+ (a_i - a_e)\frac{\partial}{\partial \lambda_\theta}\left[\lambda_\theta^2 \frac{\partial(\rho_0 W^{(2)})}{E_{\theta\theta}}\right]\frac{d\lambda_\theta}{da_i} da_i. \tag{23}$$

This can be put in the form of Eq. (6) if we identify

$$
\frac{2}{\alpha} = -\frac{p_i}{a_i} + \frac{p_e}{a_e} + \left(\frac{1}{a_i} - \frac{1}{a_e}\right)\lambda_\theta^2 \frac{\partial(\rho_0 W^{(2)})}{\partial E_{\theta\theta}}
$$
$$
+ \left(\frac{a_i}{a_e} - \frac{a_e}{a_i}\right)\frac{\partial}{\partial \lambda_\theta}\left[\lambda_\theta^2 \frac{\partial \rho_0 W^{(2)}}{\partial E_{\theta\theta}}\right].
\tag{24}
$$

The compliance α varies obviously with p_i, p_e and a_i. If only infinitesimal disturbances da_i, dp_i, du are considered, then the quantity on the right-hand side of Eq. (24) can be evaluated at the steady state and used as a constant in Eq. (11). In that case the linearized wave equation (10) applies.

Solution of the Wave Equation

To understand the nature of the phenomenon described by the differential equation (10), let us take the following mathematical approach. Let $f(z)$ be an arbitrary function of z, which is differentiable at least twice and whose second derivative is continuous for a certain prescribed region of z. Let z be a function of two variables x and t:

$$
z = x - ct,
\tag{25}
$$

where x represents the coordinate of a point on a straight line and t represents time. Now, by the rules of differentiation, we have

$$
\frac{\partial f}{\partial x} = \frac{df}{dz}\frac{\partial z}{\partial x} = \frac{df}{dz}, \qquad \frac{\partial f}{\partial t} = \frac{df}{dz}\frac{\partial z}{\partial t} = -c\frac{df}{dz},
$$
$$
\frac{\partial^2 f}{\partial x^2} = \frac{d^2 f}{dz^2}, \qquad \frac{\partial^2 f}{\partial t^2} = c^2\frac{d^2 f}{dz^2}.
\tag{26}
$$

The last line shows that the function $f(x - ct)$ satisfies the differential equation

$$
\frac{\partial^2 f}{\partial x^2} - \frac{1}{c^2}\frac{\partial^2 f}{\partial t^2} = 0,
$$

which is exactly Eq. (10). Thus Eq. (10) is solved by $p = f(x - ct)$.

Now suppose that a disturbance occurs at time $t = 0$ over a segment of the vessel as illustrated in Fig. 3.8:3. The amplitude of the disturbance is represented by $f(x)$ at $t = 0$. At a time t_1 later, the same disturbance will appear translated to the right. The value of the disturbance $f(x - ct)$ will remain constant as long as $x - ct$ has the same value; hence an increase in t requires an increase in $x = ct$. Thus the function $f(x - ct)$ represents a wave propagating to the right (in the direction of increasing x) with a speed c.

In exactly the same manner, we can show that $f(x + ct)$ satisfies the wave equation and represents a wave moving in the negative x direction with a speed c.

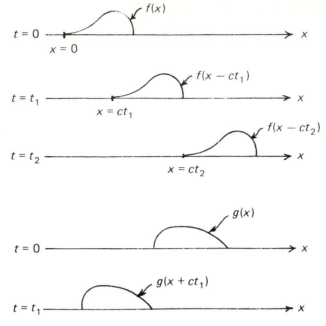

Figure 3.8:3 Wave propagation to the right and to the left.

Flow Velocity and Wall Displacement Waves

Equation (10) shows that the pressure in the elastic vessel is governed by a wave equation. Because the axial velocity u is linearly related to p through Eq. (7), and small change of the radius, a, is linearly related to changes in p through Eq. (6), (13), or (23), we see that u and a are governed by the same wave equation with the same wave speed. In other words, the p in Eq. (10) can be replaced by u and a. (Verify this by direct differentiation.) Thus disturbances in velocity and the radius of the vessel are propagated by waves of speed c, in association with the pressure wave.

We use pulse waves in arteries of the wrist, ankle, or temple to determine the heart rate. If we press very gently on the artery, we probably feel the pulsation of the radius of the artery. If we press harder, so that an area of the artery under the finger is flattened, we should feel the pressure wave in the artery. (See *Biomechanics* (Fung, 1981), p. 19, Prob 1.5.) If you use a doppler ultrasound flow meter, you will detect the velocity waves.

Our derivation of the wave equation is subjected to many simplifying assumptions. All the factors ignored in this derivation have some effect on the real wave propagation in the arteries. We shall discuss them in due course.

Relationship between the Pressure and Velocity Waves

We have argued that the pressure and velocity satisfy the same wave equation. We can show that the wave equation is satisfied by

$$p = p_o f(x - ct) + p'_o g(x + ct),$$
$$u = u_o f(x - ct) - u'_o g(x + ct), \tag{27}$$

and that by Eq. (7) or (9), the *amplitude p_o and u_o are related by the simple relationship*

$$p_o = \rho c u_o \tag{28}$$

for a wave that is moving in the positive x direction, and

$$p'_o = -\rho c u'_o \tag{29}$$

for a wave which moves in the negative x direction.

The proof is very simple. On substituting Eq. (27) into Eq. (7), carrying out the differentiation and cancelling the common factor df/dz, we obtain Eq. (28) or (29).

This important relationship shows *that the amplitude of presure wave is proportional to the product of wave speed and velocity disturbance and the fluid density, and nothing else.* This conclusion holds for progressive waves in long tubes without reflection. This, incidentally, is a general result for one-dimensional longitudinal waves, which may occur, for example, in an elastic solid rod, or in a plane compressional wave in the earth.

Examples of Series Representation of Waves (Fig. 3.8:4)

1. Consider a half-sine pulse,

$$f(x) = \sin \frac{\pi x}{L} \quad \text{for} \quad 0 \le x \le L,$$

$$f(x) = 0 \qquad \text{for} \quad x < 0, \quad x > L,$$

propagating to the right at speed c. Sketch the wave after 1 sec.

2. If at time $t = 0$ a wave is observed to have a spatial distribution

$$f(x) = \sum_{n=1}^{\infty} a_n \sin \frac{n\pi x}{L} \quad \text{for} \quad x \text{ in } (0, L) \tag{30}$$

and $f(x) = 0$ outside this interval, then at time t the solution of the wave equation (14) is

$$f(x \pm ct) = \sum_{n=1}^{\infty} a_n \sin \frac{n\pi}{L} (x \pm ct) \tag{31}$$

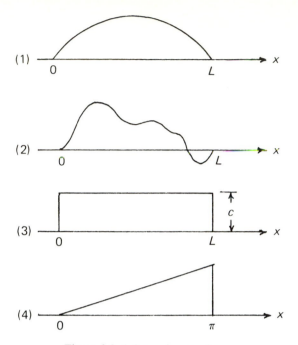

Figure 3.8:4 Several waves forms.

for $x \pm ct$ in $(0, L)$, and $f(x \pm ct) = 0$ elsewhere. The $\pm$ sign is chosen according to whether the direction of propagation is to the left $(+)$ or right $(-)$.

If a wave described by Eq. (19) propagating to the right is observed at a fixed station $x = 0$, then the time sequence is

$$f(-ct) = -\sum_{n=1}^{\infty} a_n \sin \frac{n\pi c}{L} t. \tag{32}$$

Each term in Eq. (19) is a *harmonic* of the wave. The nth is called the *nth harmonic*. The factor $n\pi c/L$ is the *frequency* (or more precisely, *circular frequency*) of the nth harmonic of the pulse wave. Equations (18), (19), and (20) embody the idea of Fourier analysis of pulse waves. If the wave speed c and the direction of propagation are known, then it is sufficient to observe the wave either at one time or at one station, and use Eq. (19) to predict its amplitude and phase at any location and time. One can use the half-range Fourier sine series as in Eqs. (18) and (20), the half-range Fourier cosine series, the full-range Fourier series, series of other orthogonal functions, such as Legendre polynomials, Bessel functions, Chebyshev polynomials, or the ordinary power series.

3. Show that a square wave of amplitude c in the region $0 < x < L$ can be represented by

$$f(x) = c = \frac{4c}{\pi} \left(\sin \frac{\pi x}{L} + \frac{1}{3} \sin \frac{3\pi x}{L} + \frac{1}{5} \sin \frac{5\pi x}{L} + \cdots \right) \tag{33}$$

whereas one in the region $-L/2 < x < L/2$ can be represented by

$$f(x) = c = \frac{4c}{\pi} \left(\cos \frac{\pi x}{L} - \frac{1}{3} \cos \frac{3\pi x}{L} + \frac{1}{5} \cos \frac{5\pi x}{L} - \cdots \right). \tag{34}$$

Both of these formulas hold for the open intervals indicated. At the ends $x = 0$ and L, Gibbs phenomenon occurs: the value represented by the series oscillates about c.

4. Show that a triangular wave $f(x) = x$ in $-\pi < x < \pi$ can be represented as

$$f(x) = x = 2 \left(\sin x - \frac{\sin 2x}{2} + \frac{\sin 3x}{3} - \frac{\sin 4x}{4} + \cdots \right) \tag{35}$$

whereas in $0 \le x \le \pi$, inclusive, we have

$$f(x) = x = \frac{\pi}{2} - \frac{4}{\pi} \left(\cos x + \frac{\cos 3x}{3^2} + \frac{\cos 5x}{5^2} + \frac{\cos 7x}{7^2} + \cdots \right). \tag{36}$$

Note the difference in rate of convergence of the series which represent the same function.

5. The choice of the series expansions, as illustrated in the examples above, is arbitrary, but there are beautiful theorems, such as the following. If one chose to represent a function in the range $-1 \le x \le 1$ by a series of so-called *ultraspherical polynomials* (Szegö, 1939), which includes powers of x, Legendre polynomials, Chebyshev polynomials, and others, then, as Lanczos (1952) has shown, *if the series is truncated at n terms, the estimated error of an expansion into Chebyshev polynomials is smaller than that of any other expansion into ultraspherical polynomials. While the expansion into powers of x (Taylor series) gives the slowest convergence, the expansion into Chebyshev polynomials gives the fastest convergence.*

In case the reader is not familiar with Chebychev polynomials, let him be reminded that it is nothing but the simple trigonometric function $\cos k\theta$, but expressed in the variable

$$x = \cos \theta.$$

Thus, the Chebyshev polynomial $T_k(x)$ is

$$T_k(x) = \cos(k \arccos x). \tag{37}$$

What is meant by the theorem above is that if a function $f(x)$ of bounded variation is expanded into a series

$$f(x) = \tfrac{1}{2}c_0 + c_1 T_1(x) + c_2 T_2(x) + \cdots + c_n T_n(x) + \eta_n(x), \tag{38}$$

then the maximum value of the remainder η_n is smaller than that of any other expansions in which $T_k(x)$ is replaced by other ultraspherical polynomials. If the expansion (38) is rearranged into an ordinary power series of the form

$$f(x) = b_0 + b_1 x + b_2 x^2 + \cdots + b_n x^n + \eta_n'(x) \tag{39}$$

then the coefficients b_i decrease much slower than the coefficients c_i as i increases and the maximum of the remainder $\eta_n'(x)$ is greater than that of $\eta_n(x)$. In fact, the convergence of the power series in Eq. (39) is the slowest among all expansions in ultraspherical polynomials.

This theorem shows that an orthogonal expansion of $f(x)$ into the polynomials $T_k(x)$ yields an expansion that for the same number of terms represents $f(x)$ with greater accuracy than the expansion into any other sets of orthogonal functions (this includes the Legendre polynomials, which give a better average error but a worse maximum error in the given range).

6. An example of an actual application of Fourier series to the analysis

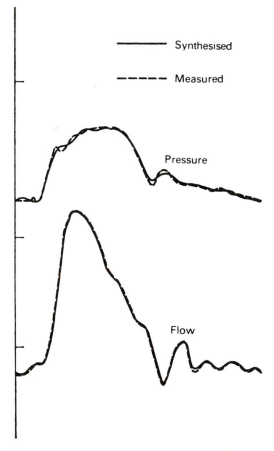

Figure 3.8:5 An example of Fourier series representation of pressure and flow waves in the ascending aorta. The experimental wave form is analyzed into a Fourier series with 10 harmonics. The series is then summed and plotted, showing good agreement with experimental data. From McDonald (1974), by permission.

of pulse waves is shown in Fig. 3.8:5. The experimental data on pressure and flow in the ascending aorta of a dog are shown by dotted curves. These curves are analyzed into a Fourier series with a constant term and 10 harmonics (with frequencies up to about 20 Hz). The solid curves represent the Fourier series. It is shown that the accuracy of the 10-harmonic approximation is acceptable. Further away from the heart, the wave forms are smoother and can be adequately described by fewer harmonics.

3.9 Progressive Waves Superposed on a Steady Flow

We must be careful to say that the results derived so far apply to a straight, cylindrical, elastic tube filled with liquid which is not flowing. The reason we assume that there is no flow is because flow requires a pressure gradient, and variable pressure in an elastic tube will induce variable strain that will cause the tube to taper, and its wall material will have variable incremental Young's modulus because the elasticity of the blood vessel wall is nonlinear. The Young's modulus of the blood vessel is almost proportional to the tensile stress acting in the vessel wall.

If the resulting taper is small and the variation of incremental Young's modulus is negligible, then the equations of Sec. 3.8 are applicable to tubes carrying a steady flow, provided that we adopt a coordinate system that moves with the undisturbed flow, and interpret u as the perturbation velocity superposed on the steady flow and c as the speed of perturbation wave relative to the undisturbed flow. The proof is as follows:

Let U be the velocity of the undisturbed flow, and u the small perturbation superposed on it. Treating u as an infinitesimal quantity of the first order, we see that the equation of motion, Eq. (3.8:2), can be linearized into

$$\frac{\partial u}{\partial t} + U\frac{\partial u}{\partial x} = -\frac{1}{\rho}\frac{\partial p_i}{\partial x}. \tag{1}$$

This can be reduced to Eq. (3.8:7) by introducing a transformation of variables from x, t to x', t':

$$x' = x - Ut, \qquad t' = t. \tag{2}$$

From (2) we have

$$\frac{\partial}{\partial t} = \frac{\partial}{\partial t'}\frac{\partial t'}{\partial t} + \frac{\partial}{\partial x'}\frac{\partial x'}{\partial t} = \frac{\partial}{\partial t'} - U\frac{\partial}{\partial x'},$$

$$\frac{\partial}{\partial x} = \frac{\partial}{\partial t'}\frac{\partial t'}{\partial x} + \frac{\partial}{\partial x'}\frac{\partial x'}{\partial x} = \frac{\partial}{\partial x'}. \tag{4}$$

Hence, a substitution into Eq. (1) reduces it to

$$\frac{\partial u}{\partial t'} = -\frac{1}{\rho}\frac{\partial p}{\partial x'}, \tag{5}$$

which is exactly Eq. (3.8:7) in the new coordinates.

The equation of continuity, Eq. (3.8:1), now becomes

$$\frac{\partial a_i}{\partial t} + U\frac{\partial a_i}{\partial x} + \frac{a_i}{2}\frac{\partial u}{\partial x} = 0 \tag{6}$$

when πa_i^2 is substituted for A, a_i being the inner radius of the tube, $U + u$ is substituted for u, and the equation is linearized for small perturbations. Under the transformation Eq. (2), and using Eq. (5), Eq. (6) becomes

$$\frac{\partial a_i}{\partial t'} + \frac{a_i}{2}\frac{\partial u}{\partial x'} = 0, \tag{7}$$

which is exactly Eq. (3.8:8).

The pressure–radius relationship, Eq. (3.8:5), (3.8:6), (3.8:13), or (3.8:23), is independent of reference coordinates; thus Eq. (3.8:9) is unchanged when t is replaced by t'. Thus all the basic equations are unchanged. Equations (5) and (7) govern the fluid and Eq. (3.8:9) governs the tube and fluid interaction, i.e., the boundary conditions. By eliminating u, the same wave equation (3.8:10) is obtained, except that the independent variables are replaced by x' and t'. But x' and t' are the distance and time measured in the moving coordinates which translate with the undisturbed flow. Thus what we set out to prove is done.

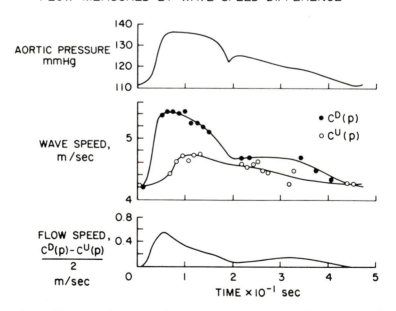

FLOW MEASURED BY WAVE SPEED DIFFERENCE

Figure 3.9:1 Wave speeds measured upstream and downstream in the aorta of a dog. Top: Natural pulse wave. Middle: Upstream wave speed (open symbols) and downstream wave speed (closed symbols) measured at different instants of the cardiac cycle. The upstream and downstream data correspond to two heartbeats a few seconds apart but with matching pressure patterns. Bottom: Mean flow velocity U. From Anliker, M. (1972), by permission.

Experimental evidence of this result is shown in Fig. 3.9:1. Anliker and Histand (1972) installed two electromagnetic wave generators at two stations along the dog's aorta and recorded the pressure fluctuations at two points between the two wave generators. A short train of high-frequency waves generated by the upstream wave generator will propagate downstream with a theoretical velocity

$$c^D = c + U, \tag{8}$$

which can be determined experimentally by the arrival times of the wave train at the two recording stations. On the other hand, if the wave train were generated by the downstream generator and propagated upstream the theoretical wave speed would be

$$c^U = c - U, \tag{9}$$

which again can be determined experimentally. From Eqs. (8) and (9) we have

$$U = \tfrac{1}{2}(c^D - c^U). \tag{10}$$

In Fig. 3.9:1, c^D, c^U, and U are shown during a cardiac cycle. The flow velocity U can also be measured by a flow gauge, and as Anliker stated, a good agreement was obtained.

3.10 Nonlinear Wave Propagation

A more general solution of Eqs. (1), (2), (3) of Sec. 3.8 is given by Riemann's method of characteristics. See, for example, Lighthill (1978), Sec. 2.8. Adding $\pm c/A$ times Eq. (1) of Sec. 3.8 to Eq. (2) of Sec. 3.8, one can show that on the characteristic curves defined by

$$dx/dt = u \pm c, \tag{1}$$

the quantities (Riemann invariants)

$$R_{\pm} = \frac{1}{2}\left[u \pm \int_{A_0}^{A} \frac{c}{A} dA \right] \tag{2}$$

are constants, where A_0 is the undisturbed area and c is the velocity

$$c^2 = \frac{A}{\rho} \frac{dp}{dA}. \tag{3}$$

Thus nonlinear waves are propagated in the $\pm x$ directions with speeds $u \pm c$. The linearized theory presented in Sec. 3.8 results if the condition $c \gg u$ is imposed.

The general solution, Eq. (2), can be used to investigate the effect of some of the simplifying assumptions used in the preceding section. It has been used by Pedley (1980, pp. 79–87) to investigate the formation shock waves in blood vessels.

The method of characteristics is one of the most important devices to investigate nonlinear wave propagation. See Lighthill (1978), and Skalak (1966, 1972) for in-depth reviews of this subject. Lambert (1958) averaged the equations of motion and continuity over the arterial cross-section to obtain uniaxial equations. Van der Werff (1973) introduced a special method to handle periodic conditions. Atabek (1980) combined the characteristics method with Ling and Atabek's (1972) "local flow" analysis to predict velocity profiles of the flow and waves in a segment from known pressure and pressure gradient at the proximal end of the segment. Atabek's detailed comparison between calculated results and those from animal experiments shows the importance of the effects of nonlinearity from various sources (see Sec. 3.16 *infra*); and he concludes that these effects are not yet fully understood.

Problem

3.13 We know that the blood vessel wall does not obey Hooke's law. Use the information on the pseudo-elasticity and viscoelasticity of the arteries presented in *Biomechanics* (Fung, 1981, chap. 8), derive an expression for the wave speed in arteries.

Devise a theory of your own to handle the viscoelasticity of the blood vessel wall in the problem of pulse wave propagation. Discuss the effect of viscoelasticity in detail.

3.11 Reflection and Transmission of Waves at Junctions

So far we have discussed propagation of axisymmetric disturbances in an infinitely long, straight, cylindrical, elastic tube filled with an incompressible nonviscous liquid. Our results are simple and interesting, but they are true only if all the idealizing qualifiers hold. Real arteries do not obey these qualifiers: they are short, tapered, branching, and filled with a viscous fluid. They are sometimes curved. Their walls are nonlinearly viscoelastic. It turns out that the effect of nonlinear viscoelasticity on wave propagation is not so severe; neglecting the blood viscosity is often acceptable for the wave propagation problem because the frequency parameter (Sec. 3.7) α or N_w is sufficiently large (we will discuss these factors later), but the "infinitely long" assumption must be removed.

A tube of finite length must have two ends. When waves of pressure and velocity reach an end they must conform to the end conditions. As a result the waves will be modified. To clarify the situation, consider first a single junction, as shown in Fig. 3.11:1, where a tube branches into two daughters. A wave traveling down the parent artery will be partially reflected at the junction and partially transmitted down the daughters. Now, at the junction, the conditions are:

(a) The pressure is a single-valued function.
(b) The flow must be continuous.

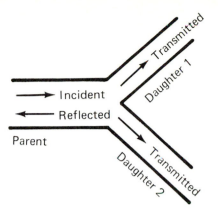

Figure 3.11:1 A bifurcating artery.

Express this mathematically: let p_I denote the oscillatory pressure associated with the incident wave, p_R that associated with the reflected wave, and p_{T_1} and p_{T_2} those associated with the transmitted waves in the two daughter tubes; then accordint to (a) we must have

$$p_I + p_R = p_{T_1} = p_{T_2}. \tag{1}$$

Similarly, let $\dot{Q}$ denote the volume-flow rate, and let the subscripts I, R, T_1, T_2 refer to the various waves as before; then, according to (b) we must have

$$\dot{Q}_I - \dot{Q}_R = \dot{Q}_{T_1} + \dot{Q}_{T_2}. \tag{2}$$

The left-hand side of Eq. (2) represents the flow out of the parent tube and the right-hand side represents the flow into the daughters. But $\dot{Q}$ is just the product of the cross-sectional area A and the mean velocity u. We have already learned the relationship between u and p in Sec. 3.8. Hence, using Eq. (3.8:28) and Eq. (3.8:29) we obtain the flow–pressure relationship:

$$\dot{Q} = Au = \pm \frac{A}{\rho c} p. \tag{3}$$

Here ρ is the density of the blood and c is the wave speed. The $+$ sign applies if the wave goes in the direction of positive x-axis; the $-$ sign applies if the wave goes the other way. The quantity $\rho c / A$ is an important characteristic of the artery, and is called the *characteristic impedance* of the tube, and is denoted by the symbol Z:

$$Z = \frac{\rho c}{A}. \tag{4}$$

Z is the ratio of oscillatory pressure to oscillatory flow when the wave goes in the direction of positive x-axis:

$$Z = \frac{p}{\dot{Q}}, \qquad Z\dot{Q} = p, \tag{5}$$

analogous to the resistance in an electric circuit:

$$R = \frac{V}{I}, \qquad RI = V, \tag{6}$$

connecting the voltage V and current I. Z has the physical dimensions $[ML^{-4}T^{-1}]$, and can be measured in the units kg m^{-4} sec^{-1}. With the Z notation, Eq. (2) can be written as

$$\frac{p_I - p_R}{Z_0} = \frac{p_{T_1}}{Z_1} + \frac{p_{T_2}}{Z_2}. \tag{7}$$

Solving Eqs. (1) and (7) for the p's, we obtain

$$\frac{p_R}{p_I} = \frac{Z_0^{-1} - (Z_1^{-1} + Z_2^{-1})}{Z_0^{-1} + (Z_1^{-1} + Z_2^{-1})} = \mathscr{R} \tag{8}$$

and

$$\frac{p_{T_1}}{p_I} = \frac{p_{T_2}}{p_I} = \frac{2Z_0^{-1}}{Z_0^{-1} + (Z_1^{-1} + Z_2^{-1})} = \mathscr{T}. \tag{9}$$

The right-hand sides of Eqs. (8) and (9) shall be denoted by $\mathscr{R}$ and $\mathscr{T}$, respectively. Hence the amplitude of the reflected pressure wave at the junction is $\mathscr{R}$ times that of the incident wave, the amplitude of the transmitted pressure waves at the junction is $\mathscr{T}$ times the incident wave. The amplitude of the reflected velocity wave is, however, equal to $-\mathscr{R}$ times that of the incident velocity wave, because the wave now moves in the negative x-axis direction, and according to Eqs. (3.8:28) and (3.8:29), there is a sign change in the relation between u and p depending on whether the waves move in the $+$ or $-$ x-axis direction.

The meaning of $\mathscr{R}$ and $\mathscr{T}$ can be clarified further by considering the transmission of energy by pressure waves. Imagine a cross section of the tube. The normal stress acting on this section is the pressure p. The force is p times the area, A. The fluid pushed by this pressure moves at a velocity u. The rate at which work is done is therefore the product pAu. But $Au = \dot{Q}$ and $\dot{Q} = p/Z$. Therefore the rate of work done is

$$\dot{W} = p\dot{Q} = p^2/Z. \tag{10a}$$

This is the rate of transmission of mechanical energy through the cross section. Now, at the junction of a bifurcating vessel, the rate of energy transmission of the incident wave is p_I^2/Z_0, whereas that of the reflected wave is

$$\frac{p_R^2}{Z_0} = \frac{(\mathscr{R}p_I)^2}{Z_0} = \mathscr{R}^2 \frac{p_I^2}{Z_0}. \tag{10b}$$

Hence the ratio of the rate of energy transmission of the reflected wave to that of the incident wave is $\mathscr{R}^2$. For this reason $\mathscr{R}^2$ is called the *energy reflection coefficient.* Similarly, the rate of energy transfer in the two transmitted waves, compared with that in the incident wave, is

$$\frac{Z_1^{-1} + Z_2^{-1}}{Z_0^{-1}} \mathcal{T}^2,$$ (10c)

which is called the *energy transmission coefficient.*

We can express the waves more explicitly as follows. Let the incident wave be

$$p_I = p_0 f(t - x/c_0).$$ (11)

Let the junction be located at $x = 0$, so that x is negative in the parent tube and positive in the daughter tubes; then at the junction, $x = 0$, the pressure of the incident wave is

$$p_I = p_0 f(t).$$

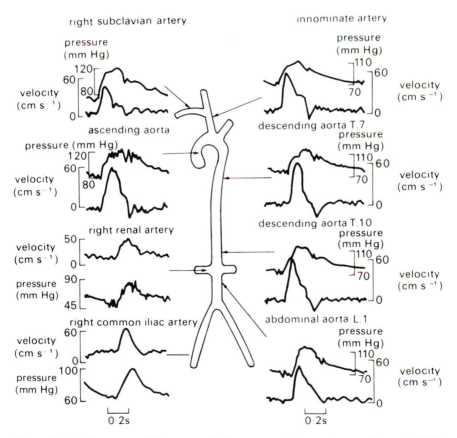

Figure 3.11:2 Pressure and flow waves in human arterial tree. From Mills et al. (1970) Pressure-flow relationships and vascular impedance in man. *Cardiovascular Res.* **4**: 405–417, by permission.

The reflectional and transmitted waves are, therefore,

$$p_R = \mathscr{R} p_0 f(t + x/c_0),$$
$$p_{T_1} = \mathscr{T} p_0 f(t - x/c_1), \tag{12}$$
$$p_{T_2} = \mathscr{T} p_0 f(t - x/c_2).$$

Here c_0, c_1, c_2 are the wave speeds in the respective tubes. Note that $p_{T_1} = p_{T_2}$ at the junction, $x = 0$ (see Eq. (1)), but c_1 may be different from c_2. The resultant disturbance in the parent tube is

$$p = p_I + p_R = p_0 f(t - x/c_0) + \mathscr{R} p_0 f(t + x/c_0). \tag{13}$$

The corresponding flow disturbance in the parent tube is, according to Eq. (3) and taking the direction of propagation into account,

$$\dot{Q} = \frac{A p_0}{\rho c_0} f(t - x/c_0) - \mathscr{R} \frac{A p_0}{\rho c_0} f(t + x/c_0). \tag{14}$$

A comparison of Eqs. (13) and (14) shows that with reflection, the pressure and flow wave forms are no longer equal.

Inequality of pressure and flow wave forms is a common feature of pulse waves in arteries (see Fig. 3.11:2), indicating the effect of reflection at branches.

Problems

3.14 Consider the case in which a parent tube gives rise to three daughter tubes at a junction. Show that $\mathscr{R}$ and $\mathscr{T}$ are given by expressions similar to Eqs. (8) and (9), except $Z_1^{-1} + Z_2^{-1}$ should be replaced by $Z_1^{-1} + Z_2^{-1} + Z_3^{-1}$ (Fig. P3.14).

3.15 Under what condition is the reflected wave zero? State the condition $\mathscr{R} = 0$ in terms of the physical parameters of the tubes.

Note. When $\mathscr{R} = 0$ the junction is said to be one at which the *impedances* are matched (Fig. P3.15).

A parent tube gives out a small daughter branch (Fig. P3.16). What are reflection and transmission characteristics ($\mathscr{R}$ and $\mathscr{T}$) at the junction?

Under what condition would a wave be totally reflected ($\mathscr{R} = 1$) (Fig. P3.17)?

If the impedance of a parent tube is perfectly matched to the daughter tubes at a junction so that $\mathscr{R} = 0$, show that $\mathscr{T} = 1$ and the transmission coefficient given in Eq. (10c) is 1. Show that $1 + \mathscr{R} = \mathscr{T}$.

3.16 Consider a bifurcating artery (Fig. 3.11:1). The functions $\mathscr{T}$ (Eq. 9) and $\mathscr{R}$ are called, respectively, the *transmission* and the *reflection coefficient* (without the word "energy"). In the special case in which the two daughter branches are of equal size and the wave speed c is the same in the parent and daughter branches, $\mathscr{R}$ and $\mathscr{T}$ are functions of the "area ratio", $(A_1 + A_2)/A_0$, i.e., the ratio of the

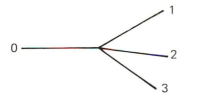

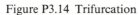

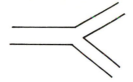

Figure P3.14 Trifurcation

Figure P3.15 Matched impedance.

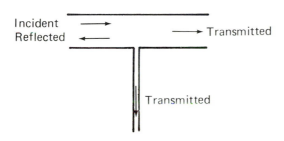

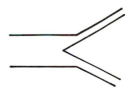

Figure P3.16 A small daughter branch.

Figure P3.17 Total reflection.

combined area of the branches to the area of the parent tube. Derive expressions of $\mathscr{R}$ and $\mathscr{T}$ in terms of the area ratio and sketch curves to show the variation of $\mathscr{R}$ and $\mathscr{T}$ with the area ratio.

   Note: Cf. Atabek (1980), p. 302, in which the viscosity of the blood and viscoelasticity of the vessel wall are considered (see Sec. 3.15 *infra*), while the motion is limited to be simple harmonic (see p. 123). Our results, Eqs. (4)–(10c), are derived for inviscid fluid in elastic tube. Whereas the wave speed c is a real number in Eq. (4), it is a complex number in Atabek (see Sec. 3.15). Figure 7.16 of Atabek (1980) shows that there is a minor dependence of the magnitude of $\mathscr{R}$ and $\mathscr{T}$ on the Womersley number (α), and a sudden change of the phase angle of $\mathscr{R}$ (from 0 to 180°) when the area ratio exceeds about 1.2–1.4.

3.17 Design an instrument to measure pulse waves noninvasively at some conveniently located arteries such as the radial artery at the wrist. What can you measure? Pressure? Force? Velocity? What significant use can be made of such measurements? (Cf. Sec. 3.18).

3.18 There are several machines in clinical use which apply pressure or vacuum on arteries of the arms or legs in a suitable periodic manner to serve as heart assist devices. One machine works on veins to reduce the threat of thrombosis. Invent one yourself, and explain why is it good.

Harmonic Waves

Oscillations that are sinusoidal in time and space are called harmonic waves. For example, a pressure wave

$$p = p_0 \cos\left\{\omega\left(t - \frac{x}{c_0}\right)\right\} = p_0 \cos\left(\omega t - \frac{2\pi x}{\lambda}\right) \tag{15}$$

$$= p_0 \cos\left\{\frac{2\pi}{\lambda}(x - c_0 t)\right\}.$$

is a harmonic progressive wave. Here ω is the *circular frequency* (unit: rad/sec), $\omega/2\pi$ is the *frequency* (unit: Hz), λ is the *wave length*, (unit: m). They are related by

$$\lambda = \frac{c_0}{(\omega/2\pi)}, \qquad \frac{\omega}{2\pi} = \frac{c_0}{\lambda}. \tag{16}$$

Thus the wave length is the wave speed divided by frequency, or the distance traveled per cycle. The wave speed is the product of frequency and wave length.

For harmonic waves, a convenient mathematical device is the *complex representation*. This is based on the relation

$$e^{iz} = \cos z + i \sin z, \tag{17}$$

where $i = \sqrt{-1}$, e is the exponential function, and z is a real variable. Thus $\cos z$ is the real part of e^{iz} and $\sin z$ is the imaginary part of e^{iz}. We can write Eq. (15) as

$$p = \mathcal{R}\ell\{p_0 e^{i\omega(t - x/c_0)}\}. \tag{18}$$

the symbol $\mathcal{R}\ell$ means the real part of the complex quantity. A great advantage of the complex representation is that in Eq. (18) p_0 does not have to be limited to a real number. If p_0 is a complex number,

$$p_0 = a + ib = P e^{i\phi},$$

$$P = \sqrt{a^2 + b^2}, \qquad \phi = \tan^{-1}\frac{b}{a};$$

then Eq. (18) means

$$p = a \cos\{\omega(t - x/c_0)\} - b \sin\{\omega(t - x/c_0)\} \tag{19}$$

$$= P \cos\{\omega(t - x/c_0) + \phi\}.$$

Hence P is the *amplitude* and ϕ is the *phase angle* of the wave. Similar expressions can be written for the flow rate and for waves traveling in the opposite direction. It is conventional to omit the symbol $\mathcal{R}\ell$, so that whenever a complex number is used to represent a physical quantity, it is assumed that its real part is being used.

We shall use this method to discuss multiple reflections below.

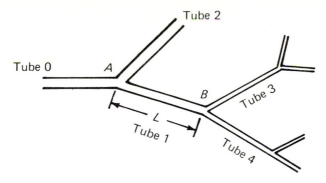

Figure 3.11:3 Multiple reflection sites of an artery with two branching junctions.

Problem

3.19 Consider energy transmission. We have shown in Eq. (10) that the rate of energy transmission in a progressive wave is

$$W = Ap \cdot u = p \cdot \dot{Q} = p^2/Z.$$

If p is a harmonic wave, show that this is

$$W = \mathscr{R}\ell p \cdot \mathscr{R}\ell \dot{Q} = (\mathscr{R}\ell p)^2/Z$$

and is not equal to $\mathscr{R}\ell(p^2)/Z$. This important example shows that one has to be careful in using the complex representation.

Show that if p is given by Eq. (15) the average value of W over a period is

$$W = \tfrac{1}{2}p_0^2/Z.$$

Multiple Reflections

Waves in more complex systems of tubes can be analyzed by repeated application of the results presented above. For example, in the double junction illustrated in Fig. 3.11:3, a wave reflected once at junction B is reflected a second time at junction A, and so on. The amplitude of the reflected and transmitted waves on each occasion are determined by the characteristics of the junction.

To see what is going on, let us consider a continuous harmonic excitation and write out in detail the perturbations in the segment AB. Let the origin of the x-axis be taken at A. Let the first wave transmitted through A be

$$p_1 e^{i\omega(t-x/c_0)}. \tag{20}$$

At B, where $x = L$, the pressure due to this wave is

$$p_1 e^{i\omega(t-L/c_0)}.$$

Here the wave is reflected. Let the reflection parameter be denoted by $\mathscr{R}_{10}$ Then the reflected wave is.

$$\mathscr{R}_{10}p_1 e^{i\omega(t-L/c_0+(x-L)/c_0)} \tag{21}$$

When this wave reaches A, the pressure is

$$\mathscr{R}_{10}p_1 e^{i\omega(t-2L/c_0)}.$$

This wave is reflected at A. To calculate the reflection parameter we must treat the segment AB as the parent tube and tubes 0 and 2 as daughters. Let the reflection parameters be denoted by $\mathscr{R}_{01}$. Then the reflected wave is

$$\mathscr{R}_{01}\mathscr{R}_{10}p_1 e^{i\omega(t-2L/c_0-x/c_0)}.$$

The process continues. The pressure perturbation in the tube AB is the sum of all these waves.

But the story cannot end here. At the ends A and B the waves do not just bounce back and forth; they are also transmitted into the vessels beyond them, to segments 0, 2, 3, 4, etc. These transmitted waves will be reflected at the junctions further away and will come back to segment AB. The total picture will not be known until the entire system is accounted for.

In practice, if the impedance is reasonably well matched the series converges rapidly.

Standing Waves

The reflection and trapping of waves are related to the phenomenon of resonance. Consider a particular condition in which the tube AB is closed at both ends so that $\mathscr{R}_{10}$ and $\mathscr{R}_{13}$ are both equal to 1. In this case the sum of the first two waves, Eqs. (20) and (21), becomes, with Eq. (16),

$$e^{i(\omega t-2\pi x/L)} + e^{i[\omega t-2\pi L/\lambda+2\pi(x-L)/\lambda]}.$$

The sum of every two succeeding terms is similar, differing only in phase angle. In the special case in which the tube length is equal to the half wave length,

$$L = \frac{\lambda}{2}, \tag{22}$$

the sum above becomes (because $e^{-i2\pi}$ is equal to 1)

$$e^{i\omega t}\{e^{-i2\pi x/L} + e^{i2\pi x/L}\} = 2e^{i\omega t}\cos\frac{2\pi x}{L}. \tag{23}$$

Thus, in this case the oscillation is a standing wave, and the motion is a *resonant vibration*. This occurs at a frequency of

$$\frac{\omega}{2\pi} = \frac{c_0}{\lambda} = \frac{c_0}{2L} = \frac{1}{2L}\sqrt{\frac{Eh}{2\rho a}}, \tag{24}$$

which is said to be the *fundamental frequency* of natural vibration; Eq. (23) is said to be the *fundamental mode*. If a system is excited at a resonance frequency, the amplitude of vibration can only be limited by damping.

Higher modes are obtained if $L = \lambda/(2n)$, where n is an integer, in which case the mode shape is $\cos 2\pi nx/L$ and the frequency is n times the fundamental.

Real use of this concept is limited. The vibration mode and natural frequency depends on the end conditions. Any change of the end conditions changes the modes. The mode (23) corresponds to a tube with closed ends. Open the ends and the mode is changed.

3.12 Effect of Frequency on the Pressure–Flow Relationship at Any Point in an Arterial Tree

The complex branching pattern of the arteries tells us at once that multiple reflections of pulse waves must be a major feature of blood flow. The different pressure and flow profiles quoted in the preceding section support this statement, because, if it were not for the reflections, the pressure and flow waves would have similar profiles. But if reflection is important, then the flow and pressure relationship at any given site in the artery must depend on how the multiple reflections at the bifurcation points are seen at this site, how far away the bifurcation points are, and how long it takes for each wave to travel from a bifurcation point to that site. At any given time, the pressure and flow at a given site is the sum of the newly arrived waves and the retarded waves of reflection from earlier fluctuations. This means that the pressure—flow relationship is frequency dependent.

To express the frequency-dependent characteristics of an arterial tree, it is customary to consider each harmonic of the pulse wave separately and write, at a given site and a given frequency, the ratio of pressure to flow:

$$\frac{p}{Q} = Me^{i\theta} = Z_{\text{eff}}. \tag{1}$$

p and Q are represented by a complex numbers multiplied by $e^{i\omega t}$. Their ratio is, of course, a complex number, and is called the *input impedance* or *effective impedance*. Its modulus, M, is the ratio of the amplitudes of pressure and flow, whereas its argument, θ, is the phase lag of flow-rate oscillation behind the pressure oscillation.

The input impedance of the human arterial tree can be obtained by analyzing the measured pressure and velocity waves at a given site (e.g., one of those illustrated in Fig. 3.11:2) by Fourier series (e.g., Fig. 3.8:4), and compute the ratio of the corresponding complex-valued harmonics. An example of experimental input impedance measured in the ascending aorta is shown in Fig. 3.12:1 which was taken from the same set of measurements as the wave forms shown in Fig. 3.11:2. There is a minimum of M at a

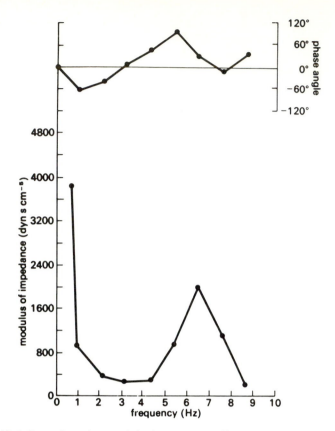

Figure 3.12:1 Input impedance of the human ascending aorta. The phase angle and modulus are plotted against the wave frequency. The single minimum of the modulus suggests that there is a single effective reflection site at the level of aortic bifurcation. From Mills et al. (1970) Pressure–flow relationships and vascular impedance in man. *Cardiovase. Res.* **4**: 405–417, by permission.

frequency of 3 Hz, and calculation shows that this implies the presence of a major reflection site roughly at the level of the aortic bifurcation. Measurements at different sites in the aorta lead to the same conclusion.

The input (or effective) impedance is not the same as the characteristic impedance of the tube in which the measurements are made. Don't use the word "impedance" without telling the reader what impedance you mean.

To recapitulate: The ratio of pressure to flow at any point is called the *effective impedance*. The effective impedance at a point A (see, for example, Fig. 3.11:3) is called the *input impedance* of the system distal to A.

This terminology comes from electric circuit theory. If a circuit is connected to a voltage source, and we want to know if the system can be operated successfully, we often need to know only the input impedance that the circuit offers to the source. Similarly, if we want to couple the arterial system to the heart, we need to know the input impedance of the arterial system at the aortic valve. If we want to know the function of the kidney, we want to know the input impedance of the kidney at the point where the renal artery branches from the abdominal aorta.

Examples

1. *Input Impedance of a Branching Artery* (Refer to Fig. 3.11 : 3). Consider an artery AB (segment 1) which branches into segments 3 and 4. Let a pressure wave $p_I e^{i\omega t}$ be imposed at the terminal A. A pressure wave $p_I e^{i\omega(t-x/c_1)}$ propagates to the right. When it reaches B at time $t = L/c_1$, it is reflected as a pressure wave

$$p_R e^{i\omega[t-L/c_1-(L-x)/c_1]}, \tag{2}$$

propagating toward A, and transmitted into segments 3 and 4 as progressive waves

$$p_{T_3} e^{i\omega(t-L/c_1-x_3/c_3)}, \qquad p_{T_4} e^{i\omega(t-L/c_1-x_4/c_4)}, \tag{3}$$

respectively, where x_3, x_4 are distances measured from point B. Since the pressure at B is single valued, we have, on substituting $x = L$, $x_3 = x_4 = 0$ (at B) and cancelling the factors $e^{i\omega(t-L/c_1)}$ throughout,

$$p_I + p_R = p_{T_3} = p_{T_4}. \tag{4}$$

The flows associated with the incident and reflected waves in segment 1 are obtained by dividing the pressure waves with the characteristic impedance Z_1 of that segment. The flows into branches 3 and 4 are obtained by dividing the pressures at point B by the effective impedances $Z_{3\,\text{eff}}$ and $Z_{4\,\text{eff}}$, respectively. Hence, on equating the inflow with outflow at B and again cancelling the factor $\exp[i\omega(t - L/c_1)]$,

$$\frac{1}{Z_1}p_I - \frac{1}{Z_1}p_R = \frac{p_{T_3}}{Z_{3\,\text{eff}}} + \frac{p_{T_4}}{Z_{4\,\text{eff}}}. \tag{5}$$

These equations are the same as those of Sec. 3.11, except that Z_3 and Z_4 are replaced by effective impedances. By solving these equations for p_R, p_{T_3}, and p_{T_4} as before, we obtain

$$\frac{p_R}{p_I} = \mathscr{R}_{\text{eff}}, \qquad \frac{p_{T_3}}{p_I} = \frac{p_{T_4}}{p_I} = \mathscr{T}_{\text{eff}}, \tag{6}$$

where

$$\mathscr{R}_{\text{eff}} = \frac{Z_1^{-1} - (Z_{3\,\text{eff}}^{-1} + Z_{4\,\text{eff}}^{-1})}{Z_1^{-1} + (Z_{3\,\text{eff}}^{-1} + Z_{4\,\text{eff}}^{-1})}, \qquad \mathscr{T}_{\text{eff}} = 1 + \mathscr{R}_{\text{eff}}. \tag{7}$$

Note that this result is the same as that of Sec. 3.11 except for a change in notation and interpretation. In Sec. 3.11 we speak of progressive waves going through the bifurcation point B, anticipating the waves to be reflected at other points of bufurcation but discussing the situation at B before any of the reflected waves arrive at B. In the present section we consider periodic oscillations and allow the waves to be reflected and transmitted as the system permits and demands, and find that a progressive wave is reflected at a junction with a complex amplitude ratio $\mathscr{R}_{\text{eff}}$ when the characteristic impedances used in Sec. 3.11 are replaced by the effective impedances of the downstream branches.

Now, back at point A, where $x = 0$, let us assume that the reflected wave passes through without further reflection. Then the pressure and flow are

$$p_A = p_I e^{i\omega t} + p_R e^{i(\omega t - 2L\omega/c_1)} = p_I e^{i\omega t}(1 + \mathscr{R}_{\text{eff}} e^{-2i\omega L/c_1}), \tag{8}$$

$$Q_A = \frac{p_I}{Z_1} e^{i\omega t} - \frac{p_R}{Z_1} e^{i(\omega t - 2L\omega/c_1)} = p_I e^{i\omega t} \frac{1}{Z_1}(1 - \mathscr{R}_{\text{eff}} e^{-2i\omega L/c_1}). \tag{9}$$

Using Eq. (1), we obtain, finally, the ratio of p_A to Q_A, which is the input impedance at A:

$$\frac{p_A}{Q_A} = Z_{1\,\text{eff}} = Z_1 \frac{1 + \mathscr{R}_{\text{eff}} e^{-2i\omega L/c_1}}{1 - \mathscr{R}_{\text{eff}} e^{-2i\omega L/c_1}}. \tag{10}$$

We can recast the final result in a different form. On substituting Eq. (7) for $\mathscr{R}_{\text{eff}}$ into Eq. (10), multiplying both the numerator and denominator by $(Z_1^{-1} + Z_{3\,\text{eff}}^{-1} + Z_{4\,\text{eff}}^{-1}) e^{i\omega L/c_1}$, and noting that for any α,

$$\frac{e^{i\alpha} + e^{-i\alpha}}{2} = \cos\alpha, \qquad \frac{e^{i\alpha} - e^{-i\alpha}}{2} = i\sin\alpha, \tag{11}$$

we obtain the important result

$$Z_{1\,\text{eff}}^{-1} = Z_1^{-1} \frac{(Z_{3\,\text{eff}}^{-1} + Z_{4\,\text{eff}}^{-1}) + iZ_1^{-1}\tan(\omega L/c_1)}{Z_1^{-1} + i(Z_{3\,\text{eff}}^{-1} + Z_{4\,\text{eff}}^{-1})\tan(\omega L/c_1)}. \tag{12}$$

By repeated use of this equation, we can obtain the effective impedance at any point, i.e., the relationship between the oscillatory pressure and flow rate at that point, from their values at the distal ends.

The factor $\omega L/c_1$ is equal to $2\pi L/\lambda$, where λ is the wavelength $2\pi c_1/\omega$, If $\omega L/c_1 = n\pi$ (n an integer), then $\tan(\omega L/c_1) = 0$ and

$$Z_{1\,\text{eff}}^{-1} = Z_{3\,\text{eff}}^{-1} + Z_{4\,\text{eff}}^{-1}. \tag{13}$$

Thus, if the arterial length L is much smaller than the wavelength, then $n \to 0$ and the formula above shows that the artery may be considered as part of the junction and there is no change of pressure–flow relationship in that segment.

On the other hand, if $\omega L/c_1$ is equal to an odd multiple of $\pi/2$, i.e., if L is equal to an odd multiple of quarter wavelengths, then $\tan(\omega L/c_1) = \infty$ and

$$Z_{1\,\text{eff}}^{-1} = \frac{Z_1^{-2}}{Z_{3\,\text{eff}}^{-1} + Z_{4\,\text{eff}}^{-1}}. \tag{14}$$

In this case, if Z_1^{-1} is smaller (or greater) than $Z_{3\,\text{eff}}^{-1} + Z_{4\,\text{eff}}^{-1}$, then $Z_{1\,\text{eff}}^{-1}$ is smaller (or greater) than Z_1^{-1}.

2. *Reverberative Reflections in an Artery.* Consider an artery with two sites of reflection, A and B (see Fig. 3.11:3). A pressure wave $p_o e^{i(\omega t - kx)}$ enters at A. At B it is reflected with a change of amplitude. The reflected wave, on arriving at A, is reflected again, and so on. Let the ratio of the complex amplitude of the reflected wave to that of the incident wave be denoted by $\mathcal{R}_1$ at A and $\mathcal{R}_2$ at B (the subscripts "eff" being omitted for simplicity). Then, at a station at a distance x from A, and at time t, the pressure is

$$p(x, t) = p_o e^{i\omega(t - x/c)} + \mathcal{R}_2 p_o e^{i\omega[(t - L/c) - (L - x)/c]}$$
$$+ \mathcal{R}_1 \mathcal{R}_2 p_o e^{i\omega[(t - 2L/c) - x/c]} \tag{15}$$
$$+ \mathcal{R}_1 \mathcal{R}_2^2 p_o e^{i\omega[(t - 3L/c) - (L - x)/c]} + \cdots.$$

We now assemble terms which represent waves going to the right and, separately, those representing waves going to the left. We obtain

$$p(x, t) = p_o e^{i\omega(t - x/c)}[1 + \mathcal{R}_1 \mathcal{R}_2 e^{-i2\omega L/c} + \cdots]$$
$$+ \mathcal{R}_2 p_o e^{i\omega(t - 2L/c + x/c)}[1 + \mathcal{R}_1 \mathcal{R}_2 e^{-i2\omega L/c} + \cdots]. \tag{16}$$

Using the summation formula

$$1 + \alpha + \alpha^2 + \alpha^3 + \cdots = \frac{1}{1 - \alpha}, \tag{17}$$

for whatever α, we obtain an important formula

$$p(x, t) = \frac{p_o e^{i\omega(t - x/c)} + \mathcal{R}_2 p_o e^{i\omega(t - 2L/c + x/c)}}{1 - \mathcal{R}_1 \mathcal{R}_2 e^{i2\omega L/c}}. \tag{18}$$

This is a general result. Now, consider the special case of total reflection at the two ends, $\mathcal{R}_1 = \mathcal{R}_2 = 1$. Then

$$p(x, t) = p_o e^{i\omega t} \frac{e^{-i\omega x/c} + e^{-i2\omega L/c} e^{i\omega x/c}}{1 - e^{-i2\omega L/c}}. \tag{19}$$

If we multiply the numerator and denominator with $e^{i\omega L/c}$ and use Eqs. (11), we obtain

$$p(x, t) = p_o e^{i\omega t} \frac{\cos \omega (L - x)/c}{i \sin (\omega L/c)}, \tag{20}$$

which represents a "standing" wave. The wave is "standing" because it does not propagate.

The amplitude of the standing wave will tend to infinity if the denominator

$\sin(\omega L/c)$ tends to zero; then the oscillation is said to "resonate." This occurs if

$$\frac{\omega L}{c} = n\pi \quad \text{or} \quad L = n\frac{\lambda}{2} \quad (n = 1, 2, \ldots), \tag{21}$$

i.e., if the length of the segment equals an integral multiple of half-wave-length.

Problems

3.20 When the frequency tends to zero, show that the phase angle θ tends to zero and the modulus M tends to a constant. With suitable assumptions with regard to an arterial tree at the peripheral end (microcirculation), derive an expression for M as the frequency tends to zero.

 Note. That the dynamics modulus of input impedance can be much smaller than the static impedance (resistance at zero frequency) is of great importance and interest. Compare this with some of our daily experiences. We can often shake a small tree if we do it at a right frequency, whereas the tree would not deflect very much if the same force is applied statically. In the circulation system, this means that we can get blood to move with much smaller driving pressure when it is done dynamically.

3.21 Explain why can we extract information on input impedance from measurements such as those illustrated in Fig. 3.11:2. One may use the Fourier analysis approach (Sec. 3.8, Example 2). Express both the pressure and flow wave forms in Fourier series, and then compare with the complex representation of waves discussed in Sec. 3.11.

3.22 In Sec. 3.8, Example 5, we extolled Chebyshev polynomials as the basis of gen-eralized Fourier series. Can you develop a formal theory of input impedance in terms of Chebyshev polynomials? What difficulty is there?

3.13 Pressure and Velocity Waves in Large Arteries

The pressure and flow waves in arteries are generated by the heart. The conditions at the aortic valve and the capillary blood vessels are the end conditions of the arterial system. Major features are explainable by the simple analysis presented in previous sections, but many details deserve attention.

 Figure 3.13:1 shows simultaneous recordings of the pressure in the left ventricle and in the ascending aorta immediately downstream from the aortic valve. When heart contracts, pressure rises rapidly in the ventricle at the beginning of systole, and soon exceeds that in the aorta, so that the aortic valve opens, blood is ejected, and aortic pressure rises. During the early part of the ejection, ventricular pressure exceeds aortic pressure. About half-way through ejection, the two pressure traces cross, and an adverse

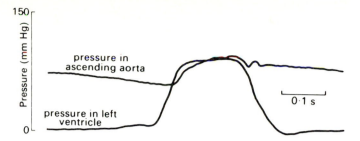

Figure 3.13:1 Pressure in the left ventricle and ascending aorta of the dog. From Noble, (1968) The contribution of blood momentum to left ventricular ejection in the dog *Circulation Res.* **23**: 663–670. Reproduced by permission of the American Heart Association.

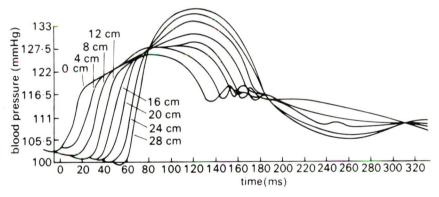

Figure 3.13:2 Simultaneous blood pressure records made at a series of sites along the aorta in the dog, with distance measured from the beginning of the descending aorta. From Olson, R. M., (1968) Aortic blood pressure and velocity as a function of time and position. *J. Appl. Physiol.* **24**: 563–569. Reproduced by permission.

pressure gradient faces the heart. The flow and pressure start to fall. Then a notch in the aortic pressure record (the *dicrotic notch*) marks the closure of the aortic valve. Thereafter the ventricular pressure falls very rapidly as the heart muscle relaxes: the aortic pressure falls more slowly, with the elastic vessel serving as a reservoir. The major feature of the pressure wave in the aorta is explained by the windkessel theory (Sec. 2.1 in Chap. 2), but the details can only be determined when all the waves are accounted for.

The change of pressure wave with distance from the aortic valve is shown in Fig. 3.13:2. First we see a shift of the profile to the right, suggesting a wave propagation. We also see a steepening and increase in amplitude, while the sharp dicrotic notch is gradually lost. This increase of systolic pressure with distance from the heart in a tapered tube is a dynamic phenomenon in an elastic branching system. In a steady flow in a rigid tube of similar

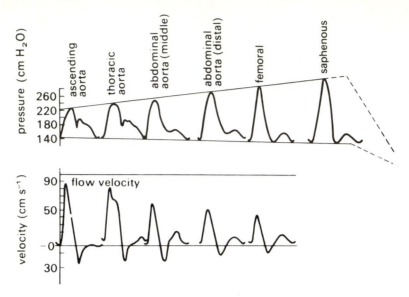

Figure 3.13:3 Pressure and velocity waves at different sites in the arteries of a dog. From McDonald (1974), by permission.

taper the pressure must go down in the direction of flow unless there is deceleration. In the present case, however, the *mean* value of the pressure, averaged over the period of a heartbeat, still decreases with increasing distance from the aortic valve. It is difficult to see it in Fig. 3.13:2 because the fall in mean pressure is only about 4 mm Hg (0.5 kPa) in the whole length of the aorta, while the amplitude of the pressure oscillation between systole and diastole nearly doubles.

This process of amplification of the pressure pulse continues into the branches of the aorta, as illustrated in Fig. 3.13:3. In the dog, it continues to about the third generation of arterial branches. Thereafter both the oscillation and the mean pressure decrease gradually downstream along the arterial tree until it reaches the level of microcirculation.

Figure 3.13:3 also shows the variation of the flow velocity along the aorta. That the pressure and velocity waves are different is an indication of reflection of waves at junctions. The velocity waves do not steepen with distance, nor does the peak systolic velocity increase downstream.

3.14 The Effects of Geometric Nonuniformity

One of the simplifying assumptions made in the preceeding sections is that the tube is circular and cylindrical in shape and is straight. Real blood vessels are often curved and of variable cross section. The nonuniform cross-

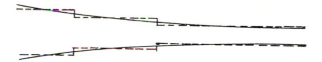

Figure 3.14:1 Approximation of a tapered blood vessel by a stepwise tapered tube.

sectional area is associated with branching (see Sec. 3.1) and elastic deformation of the vessel wall in response to a nonuniform pressure (with a finite gradient) (see Sec. 3.4). The taper is generally very mild and it is possible to evaluate its effect approximately without extensive calculations.

The Effect of Taper on Steady Flow

A smoothly tapered tube may be approximated by a stepwise tapered tube as shown in Fig. 3.14:1. A rough estimation of the pressure–flow relationship for a steady flow in such a tube can be obtained by using the Poiseuille formula (Ec. 3.2:17) for each segment of the tube. We have used this method in Sec. 3.4.

The Effect of Taper on Wave Propagation

Let a smoothly tapered tube be approximated by a stepwise tapered tube, as shown in Fig. 3.14:1. Each site of step change may be regarded as a junction of two tubes and the method of analysis presented in Sec. 3.11 can be applied. We have learned in Sec. 3.11 that the rate of energy transfer in a reflected wave is proportional to the square of $\mathcal{R}$, and therefore if $\mathcal{R} \ll 1$ it is quite negligible. $\mathcal{R}$, in this case, as is given in Eq. (3.11:8), is proportional to the difference in cross-sectional areas of the two segments divided by the sum of the cross-sectional areas, and is obviously very small if the taper is mild. $\mathcal{R}^2$ is another order of magnitude smaller. Therefore we conclude that very little energy is reflected as the wave travels along a slowly varying tube, and we may analyze the wave's development as if all the energy were transmitted.

The rate of transfer of energy in a progressive wave across any cross section of a vessel is shown in Eq. (3.11:10) to be equal to p^2/Z, the square of the oscillatory pressure divided by the characteristic impedance of the tube. If all the energy is transmitted, then p^2/Z is a constant and we have

$$p = \text{const.} \cdot Z^{1/2}. \tag{1}$$

Thus, in a gradually tapering artery, the amplitude of the pressure wave is proportional to the square root of the characteristic impedance. Since the characteristic impedance is $\rho c/A$, we see that Z increases as A decreases if

ρc were constant. Hence the amplitude of the pressure wave increases as the wave propagates down a tapering tube with decreasing cross section. The amplitude of the aortic *flow* pulse, proportional to p/Z (Eq. (3.11:5)), will correspondingly decrease, being proportional to $Z^{-1/2}$.

These predicted features are evident in the records shown in Figs. 3.13:2 and 3.13:3. However, a quantitative comparison of the predictions with the experimental results shows that the peaking is overestimated by the theory. One of the reasons for this is the neglecting of viscous effects of the blood and blood vessel, the other reason is the inaccuracy of the theory. The theory is more accurate if the taper is small. But how small is small? To answer this question one should turn to mathematics. We can reduce the general equations of motion and boundary conditions to a dimensionless form. Then we recognize two characteristic lengths: the tube radius and the wave length. For the taper, the proper dimensionless parameter is the rate of change of tube radius per unit wave length. If this rate is not very small, the theory is not very accurate. Let $\xi = x/\lambda$, where x is the axial coordinate and λ is the wave length, and let $D_r = D/D_0$, the ratio of the blood vessel at x to that at the entry section $x = 0$. Then what is said above means that the effect of taper is to be judged by the derivative $dD_r/d\xi$. Now

$$\frac{dD_r}{d\xi} = \frac{dD_r}{dx}\frac{dx}{d\xi} = \lambda\frac{dD_r}{dx} = \frac{\lambda}{D_0}\frac{dD}{dx}. \tag{2}$$

Hence the effective taper is the product of the wavelength λ, expressed in tube diameter at the entry, and the rate of change of the diameter dD/dx.

Now, in the case of the aorta, the wavelength of the first few harmonics is longer than the length of the aorta, and the effective taper $dD_r/d\xi$ may be fairly large by virtue of large values of λ/D_0. For these harmonics the inaccuracy of the simple theory may have led to the overestimation of the peaking mentioned above.

Problem

3.23 The cross-sectional area of the abdominal aorta is about 40% of the area of the thoracic aorta. The Young's modulus is about twice that of the thoracic aorta. Show that the ratio of the characteristic impedances in these aorta is 3.5 and the pressure pulse amplitude in the abdominal aorta is expected to be 85% higher than that in the thoracic aorta. How much additional increase in pressure pulse amplitude is expected because of the reflection of the wave at the iliac junction?

The Entrance Region

In the simple solution discussed in Sec. 3.2 and 3.8, and even in the general solution to be considered in Sec. 3.15, we do not specify the velocity and pressure distribution at the ends of the tube. We found solutions which satisfy the differential equations and boundary conditions on the wall of the blood vessel. These solutions are valid if the distribution of pressure and velocity over the cross sections at the ends of the tube were exactly as specified by the mathematical expressions. Any deviation from these ideal conditions will call for a modification of the solution. In reality, the aorta is joined to the heart, small arteries are joined to larger arteries, and the end conditions practically never agree exactly with those specified by the simple solutions. Therefore, a modification is almost always required.

In steady flow, the Navier–Stokes equations belong to the so-called "elliptical" type of equations in the theory of partial differential equations. In equations of this type all the partial derivatives of the highest order have the same sign. Elliptic equations have the property that any "self-equilibrating" local changes in boundary conditions (no net flow, no net force) over a small area will influence the solution only in the immediate neighborhood of the changed area, in the sense that the influence will die out as the distance from the changed area increases (St.-Venant's Principle). Applying this general property to the specific problem at hand, we conclude that if the net inflow and net pressure force remain the same, any changed boundary conditions at the ends of the tube will cause changes in the solution only in the immediate neighborhood of the ends. Therefore, any redistribution of velocity and pressure at the entry section without changing the resultant flow and force will affect only the "entrance region."

Consider the following example. A circular cylindrical tube is attached to a large reservoir which contains a Newtonian fluid. In the presence of a steady pressure gradient, the fluid flows into the tube. Far away from the entry section the velocity profile is parabolic. At the entry section, it is a good approximation to consider the velocity as uniformly distributed. Now we ask: How fast does the velocity profile change from the uniform distribution at the entry section to the parabolic (Poiseuillean) profile downstream?

The answer depends on the Reynolds number of flow. Results of a detailed analysis is presented in Fig. 3.14:2. The Reynolds number, N_R, is defined as

$$N_R = \frac{\rho a U}{\mu}, \tag{3}$$

where ρ is the fluid density, a is the tube radius, U is the averaged speed of flow over the cross section of the tube, and μ is the viscosity of the fluid. The velocity in the axial direction is denoted by u, that in the radial direction is denoted by v. In the figure, the dimensionless velocities u/U and v/U are plotted as functions of radial distance r/a, and axial distance, x/a. It is seen that the effect of the entry flow is well limited to the region $0 \le x/a < 30$ for the Reynolds numbers considered. It is interesting to note that the maximum value of radial component of velocity takes place about at $x/a = 0.2$ and $r/a = 0.7$. The maximum value of the radial component of velocity is about 30% of the mean speed of flow for Reynolds numbers less than 1. This ratio becomes about 0.1 for the case of Reynolds number equal to 50. Therefore,

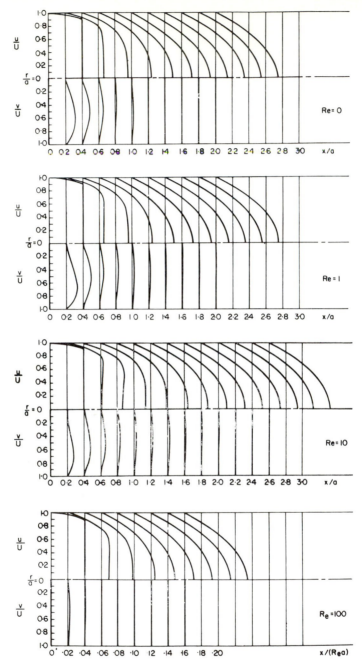

Figure 3.14:2 Examples of entry flow into a circular cylindrical tube from a reservoir. The flow in the entry region is seen to depend on the Reynolds number. u is axial velocity. v is radial velocity. U is the mean flow velocity in the tube. Distance downstream from the entry section is expressed in terms of the tube radius a. From Lew and Fung (1970), by permission.

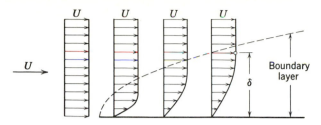

Figure 3.14:3 Velocity distribution in the boundary layer in the neighborhood of the leading edge of a flat plate.

the radial component of the velocity is not negligibly small compared to the axial component of velocity in the intermediate range of Reynolds numbers.

Boundary Layer Growth in the Entry Region when the Reynolds Number is Much Larger than 1

When blood flows from a vessel into a branch, (Fig. 3.11:1), the new branch introduces new wall surfaces on which frictional force acts through viscosity, dissipates energy, and slows down the fluid in the neighborhood of the wall. If the Reynolds number, N_R, is much greater than 1, then the principal influence of the wall friction is limited to a thin layer next to the wall, called "boundary layer." (See a book on fluid mechanics, e.g., Schlichting (1968), Fung (1977, p. 279–282) for a brief derivation which shows that the boundary layer thickness is of the order of $1/\sqrt{N_R}$.) The thickness of the boundary layer increases as the distance from the leading edge of the new wall increases. A simple derivation of a law of the growth of the boundary layer thickness when the Reynolds number is large is as follows:

Consider a flat plate introduced into a uniform flow of speed U (Fig. 3.14:3). At a station x from the leading edge of the plate, the velocity profile is illustrated in the figure. Consider the balance of the inertial forces and viscous forces acting on a small rectangular element of fluid in the boundary layer. The shear stress on the surface $dxdz$ is $\mu(\partial u/\partial y)dxdz$. This shear is variable with the depth y. In an element of thickness dy the net viscous force is

$$\mu\frac{\partial}{\partial y}\left(\frac{\partial u}{\partial y}\right)dydxdz. \tag{4}$$

This is balanced by the inertial force, which is equal to the mass $\rho dxdydz$ times the convective acceleration $u(\partial u/\partial x)$:

$$\rho u\frac{\partial u}{\partial x}dxdydz. \tag{5}$$

Hence, on equating Eqs. (4) and (5), we have

$$\rho u \frac{\partial u}{\partial x} = \mu \frac{\partial}{\partial y}\left(\frac{\partial u}{\partial y}\right). \tag{6}$$

To get an estimate of the magnitude of these terms when the Reynolds number is large ($\gg 1$) so that the boundary layer thickness δ is small, note that u varies from 0 to U when y changes from 0 to δ. Hence $\partial u/\partial y$ is of the order of magnitude of U/δ, and the right-hand side of Eq. (6) is proportional to $\mu U/\delta^2$. Similarly, the left-hand side is proportional to $\rho U^2/x$ because u varies from U to a small fraction of U when x is varied from 0 to x. Hence we have

$$\rho \frac{U^2}{x} = K^2 \mu \frac{U}{\delta^2}, \tag{7}$$

where K is some constant. Solving for δ, we obtain the important result that

$$\delta = K \sqrt{\frac{\mu x}{\rho U}}. \tag{8}$$

Thus the boundary layer thickness δ increases with $\sqrt{x}$. The boundary layer is shaped like a parabola. Theory and experiments show that the constant K is equal to 4.0 when the boundary layer thickness is defined as the height at which the velocity is 95% of the free stream value.

This result is very useful. It tells us in a general way how the boundary layer grows, and therefore, of course, how the shear stress is distributed. The sher stress on the wall is given by

$$\mu \frac{\partial u}{\partial x} \sim \mu \frac{U}{\delta} \sim \sqrt{\frac{\mu \rho U^3}{x}}. \tag{9}$$

Thus, the shear stress is large at the leading edge, and decreases as $x^{-1/2}$ when x increases. Hence, in a bifurcating artery, we expect the shear stress to be high at the tip of the new branches. If high shear stress is conducive to atherosclerosis, then this identifies the regions to watch.

This analysis is applicable to large arteries and to gas flow in trachea and large bronchi. For small vessels, whose Reynolds number approaches 1 or less, a more accurate analysis is needed. Results of such an analysis by Lew and Fung (1970) for the entry flow in Reynolds number range 0 to 100 have been presented in Fig. 3.14:2 and discussed earlier. Other references are given in the paragraphs to follow.

Inlet Length

For an entry flow into a circular cylindrical tube with a uniform axial velocity at the entry section, it is common to define an "inlet length" as a distance through which the velocity has redistributed itself approximately into a

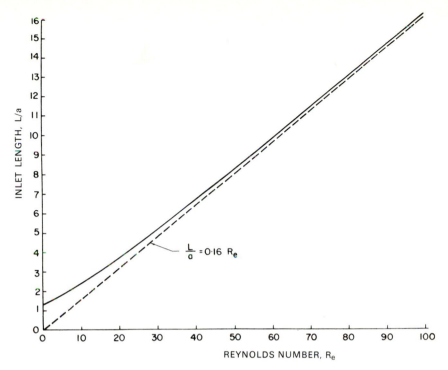

Figure 3.14:4 Change of inlet length *vs* Reynolds number in entry flow into a circular cylindrical tube from a reservoir. From Lew and Fung (1970), by permission.

parabolic profile. Since the approach to parabolic profile is asymptotic, there is no unique definition of inlet length. Boussinesq (1891) defined an *inlet length* as the distance from the entry section to a point where the deviation from parabolic profile is less than 1%. He obtained the result that the inlet length, L, is equal to $0.26a\,N_R$. With the same definition, Schiller (1922) obtained an inlet length of $0.115a\,N_R$, whereas Targ (1951) obtained the result

$$\frac{L}{a} = 0.16\,N_R. \tag{10}$$

Lew and Fung (1970) showed that Targ's result is quite good for Reynolds numbers greater than 50. For smaller Reynolds numbers, however, Eq. (10) does not apply. When the Reynolds number tends to zero, the inlet length tends to a constant $1.3a$. This is shown in Fig. 3.14:4. The low Reynolds number case is applicable to microcirculation. In the capillary blood vessels the Reynolds number is in the range 10^{-4} to 10^{-2}, and the inlet length is about 1.3 times the tube radius.

Entry Region in Oscillatory Flow

If there is an oscillation superposed on a steady flow, the entry region is also transient. Let us consider the case of large Reynolds number. The transient oscillation generates a boundary layer whose thickness is estimated in Sec. 3.7 to be proportional to $(v/\omega)^{1/2}$, where v is the kinematic viscosity and ω is the angular frequency. More detailed analysis yields a thickness equal to

$$\delta_1 = 6.5\left(\frac{v}{\omega}\right)^{1/2}. \tag{11}$$

This boundary layer is created by the balance of the viscous stresses in the boundary layer against the inertial force associated with the transient acceleration $\partial u/\partial t$ in the free stream. On the other hand, in the preceding section it is shown that the interaction of the viscous stresses next to the solid wall against the convective acceleration $u\partial u/\partial x$ takes place in a boundary layer whose thickness grows with increasing distance from the leading edge, x, according to the formula

$$\delta_2 = 4(vx/U)^{1/2} \tag{12}$$

where U is the velocity in the free stream immediately outside the boundary layer. For an unsteady flow entering a tube both transient and convective accelerations exist, and the two boundary layers named above merge into one. Since in the resulting boundary layer the viscous stresses have to balance both of these accelerations the boundary layer thickness must be at least as thick as either δ_1 or δ_2. Now, $\delta_1 = \delta_2$ when x is equal to

$$L \doteq 2.64\frac{U}{\omega}. \tag{13}$$

For $x < L$, $\delta_1 > \delta_2$, the transient acceleration tends to dominate. For $x > L$, $\delta_2 > \delta_1$, the convective acceleration tends to dominate. Thus L is said to be an *unsteady entry length* (Caro et al., 1978, p. 321).

Problem

3.24 In the aorta of a dog, with a diameter of 1.5 cm and a mean velocity of 20 cm/sec^{-1}, a heart rate of 2 Hz ($\omega = 4\pi$) and an amplitude of the largest unsteady component of about 40 cm/sec^{-1}, show that the steady inlet length is about 36 cm and the unsteady entry length is about 10 cm. Thus the entire aorta is an entrance region.

In dog's femoral artery, $a = 0.2$ cm, $U = 10$ cm/sec^{-1}, show that the entry length is about 1.2 cm.

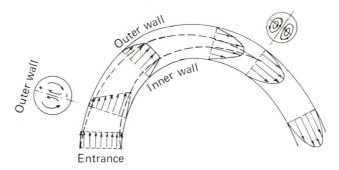

Figure 3.14:5 A sketch of entry flow into a curved pipe, showing the development of boundary layer, velocity profile, and secondary flow.

Curved Vessel

Curvature of a vessel has profound effect on flow. We may consider the physical factors as follows. Assume, as is sketched in Fig. 3.14:5, that the velocity profile is flat at the entry section. Let the Reynolds number be much larger than 1. Then in the entry region the boundary layer is very thin and the flow in the core is like that of a nonviscous fluid. In this case the velocity is higher near the inner wall, in a manner similar to a vortex flow. Further downstream the boundary layer grows. Eventually the boundary layer will reach the center of the tube. The flow is then said to be *fully developed*. In the boundary layer the centrifugal force will force the fluid toward the outer wall, and the velocity profile will be distorted, with a peak lying beyond the centerline. The pressure fields corresponding to these velocity fields are not uniform in the cross sections, and a *secondary flow* develops as sketched in the figure. This flow is called secondary because it is superimposed on the "primary" axial flow.

Secondary flow in curved tubes has been utilized by heart–lung machine builders to promote oxygenation of blood. In these machines the tubing is made of silastic, which is permeable to oxygen. When the tube is curved and blood flows in the tube and oxygen flows outside the tube, the secondary flow stirs up the blood in the tube and results in faster oxygenation.

Extensive mathematical analysis of flow in curved tubes and branched tube has been made by Pedley and is summarized in his book (Pedley, 1980).

Other Nonuniformities

Uniformity is special; nonuniformity is the rule of nature. Uniform geometry is unique; nonuniform geometry has infinite variety. In this chapter we have taken an infinitely long, straight, circular, cylinder as an idealized uniform geometry of a blood vessel and considered tapering, curvature, and entrance region as nonuniformities. There are many other important nonuniformities in arteries. For example, stenosis, or local narrowing of the vessel, has great importance in pathology. Dilatation, or local enlargement of the vessel, similarly, is important in the study of diseases. Arteries branch off like a tree. The detailed flow condition at each branching point is of interest, because at such a site there is a stagnation point where the velocity and velocity gradient are zero, and not far away is a region of a high velocity gradient. The shear stress acting on the wall is nonuniform: the highest shear stress in arteries is often reached in the neighborhood of a branching point. The lowest shear stress, zero, also occurs in this neighborhood (at the stagnation point). It turns out that atherosclerosis in man is often found to be initiated in the neighborhood of some branching points, and the implication of high or low shear stress on atherogenesis seems inescapable.

3.15 The Effects of Viscosity of the Fluid and Viscoelasticity of the Wall

At the beginning of this chapter we analyzed steady flow of a viscous fluid in a tube. In Secs. 3.8–3.12, however, we treated pulsatile flow of blood as if it has no viscosity. The major justification for this has been suggested in Sec. 3.7, namely, that in human arterial blood flow the frequency parameter α (or Womersley number N_w) is considerably larger than 1, suggesting that the major feature of pulsatile flow can be sought through the balance of pressure gradient and transient inertial forces, and that the viscous effect is significant only in a thin layer immediately next to the wall. The frequency parameter α decreases toward the periphery; it becomes much smaller than 1 in arterioles, capillaries, and venules. Hence the influence of viscosity is felt more and more as blood flows toward the peripheral vessels. In microcirculation the entire flow field is dominated by viscous stresses.

Even in large arteries, where the frequency parameter α is large, the viscosity of the fluid still has a profound influence. Viscous stresses play a dominant role in determining stability and turbulence in the arteries, in determining whether the streamline will separate (diverge) from the wall of the vessel at branching points or at segments where a sudden change in cross section occurs such as in stenosis or aneurysm.

Physically, viscosity being a dissipation mechanism (dissipating mechanical energy into heat), one expects that it would reveal itself in the attenuation (i.e., the gradual decrease in amplitude) of the velocity and pressure waves in the direction of propagation. Associated with attenuation will be phase changes. These have been found to be true. And as far as their effect on the wave propagation is concerned, the effect of viscoelastic dissipation in the vessel wall is found to be more significant than the viscous dissipation of the blood.

It would be interesting to see what type of mathematical problem results if we include viscosity of blood and viscoelasticity of the vessel wall in the pulsatile flow analysis. Consider large arteries and make the following hypotheses:

(a) The fluid is homogeneous and Newtonian.
(b) The wall material is isotropic and linearly viscoelastic.
(c) The fluid motion is laminar.
(d) The motion is so small that squares and higher-order products of displacements and velocities and their derivatives are negligible.

Then the field equations are the linearized Navier–Stokes equations for the blood, the linearized Navier's equation for the wall, and the equation of continuity. The boundary conditions are the continuity of stresses and velocities at the fluid–solid interface, and appropriate conditions on the external surface of the tube and at the ends of the tube. See the Appendix, p. 373. For an axisymmetric traveling wave in a tube of incompressible viscoelastic material, we have, for the fluid,

$$\frac{\partial v_r}{\partial t} = -\frac{1}{\rho}\frac{\partial p}{\partial r} + \nu\left(\frac{\partial^2 v_r}{\partial r^2} + \frac{1}{r}\frac{\partial v_r}{\partial r} - \frac{v_r}{r^2} + \frac{\partial^2 v_r}{\partial x^2}\right), \tag{1}$$

$$\frac{\partial v_x}{\partial t} = -\frac{1}{\rho}\frac{\partial p}{\partial x} + \nu\left(\frac{\partial^2 v_x}{\partial r^2} + \frac{1}{r}\frac{\partial v_x}{\partial r} + \frac{\partial^2 v_x}{\partial x^2}\right), \tag{2}$$

$$\frac{\partial v_x}{\partial x} + \frac{\partial v_r}{\partial r} + \frac{v_r}{r} = 0, \tag{3}$$

and, for the tube wall,

$$\frac{\rho_w}{\mu^*}\frac{\partial^2 u_r}{\partial t^2} = \frac{\partial^2 u_r}{\partial r^2} + \frac{1}{r}\frac{\partial u_r}{\partial r} - \frac{u_r}{r^2} + \frac{\partial^2 u_r}{\partial x^2} - \frac{1}{\mu^*}\frac{\partial \Omega}{\partial r}, \tag{4}$$

$$\frac{\rho_w}{\mu^*}\frac{\partial^2 u_x}{\partial t^2} = \frac{\partial^2 u_x}{\partial r^2} + \frac{1}{r}\frac{\partial u_x}{\partial r} + \frac{\partial^2 u_x}{\partial x^2} - \frac{1}{\mu^*}\frac{\partial \Omega}{\partial x}, \tag{5}$$

$$\frac{\partial u_x}{\partial x} + \frac{\partial u_r}{\partial r} + \frac{u_r}{r} = 0, \tag{6}$$

where v_x, v_r, v_θ are the velocity components of the fluid, u_x, u_r, u_θ are the displacement components of the wall, μ^* is the dynamic modulus of rigidity of the wall, and Ω is a pressure, which must be introduced since we have assumed the material to be incompressible. ν is the kinematic viscosity of the blood, μ is the coefficient of viscosity, ρ is the density of the blood, ρ_w is the density of the wall material.

The boundary conditions are, if the external surface of the tube is stress-free, and if the inner and outer radii of the tube are a and b, respectively,

$$v_r = 0 \qquad\qquad \text{at } r = 0, \tag{7}$$

$$\partial v_x/\partial r = 0 \qquad\qquad\qquad \text{at } r = 0, \qquad (8)$$

$$v_r = \partial u_r/\partial t \qquad\qquad\qquad \text{at } r = a, \qquad (9)$$

$$v_x = \partial u_x/\partial t \qquad\qquad\qquad \text{at } r = a, \qquad (10)$$

$$\mu(\partial v_r/\partial x + \partial v_x/\partial r) = \mu^*(\partial u_r/\partial x + \partial u_x/\partial r) \quad \text{at } r = a, \qquad (11)$$

$$-p + 2\mu(\partial v_r/\partial r) = -\Omega + 2\mu^*(\partial u_r/\partial r) \qquad \text{at } r = a, \qquad (12)$$

$$\mu^*(\partial u_r/\partial x + \partial u_x/\partial r) = 0 \qquad\qquad \text{at } r = b, \qquad (13a)$$

$$-\Omega + 2\mu^*(\partial u_r/\partial r) = 0 \qquad\qquad\qquad \text{at } r = b. \qquad (13b)$$

The solution that satisfies the boundary conditions (7) and (8) may be posed in the following form*:

$$v_x = -\sum_{n=0}^{N} i\{A_1\gamma_n J_0(i\gamma_n r) + A_2\kappa_n J_0(i\kappa_n r)\} \exp i(n\omega t - \gamma_n x), \qquad (14)$$

$$v_r = -\sum_{n=0}^{N} i\gamma_n\{A_1 J_1(i\gamma_n r) + A_2 J_1(i\kappa_n r)\} \exp i(n\omega t - \gamma_n x), \qquad (15)$$

$$p = \sum_{n=0}^{N} A_3 J_0(i\gamma_n r) \exp i(n\omega t - \gamma_n x), \qquad (16)$$

$$u_r = \sum_{n=0}^{N} -i\gamma_n\{A_4 J_1(k_n r) + B_4 Y_1(k_n r) + A_5 J_1(i\gamma_n r) + B_5 Y_1(i\gamma_n r)\}$$
$$\cdot \exp i(n\omega t - \gamma_n x), \qquad (17)$$

$$u_x = \sum_{n=0}^{N} -\{k_n A_4 J_0(k_n r) + k_n B_4 Y_0(k_n r) + i\gamma_n A_5 J_0(i\gamma_n r) + i\gamma_n B_5 Y_0(i\gamma_n r)\}$$
$$\cdot \exp i(n\omega t - \gamma_n x), \qquad (18)$$

$$\Omega = \sum_{n=0}^{N} \{A_6 J_0(i\gamma_n r) + B_6 Y_0(i\gamma_n r)\} \exp i(n\omega t - \gamma_n x), \qquad (19)$$

where ω is the angular frequency, n is the harmonic number, γ_n is the propagation constant of the nth harmonic, N is a constant, the A's and B's are complex constants, J_0 and J_1 are Bessel functions of the first kind, Y_0 and Y_1 are Bessel functions of the second kind, and

$$\kappa_n^2 = (in\omega/v) + \gamma_n^2, \qquad k_n^2 = n^2\omega^2\rho_w/\mu^* - \gamma_n^2. \qquad (20)$$

$$A_1 = (i/n\omega\rho)A_3, \qquad A_6 = n^2\omega^2\rho_w A_5, \qquad B_6 = n^2\omega^2\rho_w B_5. \qquad (21)$$

When these solutions are substituted into the boundary conditions (9)–(13) six linear, homogeneous, and simultaneous equations in six unknown

---

* In a strict notation the A's and B's should have a subscript n because their values may be different for each n.

coefficients A_1, A_2, ..., B_5 are obtained. For a nontrivial solution the determinant of the coefficients of A_1, A_2, ..., B_5 must vanish. This determinantal equation,

$$\Delta(\gamma_n, \kappa_n, k_n, \mu, \mu^*, a, b) = 0, \tag{22}$$

is the frequency equation for the pulse wave. If $\gamma_n = \beta + i\alpha$ is solved with other parameters assigned, then β is the *wave number*, α is the *attenuation coefficient*, and $C_p = \omega/\beta$ is the *phase velocity*.

The dynamic elastic modulus of the vessel wall, μ^*, is a complex number if the wave motion is represented by complex exponential functions listed in Eqs. (14)–(19). Since μ^* is complex, the solution γ_n is almost certain to be complex also, thus yielding the attenuation coefficient in association with each characteristic wave number.

It is evident that extensive numerical calculations are necessary to obtain detailed information.

One thing that becomes evident from the general equations is that Eq. (22) has many solutions. One of them is akin to the *flexural mode* discussed in Sec. 3.8, and is an improvement of that solution. All the others are new modes not considered before in this book. These include *longitudinal modes*, in which the principal motion consists of motion of the vessel wall in the longitudinal direction, *torsional modes*, in which the principal motion is the torsional oscillation of the vessel wall, and higher modes of these three types with higher frequencies, shorter wavelengths and different attenuation. Many of these theoretical wave types have been found in *in vivo* measurements.

A general reader would probably have little interest in the numerical details; hence we shall refer him to the original papers. Furthermore, it is possible to relax some or all of the simplifying assumptions listed earlier and to study mathematically the arterial blood flow problem in greater depth. A great deal has been published. A list of historically important papers is presented in Table 3.15:1. More recent references are given in the Bibliography at the end of the chapter. Pedley (1980) has given a thorough review of recent advances in the theory of blood flow in large arteries.

3.16 The Influence of Nonlinearities

Of all the effects, the most difficult one to evaluate is the effect of nonlinearities. In the Euler's equation (p. 372) the convective acceleration term, $u_j(\partial u_i/\partial x_j)$, is nonlinear, and it is the principal difficulty of hydrodynamics. The viscous force term, $\partial\sigma_{ij}/\partial x_j$, becomes nonlinear if the constitutive equation of the fluid is non-Newtonian. Blood is non-Newtonian, the effect of nonlinear blood viscosity is especially important with regard to flow separation at points of bifurcation in pulsatile flow. In the equation governing the

TABLE 3.15:1 Summary of Contributions to Theory of Harmonic Wave Propagation in Arteries

Reference	Fluid — Inviscid	Fluid — Viscous	Wall — Membrane	Wall — Finite thickness	Wall — Elastic	Wall — Viscoelastic	Waves — Axisymmetric	Waves — Asymmetric	Waves — Number of modes	Experiments — Flexible tube	Experiments — Animal
Euler (1775)[a]	×		×		×						
Young (1808, 1809)[b]	×		×		×		×		1		
Weber and Weber (1825)[c]	×		×		×						
Resal (1876)[d]	×		×		×						
Moens (1878)[d]										×	
Korteweg (1878)[e]	×		×		×						
Lamb (1897–1898)[f]	×		×		×				2		
Joukowsky (1900)[g]	×		×							×	
Witzig (1914)		×	×		×						
Hamilton, et al. (1939)[h]											×
King (1947)	×		×		×	×	×		1		
Lambossy (1950, 1951)	×	×	×		×						
Müller (1951, 1959)										×	
Jacobs (1953)[i]		×	×		×		×		1		
Morgan and Kiely (1954)		×	×		×	×	×		1		
Morgan and Ferrante (1955)	×		×		×		×		1		
Womersley (1955a, b 1957)[j]		×			×						
Landowne (1958)[k]											×
Taylor (1959)[l]										×	
McDonald (1960, 1965)[m]				×		×	×	×			×
Klip (1962)[n]		×	×		×		×		3		
Hardung (1962)[o]		×								×	

Fry et al. (1964)[p]		×			×			×
Atabek and Lew (1966)[q]		×	×		×		2	
Rubinow and Keller (1968)[r]		×	×	×	×			
Anliker and Raman (1966)[s]	×	×	×	×			×	
Anliker and Maxwell (1966)[t]	×			×	×	×		
Cox (1968, 1970)[u]	×		×		×			×
Jones et al. (1968)[u]		×	×	×	×			

---

[a] Pressure p related to cross-sectional area s by $s = s_0 p(c + p)^{-1}$ or $s = s_0(1 - e^{-p/c})$. Euler's eqs. were solved by Lambert (1956).

[b] Derived the wave speed formula $c_0 = (hE/2a\rho)^{1/2}$, later known as Moens-Korteweg formula.

[c] Rederived Young's formula.

[d] Gave wave speed $c = $ const. $\times c_0$; const. $= 0.8, 0.9, 1.036$ depending on various conditions.

[e] Obtained $c_1 = (2a\rho/hE + \rho/K)^{-1/2}$, $\rho = $ density of fluid, $K = $ bulk modulus of fluid, c_1 is known as water-hammer speed.

[f] Derived phase velocity of long waves, c_0 and $c_2 = [E/(1 - \sigma^2)\rho_W]^{1/2}$; $\sigma = $ Poisson's ratio, $\rho_W = $ density of wall.

[g] Exhaustive treatment of water-hammer. Riemann's method. Detailed wave form analysis.

[h] Arterial waves related to stroke volume and cardiac ejection.

[i] Nonlinear elasticity. Perturbation of mean flow.

[j] Compared with experiments. Considered tethering. Branching. Variation of crosssection. Extensive theory.

[k] Induced waves in human brachial and radial arteries.

[l] Impedance method electric analog.

[m] Thorough examination of theories and experiments from the physiological point of view.

[n] Discussed experiments, extensive theory.

[o] Input impedance and reflection at ends and branches.

[p] Evaluation of parameters.

[q] Effect of prestress demonstrated.

[r] External tissues represented by 4-parameter impedance, showed significant effect. Found frequency cutoff in inviscid membrane case.

[s] Korotkov sound.

[t] Dispersion. Initial strain. Found axisymmetric waves mildly dispersive, asymmetric waves highly dispersive, frequency cutoff.

[u] Extensive parametric study. Include surrounding tissues.

blood vessel wall, the most significant nonlinearity comes from the finite strain and nonlinear viscoelasticity.

To check the effects of nonlinearity means to compare the solutions of the linearized equations and boundary conditions with those of nonlinear ones. This is usually impossible because we do not know how to solve the nonlinear problems. But engineers grapple with nonlinear problems. The vast majority of new publications in biomechanics, applied mechanics, applied mathematics and applied physics are concerned with the evaluation of nonlinear effects.

Sometimes we can discuss the effects of nonlinearity on the basis of dimensional analysis and comparison with experimental evidences. Several examples follow:

Convective Acceleration in Wave Propagation

In the wave analysis of Sec. 3.8, the local convective acceleration $u_j(\partial u_i/\partial x_j)$ is neglected against the transient acceleration $\partial u_i/\partial t$. Now, let $\tilde{u}$ represent a characteristic velocity of the disturbed flow due to wave motion, ω be the circular frequency of the wave, and c be the wave speed relative to the mean flow. Then the period of oscillation is $2\pi/\omega$, the wavelength is $2\pi c/\omega$, and the orders of magnitude of the two accelerations are

$$\text{Transient,} \quad \frac{\partial u_i}{\partial t} : \quad \frac{\tilde{u}}{(2\pi/\omega)}, \tag{1}$$

$$\text{Convective,} \quad u_j\frac{\partial u_i}{\partial x_j} : \quad \tilde{u}\frac{\tilde{u}}{(2\pi c/\omega)}. \tag{2}$$

Hence the condition that the convective acceleration is negligible compared with the transient acceleration is that (2) $\ll$ (1), i.e., if

$$\frac{\tilde{u}}{c} \ll 1. \tag{3}$$

This is approximately satisfied in large arteries, but the maximum value of $\tilde{u}/c$ is normally about 0.25, which is large enough to suggest nonlinear effects. In more peripheral arteries, $\tilde{u}$ is smaller and c is larger, and the linearity condition is better justified. In certain rare connective tissue disorders the arterial wall becomes floppy and c is so low that $\tilde{u}/c$ approaches 1. On the other hand, in conditions such as aortic value incompetence, the upstroke of the pulse wave becomes very steep, $\tilde{u}$ becomes quite large, and a nonlinear effect is expected.

The effect of convective acceleration is to increase the total acceleration so that the pressure drop is increased where the velocity is high. The pressure wave form is therefore steepened at the peak of the velocity wave and flattened at the valley.

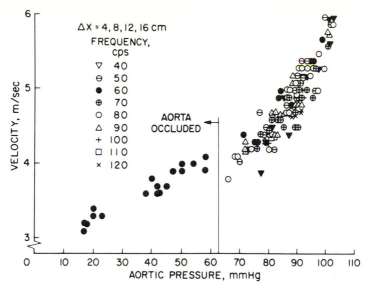

Figure 3.16:1 Relationship between the speed of sinusoidal pressure waves of various frequencies in the aorta of the dog and the instantaneous aortic pressure. In this case the diastolic pressure varied between 65 and 85 mm Hg while the systolic pressure was between 85 and 100 mm Hg. Data points corresponding to pressure below the diastolic were obtained by occluding the aorta for about 10 sec. The steeper rise of the wave speed with pressure between systole and diastole is attributed to a stiffening of the aorta with pressure and to an increase in mean flow. From Antiker, M. (1972) by permission of Prentice-Hall, Inc. Englewood Cliffs, N.J.

Effect of Nonlinear Elasticity of Vessel Wall on Wave Propagation

The incremental Young's modulus of the arterial wall increases with the tensile stress in the vessel wall. The latter increases with internal pressure. In the simple theory the Young's modulus is treated as a constant. The variation of Young's modulus causes a nonlinear effect. In order that the variation of Young's modulus be small compared with the average Young's modulus, the amplitude of pressure oscillation should be small compared with the average pressure. In fact, this ratio is normally about 0.2 in a systemic artery, again large enough to suggest a significant effect.

An increase in Young's modulus of the vessel wall increases the wave speed; see Eq. (3.8:15). Experimental evidence for this is shown in Fig. 3.16:1, which was obtained by Anliker (1971) using short trains of high-frequency pressure oscillations generated in dog's aorta and superposed on the normal pulse waves, except for the low-pressure range, as noted in the legend. The wavelength of such high-frequency oscillations is short, so that several cycles can be recorded at a downstream observation site before the reflected wave from the iliac junction returns to that site and distorts the recording. The results show that the wave speed is higher in systole than in diastole. This is due partly to the increase in the speed of the progressive waves, c, and partly to the higher mean flow velocity, $U(t)$, at systole. According to Sec. 3.10, pressure perturbations superposed on a steady flow have a velocity of propagation equal to the velocity c plus the steady flow velocity. The forward-moving wave in the artery has a velocity $U + c$. Since both U and c are higher at systole, the resultant $U + c$ is also higher at systole.

Apply the same principle to a single harmonic pressure wave. At a peak (high pressure) the velocity of propagation is higher than the mean velocity. At a valley (low pressure) the velocity is lower. The wave form, if it was initially sinusoidal, will become distorted as it is propagated downstream, the peak trying to overtake the mean, while the valley tries to lag behind. The result may be compared with the water waves over the sea. For these water waves the crest moves faster, and, if the wave amplitude is large enough, may distort the wave form so much as to cause the water to tumble over at the crest and form the "breakers." A different phenomenon caused by a similar reason is the shock wave generated by the wings of a high-speed airplane due to the compressibility of the air. Thus, one is led to expect shock waves in arteries and veins, especially in the veins which operate at a lower pressure, and hence are softer and have a lower wave speed. Countering this nonlinear effect are the shortness of the blood vessel, which does not make enough running distance to develop the steepening wave front, and the existence of numerous side branches, which would "bleed" the pressure buildup; and the viscous dissipation in the vessel wall.

Stability and Turbulence

A much more subtle nonlinear effect of convective acceleration and viscous dissipation is the creation of instability and turbulence in a flow. The phenomenon is described in Sec. 3.6. The theory of turbulence has occupied the center stage of fluid mechanics for 60 years, yet a complete understanding has not been achieved. The physiological effect of turbulence in the arterial blood flow is even less clearly understood.

Critical Comparison between Theory and Experiment

Many critical comparisons of theoretical predictions and experimental results on pulsatile blood flow in arteries have been done. The reader is referred to Atabek's review in the book by Patel and Vaishnav (1980) for a thorough discussion.

3.17 Flow Separation from the Wall

It is a well-known observation by designers of diffusers, wind tunnels, and airplanes that if the angle between the wall and the main flow direction is too large, the streamlines of the flow may detach from the wall and create a so-called "separated" region. An example is shown in Fig. 3.17:1, which shows a photograph of a water stream containing minute air bubbles which make the streamlines visible. As the channel widens in the direction of flow the velocity slows down and pressure goes up. The fluid in the boundary layer at the wall has to move against a pressure gradient, and after a certain distance the boundary layer becomes unstable and turbulent, and the stream leaves the wall and forms a jet. The "separated" region is a "dead water" region in which eddying motion occurs. A similar explanation can be given to the separated flow of a "stenosis" in a circular cylindrical tube, as shown in Fig. 3.17:2.

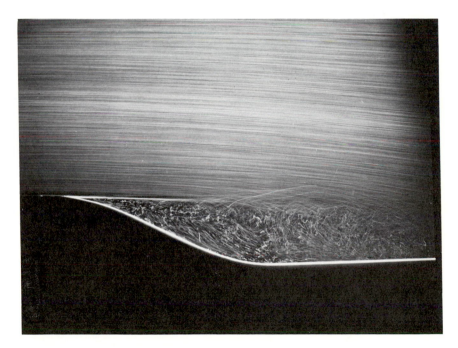

Figure 3.17:1 Flow separation from a curved wall. The laminar boundary layer has a Reynolds number of 20,000 based on distance from the leading edge (not shown). Because it is free of bubbles, the boundary layer appears as a thin dark line at the left. It separates tangentially near the start of the convex surface, remaining laminar for the distance to which the dark line persists, and then becomes unstable and turbulent. From Werlé (1974), an ONERA photograph, by permission.

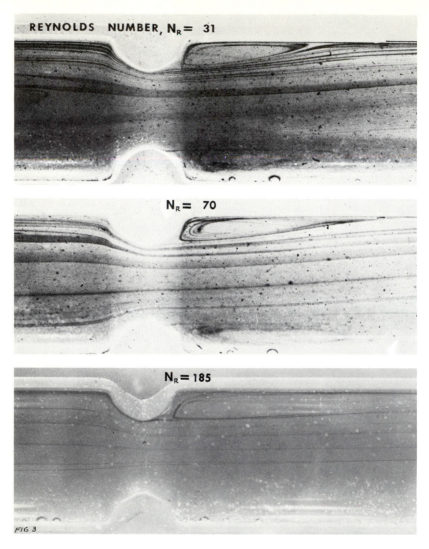

Figure 3.17:2 Flow separation in a model of stenosis in a circular cylindrical tube at Reynolds numbers of 31, 70, and 185. From Lee, J. S., and Fung, Y. C. (1971) Flow in non-uniform small blood vessels. *Microvasc Res.* **3**: 272–287, by permission.

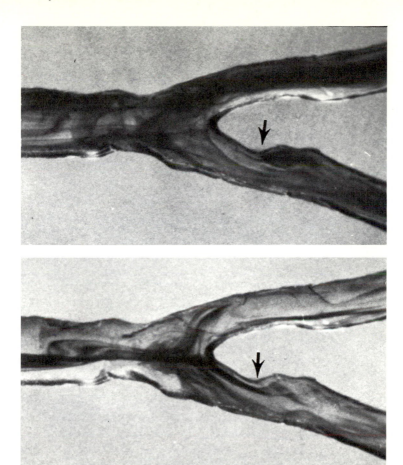

Figure 3.17:3 Flow separation distal to an atherosclerotic plaque during pulsatile flow in a mold of a human abdominal aorta. Flow was from left to right and was made visible with a dye. Separation is shown on the medial surface of the right common iliac artery (arrow). From F. J. Walburn, H. N. Sabbah, and P. D. Stein, "Flow visualization in a model of an atherosclerotic human abdominal aorta", *J. Biomechanical Engineering*, **103**: 168–170, 1981. Reproduced by permission.

In a pulsatile flow, the point of separation and the size of the separated region may vary with time. An example is shown in Fig. 3.17:3, which are photographs of flow visualization in a mold of an atherosclerotic human abdominal aorta. Separation distal to an atherosclerotic plaque (arrow) is seen in a pulsatile flow at a mean Reynolds number of 500 and a Womersley number of 8.1. The zone of separation is seen to be greater during end diastole (top) than during peak flow (bottom).

In the separated region, the fluid is more or less stagnant and the shear stress on the wall is low. This is, then, a region of low rate of mass transfer between the blood and tissue. According to Caro et al. (1969, 1971) this low shear stress and low mass transfer is implicated in atherogenesis.

3.18 Messages Carried in the Arterial Pulse Waves and Clinical Applications

Clinical applications of pulse wave studies are generally aimed at the following:

(a) To discover and explain diseases of the arteries such as atherosclerosis, stenosis, and aneurysm. To locate sites that need surgical treatment.
(b) To infer the condition of the heart.
(c) To diagnose diseases anywhere in the body.

The approach to any of these objectives is to extract information from the characteristics of the waves. The most ancient method is to use fingers as probes. Modern transducers and computers have replaced the role of the fingers, but the principle remains the same: any abnormality in the condition of the body affects pulse waves, which carry the message from distant sites.

Modern literature has concentrated mostly on objective (a), for which great accuracy is required and success has been limited. But wave analysis can be supplemented by measurements of velocity of flow by ultrasound according to doppler principle, and by measurements of sound radiation if turbulence exists. Plethysmographic measurement of the diameter of the arm or finger, (hence the cross-sectional area of the blood vessels) can supplement pressure and velocity data. Fronek (1978) has used such measurements to determine the degree of reactive hyperemia (transient dilation of arteries after being compressed for a short period). Abnormality in reactive hyperemia is related to arterial diseases.

Events in the aorta, of course, reflect the function of the heart in health and disease. Cardiac catheterization has provided the opportunity to record pulsatile pressure in all chambers of the heart and great vessels. Simultaneous measurement of phasic blood pressure and flow during clinical aortic (or pulmonary arterial) catheterization has provided the data necessary to calculate the total hydraulic power or energy required to move blood into the vascular system and to define the input impedance of the arterial system. Input impedance and hydraulic power are important factors in evaluating the function of the heart as a pump.

But the idea of extracting information from the arterial pulse waves to gain information about the heart and other organs of the body remains an ideal. If we were able to read all the messages in the arterial pulse waves, then all we need is to observe these waves in some conveniently located arteries (such as the radial artery on the wrist) in order to get the message, and the art of noninvasive diagnosis would have been moved ahead a big step.

The idea of using pulse waves for diagnosis has been with us for a long time. In China, the oldest classics on arterial pulse waves is the *Nei Jing* (內經) mentioned in Chapter 1, Sec. 1.10. It was followed by *Nan Jing* (難經, 1st or 2nd century B.C., authorship attributed to Qin Yue-Ren, 秦越人). *Jing* means classic, *Nan* means difficult as an adjective, or question as a verb). The book of Nan Jing sought to answer difficult questions, including those concerned with pulse waves. In the Eastern Han Dynasty, Chang Chi (張機, 字仲景) (probably 150–219 AD) wrote the books *The Influence of External Factors* (傷寒論) and the *Abstracts of the Golden Chest* (金匱要略), which systematically organized the Han Dynasty's 300 years' clinical experience in using pulse waves in diagnosis. Then in Tzin Dynasty (晉代), Wang Shu-He (王叔和) (201–285 AD) wrote *Mai Jing*, the *Book on Pulse Waves* (脈經). These became the classics of Chinese medicine, and their ideas and methods have been continuously developed and are used in the Orient to this day.

The presentation given in these classics are descriptive and speculative, using similes and words like floating, deep, hidden, rapid, slow, moderate, feeble, replete, full, thready, faint, weak, soft, slippery, hesitant, hollow, firm, long, short, swift, running, intermittent, uneven, taut or string tight, gigantic and tremulous to describe and classify the waves. Empirically, abnormal waves were related to disease states; but rational explanations were lacking. Clearly, the tasks of good recording, clear analysis, physiological experimentation, and rational explanation are left to the modern research workers!

References

In addition to articles referred to in the text, the following literature is listed:

Books:
Aperia (1940), Attinger (1964), Bauereisen (1971), Bergel (1972), Bohr et al. (1980), Brankov (1981), Burton (1965), Caro et al. (1978), Folkow and Neil (1971), Fung (1977, 1981), Fung et al. (1972), Knets et al. (1980), Lighthill (1975, 1978), McDonald (1960, 1974), Oka (1974), Patel and Vaishnav (1980), Pedley (1980), Poorinya and Kasyanov (1980), Rushmer (1970), Wetterer and Kenner (1968).

Classics:
Euler (1775), Frank (1899, 1926, 1930), Harvey (1628), Joukowsky (1900), Lamb (1897), Moens (1878), Resal (1876), Weber & Weber (1825), Weber (1850), Witzig (1914), Womersley (1957), Young (1808, 1809).

Surveys:
Fung (1970), Jones et al. (1971), Kenner (1972), Klip (1962), Lambossy (1950, 1951), Müller (1951, 1959), Rubinow and Keller (1972), Wiedeman (1963).

On Atherosis, Atherogenesis:
Caro et al. (1969, 1971, 1973), Nerem (1981), Nerem et al. (1972, 1974), Schneiderman et al. (1979), Oka (1981).

On Measurements and Instrumentation:
Agrawal et al. (1978), Atabek et al. (1975), Deshpande et al. (1976), Deshpande and Giddens (1980), Fry et al. (1964), Gabe (1965), Holenstein et al. (1980), Klip (1958, 1967), Ling et al. (1968, 1973), Lutz et al. (1977), Milnor and Bertram (1978), Patel et al. (1964, 1966), Young and Tsai (1973).

On Nonlinear Effects:
Atabek (1968, 1980), Atabek et al. (1975), Pedley (1980) Lambert (1958), Ling et al. (1968), Ling and Atabek (1972), Yao and Berger (1975).

On Wave Propagation:
Anliker (1972), Anliker et al. (1966, 1968, 1969, 1971, 1977), Atabek et al. (1961, 1962, 1966), Attinger (1964), Attinger et al. (1966), Branson, (1945), Cox (1968, 1970), Davis (1976), Evans (1962), Hardung (1962), Holenstein et al. (1980), Jacobs (1953), Krovetz (1965), Landowne (1958), Lee (1966), Maxwell & Anliker (1968), Mirsky (1965), Mirsky et al. (1974), Skalak (1966, 1972), Smith (1975, 1976), Stettler et al. (1980), Streeter et al. (1963), Taylor (1959, 1965, 1966), Van der Werff (1973), Weiss (1964).

On Windkessel Theory:
Aperia (1940), Elcrat and Lieberstein (1967), Freis and Heath (1964), Hamilton and Dow (1939).

Agrawal, Y., Talbot, L. and Gong, K. (1978). Laser anemometer study of flow development in curved circular pipes. *J. Fluid Mechanics* **85**: 497–518.

Anliker, M. (1972). Toward a nontraumatic study of the circulatory system. In *Biomechanics: Its Foundations and Objectives,* Prentice-Hall, Englewood Cliffs, N. J., pp. 337–379.

Anliker, M. and Maxwell, J. A. (1966). The dispersion of waves in blood vessels. In *Biomechanics* (Y. C. Fung ed.), Amer. Soc. Mech. Engrs., New York, pp. 47–67.

Anliker, M. and Raman, K. R. (1966). Korotkoff sounds at diastole—a phenomenon and dynamic instability of fluid-filled shells. *International J. of Solids and structures,* **2**: 467–492.

Anliker, M., Histand, M. B. and Ogden, E. (1968). Dispersion and attenuation of small artificial pressure waves in canine aorta. *Circulation Research* **23**: 539–551.

Anliker, M., Moritz, W. E. and Ogden, E. (1968). Transmission characteristics of axial waves in blood vessels. *J. Biomechanics* **1**: 235–246.

Anliker, M., Wells, M. K. and Ogden, E. (1969). The transmission characteristics of large and small pressure waves in the abdominal vena cava. *IEEE Trans. on Bio-Medical Eng.* **BME-16**: 262–273.

Anliker, M., Rockwell, R. L. and Ogden, E. (1971). Nonlinear analysis of flow pulses and shock waves in arteries. *Z. angew. Math. Physics* **22**: 217–246, 563–581.

Anliker, M., Casty, M., Friedli, P., Kubli, R. and Keller, H. (1977). Noninvasive measurement of blood flow. In *Cardiovascular Flow Dynamics and Measurements* (N. H. C. Hwang and N. A. Norman, eds.), Univ. Park Press, Baltimore, Md., pp. 43–88.

Aperia, A. (1940). *Hemodynamical Studies. Skandinavisches Archiv für Physiologie*, Suppl. 16 to Vol. 83.

Atabek, H. B. (1962). Development of flow in the inlet length of a circular tube starting from rest. *Z. angew. Math. Phys.* **13**: 417–430.

Atabek, H. B. (1968). Wave propagation through a viscous fluid contained in a tethered, initially stressed, orthotropic elastic tube. *Biophysical J.* **8**: 626–649.

Atabek, H. B. (1980). Blood flow and pulse propagation in arteries. In *Basic Hemodynamics and Its Role in Disease Processes* (Patel, D. J. and Vaishnav, R. N. eds.), University Park Press, Baltimore, Md., Ch. 7, pp. 255–361.

Atabek, H. B. and Chang, C. C. (1961). Oscillatory flow near the entry of a circular tube. *Z. angew. Math. Physiol.* **12**: 185–201.

Atabek, H. B. and Lew, H. S. (1966). Wave propagation through a viscous incompressible fluid contained in an initially stressed elastic tube. *Biophysical J.* **6**: 481–502.

Atabek, H. B., Ling, S. C. and Patel, D. J. (1975). Analysis of coronary flow fields in thoracotomized dogs. *Circulation Res.* **37**: 752–761.

Attinger, E. O. (1964). Flow patterns and vascular geometry. In *Pulsatile Blood Flow*, (E. O. Attinger ed.), McGraw Hill, New York, Ch. 9, pp. 179–220.

Attinger, E. O., Sugawara, H., Navarro, A. and Anne, A. (1966). Pulsatile flow patterns in distensible tubes. *Circulation Res* **18**: 447–456.

Attinger, E. O., Sugawara, H., Navarro, A., Riceeto, A. and Martin, R. (1966). Pressure-flow relations in dog arteries. *Circulation Res.* **19**: 230–246.

Bauereisen, E. (ed.) (1971) *Physiologie des Kreislaufs. Band 1. Arteriensystem, Capillarbett, Organkreislauf, Fetal-und Placentarkreislauf*, Springer-Verlag, Heidelberg.

Bergel, D. H. (ed.) (1972). *Cardiovascular Fluid Dynamics*. Vols. 1 & 2. Academic Press, New York.

Bohr, D. F., Somlyo, A. P., and Sparks, H. V., Jr. (eds.) (1980). *Handbook of Physiology, Sec. 2. The Cardiovascular System*. Vol. 2, *Vascular Smooth Muscles*, American Physiological Society, Bethesda, Md.

Boussinesq, J. (1891). Maniere dont les vitesses, se distrib. depui l'entree—Moindre longueur d'un tube circulaire, pour qu'un regime uniforme s'y etablisse. *Comptes Rendus*, **113**: 9, 49.

Brankov, G. (1981). *Osnovi Biomechaniki. (Basic Biomechanics)* Izdatelstvo "MIR", Moscow.

Branson, H. (1945). The flow of a viscous fluid in an elastic tube: a model of the femoral artery. *Bull. Math. Biophysics* **7**: 181–188.

Burton, A. C. (1965). *Physiology and Biophysics of the Circulation*. Year Book Medical Publishers, Chicago, Ill.

Caro, C. G., Fitzgerald, J. M. and Schroter, R. C. (1969). Arterial wall shear and distribution of early atheroma in man. *Nature.* **223**: 1159–1161.

Caro, C. G., Fitzgerald, J. M. and Schroter, R. C. (1971). Atheroma and arterial wall shear. *Proc. Roy. Soc. London*, B, **177**: 109–159.

Caro, C. G., and Nerem, R. M. (1973). Transport of ^{14}C-4-Cholesterol between serum and wall in the perfused dog common carotid artery. *Circulation Res.* **32**: 187–205.

Caro, C. G., Pedley, T. J., Schroter, R. C., and Seed, W. A. (1978). *The Mechanics of the Circulation*. Oxford University Press, Oxford.

Cox, R. H. (1968). Wave propagation through a Newtonian fluid contained within a thick-walled, viscoelastic tube. *Biophys. J.* **8**: 691–709.

Cox, R. H. (1970). Blood flow and pressure propagation in the canine femoral artery. *J. Biomech.* **2**: 131–150.

Davis, S. H. (1976). The stability of time-periodic flows. *Annual Review of fluid Mechanics*, **8**: 57–74.

Deshpande, M. D., Giddens, D. P., and Mabon, R. F. (1976). Steady laminar flow through modelled vascular stenosis. *J. Biomechanics* **9**: 165–174.

Deshpande, M. D. and Giddens, D. P. (1980). Turbulence measurements in a constricted tube. *J. Fluid Mechanics* **97**: 65–90.

Elcrat, A. R. and Lieberstein, H. M. (1967). Asymptotic uniqueness for elastic tube flows satisfying a windkessel condition. *Math. Biosci.* **1**: 397–411.

Euler, L. (1775). Principia pro motu sanguins per arterias determinado. *Opera posthuma mathematica et physica* anno 1844 detecta, ediderunt P. H. Fuss et N. Fuss. Petropoli, Apud Eggers et socios, Vol. 2, pp. 814–823.

Evans, R. L. (1962). Pulsatile flow in vessels whose distensibility and size vary with site. *Phys. Med. Biol.* **7**: 105–116.

Evans, R. L. (1962). A unifying approach to blood flow theory. *J. Theoretical Biophysics* **3**: 392–411.

Folkow, B. and Neil, E. (1971). *Circulation*, Oxford Univ. Press, New York.

Frank, O. (1899). Die Grundform des arteriellen pulses. *Zeitschrift für Biologie*, **37**: 483–526.

Frank, O. (1926). Die Theorie der pulswellen. *Zeitschrift für Biologie*, **85**: 91–130.

Frank, O. (1930). Schatzung des Schlagvolumens des menschlichen Herzens auf Grund der Wellen-und Weinkessel theorie. *Zeitschrift für Biologie*, **90**: 405–409.

Freis, E. D. and Heath, W. C. (1964). Hydrodynamics of aortic blood flow. *Circulation Res.* **14**: 105–116.

Fronek, A., Coel, M. and Bernstein, E. F. (1978). Post-occlusive hyperemia and the toe-pulse-reappearance time in the evaluation of arterial occlusive disease. In *Non-Invasive Diagnostic Techniques in Vascular Disease* (Bernstein, E. F. ed.), Mosby, St. Louis.

Fry, D. L., Griggs, D. M., Jr. and Greenfield, J. C. Jr. (1964). In vivo studies of pulsatile blood flow: the relationship of the pressure gradient to the blood velocity. In *Pulsatile Blood Flow* (Attinger, E. O. ed.), McGraw-Hill, New York, Chap. 5, pp. 101–114.

Fung, Y. C. (1970). Biomechanics: A survey of the blood flow problem. In *Advances of Applied Mechanics* (Yih, C. S. ed.), Academic Press, New York, Vol. II. pp. 65–130.

Fung, Y. C. (1977). *A First Course in Continuum Mechanics*. 2nd edn. Prentice-Hall, Englewood Cliffs, N.J.

Fung, Y. C. (1981). *Biomechanics: Mechanical Properties of Living Tissues*. Springer-Verlag, New York.

Fung, Y. C., Perrone, N. and Anliker, M. (1972). *Biomechanics: Its Foundations and Objectives*. Prentice-Hall, Englewood Cliffs, N.J.

Fung, Y. C., Fronek, K. and Patitucci, P. (1979). On pseudo-elasticity of arteries and the choice of its mathematical expression. *Am. J. of Physiol.*, **237**(5): H620–H631.

Gabe, I. T. (1965). An analogue computer deriving oscillatory arterial blood flow from the pressure gradient. *Phys. Med. Biol.* **10**: 407–415.

Hamilton, W. F. and Dow, P. (1939). An experimental study of the standing waves in the pulse propagated through the aorta. *Am. J. Physiol.* **125**: 48–59.

Hardung, V. (1962). Propagation of pulse waves in viscoelastic tubing. In *Handbook of Physiology*, Sec. 2, *Circulation* (W. F. Hamilton, ed.), Am. Physiological Society, Washington, D.C., Ch. 7, pp. 107–135.

Harvey, W. (1628). *Exercitatis anatomica de motu cordis et sanguinis in animalibus*. An English translation with annotations by D. C. Leake, 4th ed. Thomas, Springfield, Ill., (1958).

Holenstein, R., Niederer, P. and Anliker, M. (1980). A viscoelastic model for use in predicting arterial pulse waves. *J. Biomechanical Eng.* **102**: 318–325.

Jacobs, R. B. (1953). On the propagation of a disturbance through a viscous liquid flowing in a distensible tube of appreciable mass. *Bull. Math. Biophysics* **5**: 395–409.

Jones, E., Anliker, M., and Chang, I. D. (1971). Effects of viscosity and constraints on the dispersion and dissipation of waves in large blood vessels. I & II. *Biophysical J.* **11**, 1085–1120, 1121–1134.

Jones, R. T. (1969). Blood flow. *Annual Review of Fluid Mechanics*, **1**: 223–244.

Joukowsky, N. W. (1900). Ueber den hydraulischen Stoss in Wasserheizungsrohren. *Memoires de l'Academie Imperiale des Science de St. Petersburg*, 8 series, Vol. 9, No. 5.

Kamiya, A., and Togawa, T. (1972). Optimal branching of the vascular tree. (Minimum volume theory) *Bull. Math. Biophysics*, **34**: 431–438.

Kenner, T. (1972). Flow and pressure in the arteries. In *Biomechanics: Its Foundations and Objectives*. (Fung, Y. C., Perrone, N. and Anliker, M. eds.), Prentice-Hall, Englewood Cliffs, N.J., pp. 381–434.

King, A. L. (1947). On a generalization of the Poiseuille law. *Am. J. Physiol.* **15**: 240–242.

King, A. L. (1947). Waves in elastic tubes: velocity of the pulse wave in large arteries. *J. Appl. Phys.* **18**: 595–600.

Kivity, Y. and Collins, R. (1974). Nonlinear wave propagation in viscoelastic tubes: application to aortic rupture. *J. of Biomechanics* **7**: 1–10.

Klip, W. (1958). Difficulties in the measurement of pulse wave velocity. *Am. Heart J.* **56**: 806–813.

Klip, W. (1962). *Velocity and Damping of the Pulse Wave*. Martinus Nijhoff, Hague.

Klip, W. (1967). Formulas for phase velocity and damping of longitudinal waves in thick-walled viscoelastic tubes. *J. Appl. Physics.* **38**: 3745–3755.

Knets, E. V., Pfafrod, G. O., Saulgozis, U. J. (И. В. Кнетс, Г. О. Пфафрод, Ю, Ж. Саулгозис). Deformation and Failure of Solid Biological Tissues (Deformerovanie e Razryshenie Tverdih Biologichskeh Tkanee), Riga, "zenatne".

Korteweg, D. J. (1878). Ueber die Fortpflanzungesgeschwindigkeit des Schalles in elastischen Rohren. *Ann. der Physik. u. Chemie.* **5**(3): 525–542.

Krovetz, L. J. (1965). The effect of vessel branching on haemodynamic stability. *Phys. in Med. and Biol.* **10**: 417–427.

Kuchar, N. R. and Ostrach, S. (1966). Flows in the entrance regions of circular elastic tubes. In *Biomedical Fluid Mechanics Symposium*, Amer. Soc. Mech. Engrs., pp. 45–69.

Lamb, H. (1897–1898). On the velocity of sound in a tube, as affected by the elasticity of the walls. *Phil. Soc. of Manchester Memoirs and Proc.*, lit. A, **42**: 1–16.

Lambert, J. W. (1958). On the nonlinearities of fluid flow in nonrigid tubes. *J. Franklin Inst.* **266**: 83–102.

Lambossy, P. (1950, 1951). Apercu historique et critique sur le probleme de la propaga-
    tion des ondes dans un liquide compressible enferme dan un tube elastique. *Helv.
    Physiol. Pharm. Acta.* **8**: 209–227, **9**: 145–161.

Lanczos, C. (1952). Introduction. In *Tables of Chebyshev Polynomials.* Nat. Bureau of
    Standards, Appl. Math., Ser. 9, U.S. Govt. Printing Office, Washington, D.C.,
    pp. 7–9.

Landowne, M. (1958). Characteristics of impact and pulse wave propagation in brachial
    and radial arteries. *J. Appl. Physiol.* **12**: 91–97.

Lee, J. S. (1966). The pressure-flow relationship in long-wave propagation in large
    arteries. In *Biomechanics* (Fung, Y. C. ed.), ASME Symposium, American Society
    of Mech. Engineers, New York, pp. 96–120.

Lew, H. S., and Fung, Y. C. (1970). Entry flow into blood vessels at arbitrary Reynolds
    number. *J. Biomech.* **3**: 23–38.

Lighthill, J. (1975). *Mathematical Biofluiddynamics.* Society for Industrial and Applied
    Mathematics, Philadelphia, Pa.

Lighthill, M. J. (1978). *Waves in Fluids.* Cambridge University Press.

Ling, S. C., Atabek, H. B., Fry, D. L., Patel, D. J. and Janicki, J. S. (1968). Application
    of heated film velocity and shear probes to hemodynamic studies. *Circulation Res.*
    23: 789–801.

Ling, S. C. and Atabek, H. B. (1972). A nonlinear analysis of pulsatile flow in arteries.
    J. Fluid Mechanics **55**: 493–511.

Ling, S. C., Atabek, H. B., Letzing, W. G. and Patel, D. J. (1973). Nonlinear analysis
    of aortic flow in living dogs. *Circulation Res.* **33**: 198–212.

Lutz, R. J., Cannon, J. N., Bischoff, K. B., and Dedrick, R. L. (1977). Wall shear stress
    distribution in a model canine artery during steady flow. *Circulation Res.* **41**:
    391–399.

Matunobu, Y. and Arakawa, M. (1974). Model experiments on the post-stenotic
    dilatation in blood vessels. *Biorheology* **11**: 457–464.

Maxwell, J. A. and Anliker, M. (1968). The dissipation and dispersion of small waves
    in arteries and veins with viscoelastic wall properties. *Biophysical J.* **8**: 920–950.

McCutcheon, E. P. and Rushmer, R. F. (1967). Korotkoff sounds: An experimental
    critique. *Circulation Res.* **20**: 149–161.

McDonald, D. A. (1968). Regional pulse wave-velocity in the arterial tree (dog). *J.
    Appl. Physiol.* **24**: 73–78.

McDonald, D. A. (1960, 1974). *Blood Flow in Arteries.* Williams & Wilkins, Baltimore,
    Md. 1st ed, 1960, 2nd ed., 1974.

Milnor, W. R. and Bertram, C. D. (1978). The relation between arterial viscoelasticity
    and wave propagation in the canine femoral artery in vivo. *Circulation Res.* **43**:
    870–879.

Mirsky, I. (1965). Wave propagation in transversely isotropic circular cylinders. Part 1:
    Theory. *J. Acoust. Soc. Amer.* **37**: 1016–1025.

Mirsky, I., Ghista, D. N. and Sandler, H. (eds.) (1974). *Cardiac Mechanics: Physiolog-
    ical, Clinical, and Mathematical Considerations.* John Wiley & Sons, New York.

Moens, A. I. (1878). *Die Pulskwive.* Brill, Leiden, Netherlands.

Morgan, G. W. and Kiely, J. P. (1954). Wave propagation in a viscous liquid contained
    in a flexible tube. *J. Acoust. Soc. Amer,* **26**(3): 323–328.

Morgan, G. W. and Ferrante, W. R. (1955). Wave propagation in elastic tubes filled with streaming liquid. *J. Acoust. Soc. Amer.* **27**(4): 715–725.

Müller, V. A. (1951). Ueber die Abhängigkeit der Fortpflanzungsgeschwindigkeit und der Dämpfung der Druckwellen in dehnbaren Rohren von deren Wellenlänge. *Helvetica Physiologica et Pharma. Acta* **9**: 162–176.

Müller, V. A. (1959). Die Mehrschichtige Rohrwand als Modell für die Aorta. *Helv. Physiol. Pharmacol. Acta* **17**: 131–145.

Murray, C. D. (1926). The physiological principle of minimum work. I. The vascular system and the cost of blood volume. *Proc. Nat. Acad. Sci. U.S.A.,* **12**: 207–214. Also, *J. Gen. Physiol.* **9**: 835–841.

Nerem, R. M. (ed.) (1981). Hemodynamics in the arterial wall. *J. Biomech. Eng.* **103**: Introduction p. 171. Technical Papers pp. 172–212.

Nerem, R. M., Seed, W. A. and Wood, N. B. (1972). An experimental study of the velocity distribution and transition to turbulence in the aorta. *J. Fluid Mechanics* **52**: 137–160.

Nerem, R. M., Rumberger, J. A., Gross, D. R., Hamlin, R. L. and Geiger, G. L. (1974). Hot-film anemometer velocity measurements of arterial blood flow in horses *Circulation Res.* 34, 193–203.

Oka, S. (1974). *Rheology-Biorheology.* Syokabo, Tokyo. (In Japanese).

Patel, D. J., Greenfield, J. C. Jr., and Fry, D. L. (1964). In vivo pressure-length radius relationship of certain blood vessels in man and dog. In *Pulsatile Blood Flow* (E. O. Attinger, ed.), McGraw-Hill, New York, pp. 293–305.

Patel, D. J., and Fry, D. L. (1966). Longitudinal tethering of arteries in dogs. *Circulation Res.* **19**: 1011–1021.

Patel, D. J. and Vaishnav, R. N. (eds.) (1980). *Basic Hemodynamics and Its Role in Disease Process,* University Park Press, Baltimore, Md.

Pedley, T. J. (1980). *The Fluid Mechanics of Large Blood Vessels.* Cambridge University Press, London.

Poorinya, B. A. and Kasyanov, V. A. (1980). *Biomechanika Kropnich Krovenosnich Sosoodov Cheloveka* (*Biomechanics of Large Blood Vessels of Man*). Riga, "Zenatne".

Resal, H. (1876). Sur les petits movements d'un fluid incompressible dans un tuyau elastique. *Comptes Rendus, Academie des Sciences,* **82**: 698–699.

Rosen, R. (1967). *Optimality Principles in Biology.* Butterworth, London.

Rubinow, S. I. and Keller, J. B. (1972). Flow of a viscous fluid through an elastic tube with applications to blood flow. *J. Theo. Biol.* **35**(2): 299–313.

Rushmer, R. F. (1955, 1961, 1970). *Cardiovascular Dynamics.* Saunders, Philadelphia.

Schiller, L. (1922). Die Entwicklung der laminaren Geschwindigkeitsverteilung und ihre Bedeutung für Zahigkeitsmessungen. *Z. angew. Math. Mech.* **2**: 96–106.

Schlichting, H. (1968). *Boundary Layer Theory,* 6th ed., McGraw-Hill, New York.

Schneiderman, G., Ellis, C. G., and Goldstick, T. K. (1979). Mass transport to walls of stenosed arteries: variation with Reynolds number and blood flow separation. *Biomechanics J.* **12**: 869–878.

Skalak, R. (1966). Wave propagation in blood flow. In *Biomechanics Symposium* (Y. C. Fung, ed.), American Soc. of Mech. Engrs., New York, pp. 20–40.

Skalak, R. (1972). Synthesis of a complete circulation. In *Cardiovascular fluid Dynamics* (D. H. Bergel, ed.), Vol. 2, Chap. 19, Academic Press, New York, pp. 341–376.

Skalak, R. and Stathis, T. (1966). A porous tapered elastic tube model of a vascular bed. In *Biomechanics Symposium* (Y. C. Fung, ed.), Amer. Soc. of Mech. Engrs., New York, pp. 68–81.

Smith, F. T. (1975). Pulsatile flow in curved pipes. *J. Fluid Mechanics*, **71**: 15–42.

Smith, F. T. (1976). Pipeflows distorted by non-symmetric indentation or branching. *Mathematika*. **23**: 62–83.

Stettler, J. C., Niederer, P. and Anliker. M. (1980). Theoretical analysis of arterial hemodynamics including the influence of bifurcations. Part I. Mathematical Model and prediction of normal pulse patterns. *Annals of Biomedical Eng.* **9**: 145–164. Part II. (with Casty, M.) Comparison with noninvasive measurements of flow patterns in normal and pathological cases, *loc cit.*, 165–175.

Streeter, V. L., Keitzer, W. F. and Bohr, D. F. (1963). Pulsatile pressure and flow through distensible vessels. *Circulation Res.* **13**: 3–20.

Szegö, G. (1939). *Orthogonal Polynomials*, 4th ed. American Math. Soc. Colloquium Publication, Vol. 23.

Targ, S. M. (1951). *Basic Problems of the Theory of Laminar Flows*. Moskva. (In Russian).

Taylor, M. G. (1959). An experimental determination of the propagation of fluid oscillations in a tube with a viscoelastic wall. *Phys. Med. Biol.* **4**: 63–82.

Taylor, M. G. (1965). Wave travel in a non-uniform transmission line, in relation to pulses in arteries arteries. *Phys. Med. Biol.* **10**: 539–550.

Taylor, M. G. (1966). Use of random excitation and spectral analysis in the study of frequency-dependent parameters of the cardiovascular system. *Circulation Res.* **18**: 585–595.

Taylor, M. G. (1966). Input impedance of an assembly of randomly branching elastic tubes. *Biophysical J.* **6**: 29–51., **6**: 697–716.

Van der Werff, T. J. (1973). Periodic method of characteristics. *J. Comp. Phys.* **11**: 296–305.

Walawender, W. P. and Chen, T. Y. (1975). Blood flow in tapered tubes. *Microvas. Res.* **9**: 190–205.

Weber, E. H. and Weber, W. (1825). *Wellenlehre auf experimente begrundet*; oder, *Über die Wellen tropfbarer flüssigkeiten mit Anwendung auf die Schall-und- lichtwell.* Fleischer, Leipzig.

Weber, E. H. (1850). *Ueber die Anwendung der Wellenlehre auf die Lehre vom Kreislaufe des blutes und insbesondere auf die Pulslehre.* Berichte uber die Verhandlungen der königl sachsischen Gesellschaft der Wissenschaft zu Leipzig, Mathematisch-physische Klasse.

Weiss, G. H. (1964). On the theory of blood flow in tapered arteries. *Biorheology* **2**: 153–158.

Werlé, H. (1974). *Le Tunnel Hydrodynamique au Service de la Recherche Aérospatiale.* Publication No. 156, ONERA, France.

Wetterer, E. and Kenner, T. (1968). *Grundlagen der Dynamik des Arterienpulses.* Springer-Verlag, Berlin.

Wetterer, E., Bauer, R. D., and Busse, R. (1978). New ways of determining the propagation coefficient and the viscoelastic behavior of arteries in situ. In *The Arterial System* (Bauer, R. D. & Busse, R. ed.), Springer-Verlag, Berlin, pp. 35–47.

Wiedeman, M. P. (1963). Dimensions of blood vessels from distributing artery to collecting vein. *Circulation Res.* **12**: 375–378.

Witzig, K. (1914). *Über erzwungene Wellenbewegungen zaher, inkompressibler Flüssigkeiten in elastischen Rohren.* Inaugural Dissertation, Universitat Bern, K. J. Wyss, Bern.

Womersley, J. R. (1955). Method for the calculation of velocity, rate of flow, and viscous drag in arteries when the pressure gradient is known. *J. Physiol.* **127**: 553–563.

Womersley, J. R. (1955). Oscillatory motion of a viscous liquid in a thin-walled elastic tube-I: the linear approximation for long waves. *Phil. Mag.* **46**(Ser. 7): 199–221.

Womersley, J. R. (1957). *The mathematical analysis of the arterial circulation in a state of oscillatory motion.* Wright Air Development Center, Technical Report WADC-TR-56-614, 123pp.

Womersley, J. R. (1958). Oscillatory flow in arteries. I. The constrained elastic tube as a model of arterial flow and pulse transmission. II. The reflection of the pulse wave at junctions and rigid inserts in the arterial system. *Phys. Med. Biol.* **2**: 177–187, 313–323.

Wylie, E. R. (1966). Flow through tapered tubes with nonlinear wall properties. In *Biomechanics Sympoisum* (Fung, Y. C. ed.), Amer. Soc. Mech. Engrs., New York, pp. 82–95.

Yao, L. S. and Berger, S. A. (1975). Entry flow in a curved pipe. *J. Fluid Mechanics.* **67**: 177–196.

Young, D. F. and Tsai, F. Y. (1973). Flow characteristics in models of arterial stenosis. I. Steady flow. *J. Biomechanics*, **6**: 395–410.

Young, T. (1808). Hydraulic investigations, subservient to an intended Croonian lecture on the motion of the blood. *Phil. Trans. Roy. Soc. London*, **98**: 164–186.

Young, T. (1809). On the functions of the heart and arteries. *Phil. Trans. Roy. Soc. London*, **99**: 1–31.

Zamir, M. (1976). The role of shear forces in arterial branching. *J. General Biology* **67**: 213–222.

CHAPTER 4

The Veins

4.1 Introduction

Veins normally contain about 80% of the total volume of blood in the systemic vascular system. Any change in the blood volume in the veins will affect blood flow through the heart. The most important feature of the systemic veins is, therefore, their compliance.

In histological structure, both systemic and pulmonary veins resemble arteries. Their anatomy and material properties have been discussed in Chapter 8 of *Biomechanics: The Mechanical Properties of Living Tissues* (Fung, 1981). Compared with the arteries, there are several important differences: (1) The pressure in a vein is normally much lower than that in an artery at the same general location. (2) The veins have thin walls and some of them may be collapsed in normal function. (3) Blood flows in veins from the periphery toward the heart. (4) Many veins have valves which prevent blackflow. Veins more distal to the heart have more valves. The vena cava and the pulmonary veins have none.

Normally, the internal pressure in the vein is higher than the external pressure and the flow in the vein is similar to that in the artery. In certain situations, however, the external pressure may be raised or the internal pressure decreased to such a degree that the external pressure exceeds the internal pressure. In this situation, some vessels or parts of vessels may be collapsed. The controlling factor is the transmural pressure, Δp, which is equal to the internal minus external pressures. Since in general the internal pressure in a blood vessel falls along the length because of frictional loss, Δp falls continuously from the entry to the exit section if the external pressure remains constant. In dynamic condition, three eventualities may occur in a vein:

(a) $\Delta p > 0$ at entry, $\Delta p > 0$ at exit,

(b) $\Delta p > 0$ at entry, $\Delta p < 0$ at exit,

(c) $\Delta p < 0$ at entry, $\Delta p < 0$ at exit.

If a vein collapses whenever $\Delta p < 0$, then in case (a) the vein functions normally, and the principles discussed in the preceding chapter apply. In case (c), the vein will be collapsed and the flow will be greatly reduced. In case (b), the entry section is open and patent, but the exit section is collapsed. Case (b) is the really interesting one. How effective is the choking at the exit section to the flow? If it were very effective, the flow would stop, the pressure drop would become zero, the whole tube would have a Δp equal to that of the entry section, the conditions of (a) would then prevail, and flow would start again. But if flow starts, the pressure will drop along the tube, and the exit section will be choked again. This may lead to a dynamic phenomenon of "flutter", or a limiting steady state flow described below.

It will be shown (Sec. 4.5) that in the case (b), the flow is controlled by the choking section, but the actual value of Δp at the exit section is quite immaterial as long as it is negative. An analogy may be drawn between this and the waterfall in our landscape, or sluicing in industry or flood control: The volume flow rate in a waterfall depends on the conditions at the top of the fall, and is independent of how high the drop is. Thus, the phenomenon of flow in case (b) is described as the "waterfall" phenomenon, or as "sluicing".

The waterfall phenomenon occurs in a number of important organs: the lung, the vena cava, etc. It occurs in thoracic arteries while in resuscitation maneuvers, and in brachial arteries while measuring blood pressure by cuff and Korotkov sound. The same phenomenon occurs also in male and female urethra in micturition, and in man-made instruments such as the blood pump and the heart–lung machine. Therefore, it pays to understand it well. Accordingly, in this chapter we shall consider the concept of elastic stability (Sec. 4.2), study the pressure–area relationship of veins in partially collapsed states (Secs. 4.3, 4.4), clarify steady and unsteady flows in the veins (Secs. 4.5, 4.6, 4.7), and investigate some aspects of the dynamics of flow in collapsible tubes, such as flutter and Korotkov sound.

If the vascular waterfall phenomenon is important, we should know where the waterfalls are on the venous tree. This seemingly simple question does not have an easy answer. In Sec. 4.9 we shall show that the pulmonary veins will not collapse, i.e., they remain patent when the blood pressure is smaller than the alveolar gas pressure (i.e., Δp is negative) in the physiological range. Thus, one should not believe that every vein must collapse when Δp is negative. There are other factors to be considered, e.g., tethering, or the relationship to the neighboring structures. The pulmonary capillary blood vessels, however, will collapse to zero thickness under negative transmural pressure. Hence (Sec. 4.10), we can show that the pulmonary "waterfalls," or "sluicing gates," are located at the exit ends of capillaries where the blood enters the venules. Once this is known, the blood flow analysis is relatively easy.

4.2 The Concept of Elastic Instability

The collapsing of a vein under negative transmural pressure is a phenomenon of elastic instability, similar to the buckling of thin-walled structures such as airplane wings and fuselages, submarine hulls, and underwater pipelines. This topic is dealt with in the theory of elastic stability, an outline of which is given below.

Adjacent Equilibrium

A structure carries a certain load which causes a certain deformation. Let this system be disturbed slightly by a small additional load. If the basic load is sufficiently small, the small additional load will cause a small additional deformation, and structure will return to the basic configuration when the disturbance is removed. The structure is then said to be *stable*. If the basic load is increased beyond certain limit, it may happen that a small disturbance will cause a large deformation, and the structure will not return to the basic configuration when the disturbance is removed. The structure is then said to be *unstable*.

Let us illustrate this concept with the classical theory of *columns* (a column is a beam used to support an axial load). Leonhard Euler (1707–1783) considered a column made of a material that obeys Hook's law of elasticity, simply supported at both ends, and subjected to an end thrust as illustrated in Fig. 4.2:1(a). Under the load P, there is an axial compressive stress $-P/A$ in all sections of the column, where A is the cross-sectional area.

Let us disturb the equilibrium by imposing some infinitesimal lateral loads on the column (loads acting in the direction perpendicular to the column axis). If the column is stable, this will cause only an infinitesimal lateral deformation. If, however, the load P is so large as to cause the column to be unstable, then under the infinitesimal disturbance a finite (i.e., "large") deformation of the column will be possible. Let us consider an unstable column, and assume that under an infinitesimal lateral disturbance a finite deflection w as illustrated in Fig. 4.2:1(b) occurs. A free-body diagram of a segment of the column is shown in Fig. 4.2:1(c), in which P and M represent the thrust and bending moment in the column. Taking moment about the lower end yields a condition of equilibrium

$$M - Pw = 0. \tag{1}$$

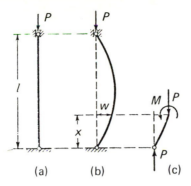

Figure 4.2:1 An Euler column used to support an axial load P. (a) Straight equilibrium configuration. (b) Deflected equilibrium configuration. (c) A free-body diagram of a portion of the column showing external and internal forces, and moments acting on the column.

The bending moment M is assumed to be directly proportional to the curvature of the column, (see Fig. 4.2:2, and Fung, 1977, Sec. 7.7), so that

$$M = -EI\frac{d^2w}{dx^2},\tag{2}$$

where E is the Young's modulus of elasticity of the material, and I is the moment of inertia of the cross-sectional area. Combining Eqs. (1) and (2) yields the differential equation

$$EI\frac{d^2w}{dx^2} + Pw = 0.\tag{3}$$

The boundary conditions for a column simply supported at both ends are

$$w = 0 \quad \text{at } x = 0 \quad \text{and} \quad x = L.\tag{4}$$

Equations (3) and (4) have an obvious solution, $w = 0$, which is the answer for a stable column. To look for a nontrivial solution for an unstable column, we note that Eq. (3) is satisfied by

$$w = c_1 \sin\sqrt{\frac{P}{EI}}x + c_2 \cos\sqrt{\frac{P}{EI}}x,\tag{5}$$

where c_1, c_2 are integration constants. The boundary conditions of Eq. (4) are satisfied if

$$c_2 = 0 \quad \text{and} \quad 0 = c_1 \sin\sqrt{\frac{P}{EI}}L.\tag{6}$$

The last equation is satisfied if

$$\sqrt{\frac{P}{EI}}L = n\pi \quad (n = 1, 2, \ldots),\tag{7}$$

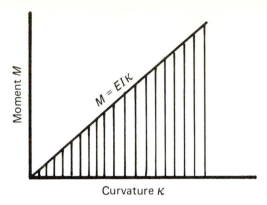

Figure 4.2:2 The relationship between bending moment and curvature of a beam (or column). This relationship is assumed to be linear in the classical theory of beams which are made of material obeying Hooke's law. It is shown as a straight line $M = EI\varkappa$ in the figure. The area under the curve (shaded) represents the work done by gradually bending the beam to the curvature $\varkappa$. The curvature is equal to $-d^2w/dx^2$ if $dw/dx \ll 1$, and if the signs of w and x are chosen as illustrated in Fig. 4.2:1(b). Then Eq. (2) applies. If dw/dx is not negligibly small compared to 1, then the exact expression for curvature should be used:

$$\varkappa = (d^2w/dx^2)[1 + (dw/dx)^2]^{-3/2},$$

i.e., if

$$P = \frac{n^2\pi^2 EI}{L^2} \qquad (n = 1, 2, \ldots).\tag{8}$$

Thus, if the load P equals the value specified by Eq. (8), the column can deform into a buckled form with

$$w = c_1 \sin\frac{n\pi x}{L}\tag{9}$$

without any lateral load. The amplitude c_1 is arbitrary. The load P given by Eq. (8) is the *critical load for neutral stability*. As the axial load P is increased gradually from zero, instability is encountered for the first time when $n = 1$, and $P = P_{cr}$.

$$P_{cr} = \frac{\pi^2 EI}{L^2},\tag{10}$$

which is known as the *Euler load*.

This method of derivation yields the critical condition, but it says nothing about what happens when P is slightly greater than P_{cr}. What happens to the column when $P \geq P_{cr}$ becomes clear if the column was slightly crooked originally: it will collapse suddenly! (See Prob. 4.2.) When $P = P_{cr}$, the deflection given by Eq. (9) will have a finite amplitude. The column cannot carry a load larger than P_{cr} unless lateral deformation is prevented by some special means.

Energy Method

An alternative method to derive the results presented above uses the concept of work and energy. Consider again the Euler column. When the column is deflected (Fig. 4.2:1(b)), there is some strain energy stored in it. To evaluate the strain energy, note that if the material obeys Hooke's law of elasticity, the bending moment is proportional to the curvature with a constant of proportionality EI (see Eq. (2)). When a segment of straight column of unit length is bent gradually to a curvature $\varkappa$, the work done on the column is stored as strain energy, and is equal to the area under the moment-curvature curve as shown in Fig. 4.2:2. Thus, the strain energy per unit length of the column is the area of the triangle, $\frac{1}{2}EI\varkappa^2$. For small deflection, the curvature $\varkappa = d^2w/dx^2$. Integrating throughout the column, we obtain the strain energy

$$V = \frac{EI}{2}\int_0^L \left(\frac{d^2w}{dx^2}\right)^2 dx. \tag{11}$$

In the meantime, the ends of the column are moved closer because the column is bent. The axial load P does the work Pu, where u is the distance the ends approached each other. The column itself, opposing P, does the work $-Pu$. To compute u, note that the vertical projection of an element of length dx in the deformed state is (Fig. 4.2:3)

$$dx\cos\frac{dw}{dx} = dx\left[1 - \frac{1}{2}\left(\frac{dw}{dx}\right)^2 + \cdots\right].$$

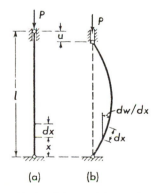

(a)   (b)

Figure 4.2:3 Euler column. (a) Straight and in equilibrium. (b) Deflected and in equilibrium.

The total vertical projection of the deformed column is, therefore,

$$L - u = \int_0^L \left[1 - \frac{1}{2} \left(\frac{dw}{dx} \right)^2 \right] dx = L - \frac{1}{2} \int_0^L \left(\frac{dw}{dx} \right)^2 dx.$$

Hence,

$$u = \frac{1}{2} \int_0^L \left(\frac{dw}{dx} \right)^2 dx. \tag{12}$$

The total energy needed to produce the deflection w is

$$V - Pu = \frac{EI}{2} \int_0^L \left(\frac{d^2w}{dx^2} \right)^2 dx - \frac{P}{2} \int_0^L \left(\frac{dw}{dx} \right)^2 dx. \tag{13}$$

It is zero if

$$P = \frac{EI \int_0^L \left(\dfrac{d^2w}{dx^2} \right)^2 dx}{\int_0^L \left(\dfrac{dw}{dx} \right)^2 dx}. \tag{14}$$

This is the value of P at which the column can deform by itself into a curve w without an external supply of energy. It signals an instability. We look for a function $w = w(x)$ which yields the smallest value of P, which is P_{cr}. Since both the numerator and denominator are quadratic in derivatives of w, the quotient does not depend on the absolute magnitude of the deflection but only on its shape.

There are several ways of finding this smallest value. We may use the calculus of variations, finding and solving the differential equation and boundary conditions for w as in the method of adjacent equilibrium. It will be found that these equations are exactly Eqs. (3) and (4). We may also assume a general expression for the unknown function $w(x)$, such as a Fourier series,

$$w(x) = \sum_{n=1}^{\infty} c_n \sin \frac{n\pi x}{L}, \tag{15}$$

which satisfies the boundary conditions, and then determine the coefficient c_n so that P from Eq. (14) becomes a minimum. When this is done, one finds that $c_n = 0$ for $n > 1$ and that c_1 is arbitrary while P becomes equal to the Euler load, Eq. (10).

Recapitulation

Both the adjacent equilibrium method and the energy method examine a disturbed basic system. In the adjacent equilibrium method, one studies the differential equation and boundary conditions governing the disturbed system, and looks for the eigenvalues at which a nontrivial solution exists. In the energy method, the problem is converted into a variational principle. Physically, one looks for a perturbed deformation that can occur in the system without additional external energy input.

It is a special merit of the energy method that one can find an approximate value of P_{cr} by introducing into Eq. (14) some plausible function $w(x)$. The approximate function $w(x)$ can be obtained often by experimental observations. Since the assumed, plausible function $w(x)$ is not necessarily the one which makes P a minimum, the approximate value of P found by this method is always higher than the correct one. The approximation can be very good if the function $w(x)$ is skillfully chosen.

Problems

4.1 In Sec. 4.1 we said that in general the internal pressure in a blood vessel falls along the length because of frictional loss. Under what conditions can exceptions to the general rule be found?

4.2 Consider a slightly crooked column with an initial deflection

$$w_0 = A \sin\frac{\pi x}{L}.$$

When the column is loaded by P (Fig. 4.2:1), an addition deflection w occurs. The bending moment in a cross section at x is then equal to $P(w_0 + w)$. The second term in Eq. (3) must be changed to $P(w_0 + w)$. Equation (4) remains valid. Find the solution. Show that when $P = P_{cr}$, the ratio c_1/A tends to ∞.

4.3 Show that the column can be strengthened if a lateral support is introduced to make $w = 0$ at some intermediate station x between 0 and L.

4.3 Instability of a Circular Cylindrical Tube Subjected to External Pressure

Now let us turn to a problem of more direct physiological interest: the collapse of a circular cylindrical tube under external pressure. The general theory of cylindrical shells is very complicated, so we shall deal explicitly with only one of the simplest cases: the deformation of a cylinder into another cylinder with a cross section of different shape. After the solution to this simple case is obtained, we shall then survey the general cases.

Consider a cylindrical tube made of a material which obeys Hooke's law of elasticity, as is shown in Fig. 4.3:1(a). Let the wall thickness be uniform, and equal to h. Assume that h is very small compared with the radius of the cylinder R. The cylinder is subjected to an internal pressure p and an external pressure p_e, and there is no force acting on the cylinder in the direction of the generating lines.

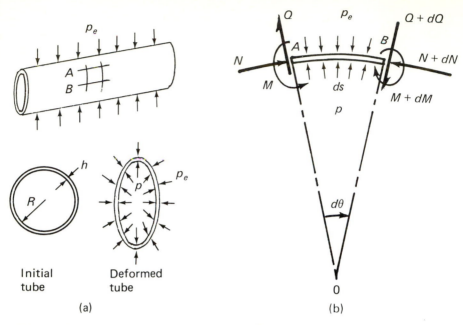

Figure 4.3:1 A circular cylinder subjected to an internal pressure p and external pressure p_e. (a) dimensions and loads. (b) forces and moments.

To visualize the forces and moments acting in the walls of the deformed tube, let us cut a small rectangular element out from the strained cylinder by two planes parallel to the tube axis and perpendicular to the middle surface of the wall, and two planes perpendicular to the cylinder axis at a unit distance apart. The isolated element is shown in Fig. 4.3:1(b) as a free body, where the points A and B are on the middle surface of the tube wall, and on planes containing generating lines. The plane of the figure is perpendicular to the tube axis. The location of the point A or B will be described by the arc length s measured in the circumferential direction from an arbitrary origin C on the middle surface of the tube wall. Let the length of the arc AB be infinitesimal and equal to ds. Let N denote the mean compressive stress resultant acting in the section at A. Let M denote the bending moment at A, which is a couple in a plane parallel to the plane of the figure. Q is the shear force per unit length across the wall, in the direction perpendicular to the middle surface of the wall. A pressure p acts on the concave side of the cylinder, and a pressure p_e acts on the convex side of the cylinder. The lines OA, OB are normal to the strained middle surface, and contain an angle $d\theta$. The forces and couple at B are $Q + dQ$, $N + dN$, and $M + dM$, respectively.

The equations of equilibrium can be obtained by considering the balance of forces and moments acting on this element. By taking moments about B and neglecting small quantities of the second order, we get

$$dM + Qds = 0,$$

from which we obtain

$$\frac{dM}{ds} = -Q. \tag{1}$$

By summing all forces in the direction BO, we get

$$Q + dQ - Q\cos d\theta - N\sin d\theta + (p_e - p)ds = 0.$$

Neglecting small quantities of the second and higher orders, we obtain

$$dQ - Nd\theta + (p_e - p)ds = 0,$$

or

$$\frac{dQ}{ds} - N\frac{d\theta}{ds} + p_e - p = 0. \tag{2}$$

The ratio $d\theta/ds$ is, of course, the curvature of the wall.

Finally, by summing all forces in the direction of $N + dN$, we obtain

$$N + dN - N\cos d\theta + Q\sin d\theta = 0,$$

or

$$\frac{dN}{ds} + Q\frac{d\theta}{ds} = 0. \tag{3}$$

Combining Eqs. (1) and (2) we obtain

$$\frac{d^2M}{ds^2} + N\frac{d\theta}{ds} = p_e - p. \tag{4}$$

Now we need an expression connecting the bending moment and wall deformation. In simple beams, the moment M is equal to EI times the change of curvature (see Eq. (4.2:2)). In the theory of plates and shells, it can be shown that a similar result holds if the wall is thin:

$$M = E'I(\varkappa - \varkappa_o), \tag{5}$$

where $E'I$ is the flexural rigidity,

$$E'I = \frac{Eh^3}{12(1 - v^2)}, \tag{6}$$

and $\varkappa$ and $\varkappa_o$ are the curvatures of the wall in the deformed and initial states. E is the Young's modulus of the material, v is the Poisson's ratio, I is the cross-sectional area moment of inertia per unit length, $h^3/12$. On introducing ξ for the change of curvature,

$$\xi = \varkappa - \varkappa_o, \tag{7}$$

Eqs. (4) and (3) can be written in the form

$$E'I\frac{d^2\xi}{ds^2} + N(\xi + \varkappa_o) = p_e - p, \tag{8}$$

$$\frac{dN}{ds} + Q(\xi + \varkappa_o) = 0. \tag{9}$$

These are differential equations governing the deformation of a cylinder into another cylinder. Let us apply them to the case in which the cylinder is initially circular with a radius of R. Then

$$\varkappa_o = \frac{1}{R} = \text{constant}. \tag{10}$$

In the basic state, the cylinder remains circular and the hoop stress is

$$N_o = (p_e - p)R. \tag{11}$$

If the pressure p_e is so large that the cylinder becomes neutrally unstable, a small deformation into a noncircular cylinder is possible. Let the change of curvature ξ be small compared with $\varkappa_o$. Then Eq. (9) can be approximated by

$$\frac{dN}{ds} = -Q\varkappa_o, \tag{12}$$

whereas Eqs. (1) and (5) yield

$$Q = -\frac{dM}{ds} = -E'I\frac{d\xi}{ds}. \tag{13}$$

Substituting Eq. (13) into Eq. (12) and integrating, we get

$$N = -\varkappa_o \int Q\,ds = E'I\varkappa_o\xi + N_o, \tag{14}$$

where N_o is a constant given by Eq. (11), because when ξ vanishes, N must be reduced to N_o. Now substituting Eq. (14) into Eq. (4), noting that $d\theta/ds = \kappa = \xi + \varkappa_o$, and neglecting the second order term ξ^2, we obtain

$$E'I\frac{d^2\xi}{ds^2} + (N_o + E'I\varkappa_o^2)\xi = 0. \tag{15}$$

The solution of this equation is

$$\xi = c\cos(ms + k), \tag{16}$$

where

$$m^2 = \frac{N_o + E'I\varkappa_o^2}{E'I}, \tag{17}$$

and c and k are arbitrary constants. Now, since the displacement must be continuous, ξ must be such that its value is repeated when s is increased by $2\pi R$, the circumference of the cylinder. Thus,

$$m2\pi R = 2n\pi, \tag{18}$$

n being an integer; that is,

$$\frac{N_o + E'I\varkappa_o^2}{E'I}R^2 = n^2,$$

or, by Eq. (10),

$$N_o = \frac{E'I}{R^2}(n^2 - 1); \tag{19}$$

and, by Eq. (11),

$$p_e - p = \frac{E'I}{R^3}(n^2 - 1). \tag{20}$$

These are the critical values of pressure at which the cylinder can deform into a shape described by Eq. (16). Here, n must be an integer. If $n = 1$, then $p_e - p = 0$ and we obtain the initial, no-load condition. As the transmural pressure $p_e - p$ is gradually increased, the cylinder becomes unstable for the first time when $n = 2$, at which the pressure equals the *critical pressure of buckling*:

$$(p_e - p)_{cr} = \frac{3EI}{R^3} = \frac{Eh^3}{4(1 - v^2)R^3}. \tag{21}$$

The corresponding shape of the buckled cross section is elliptical.

Problems

4.4 Let w be the radial displacement of the cross section of a circular cylinder as illustrated in Fig. 4.3:2. Derive an expression for the curvature of the deformed cylinder, $\varkappa$, in terms of w. It is simpler to use polar coordinates and express the radius vector $\rho = R + w$ as a function of the polar angle θ. Simplify the expression when $w \ll R$. Then use Eqs. (7), (10), (16), (18), and $n = 2$ to show that the deformed cross section is elliptical.

4.5 Discuss the deformation patterns corresponding to $n = 3$.

4.6 What is the compressive stress in the tube wall at the critical buckling condition?

4.7 Equation (6) of Sec. 3.8, $h\langle\sigma_\theta\rangle = p_i r_i - p_o r_o$, gives the average value of the circumferential stress σ_θ in terms of the external and internal pressures and radii, (p_o, p_i), and (r_o, r_i) respectively. Apply this formula to the femeral artery, the arterioles, capillaries, and venules. Use the data for h, r_0, r_i from Table 3.1:1, and p_i above atmospheric from Figs. 5.3:4 or 5.3:5. Assume the external pressure p_0 to be atmospheric (a compressive stress of about 1.013×10^5 Nm^{-2} or 1 kgf/cm^2). Show that the mean circumferential stress σ_θ is negative (compressive).

If both the external and internal pressures acting on a circular cylindrical tube are atmospheric, then the circumferential stress σ_θ is, of course, compressive and

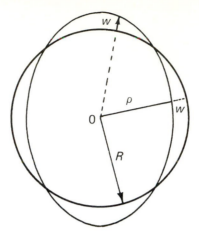

Figure 4.3:2 A circular cylinder deformed. The radial displacement w is shown.

equal to the atmospheric pressure. Would this compressive stress cause instability of the blood vessel?

Cells grown under atmospheric pressure are subjected to a compressive stress. Cells grown in deep sea are subjected to very high compressive stress. Is their stability affected?

These considerations show that a uniform hydrostatic pressure has no influence on the stability of a structure. Straightforward as it is, this point was subjected to considerable debate in the literature of 1960's.

Stability of Thin Ring under External Pressure

The foregoing reasoning applies equally well to a thin ring if E' were replaced by E, and if I were regarded as the moment of inertia of the cross section of the ring and p_e the external thrust per unit length applied to the ring. The critical value of the thrust that would cause collapse of the ring is then

$$p_e = \frac{3EI}{R^3}. \tag{22}$$

Post-buckling Behavior of Uniform Circular Tube

So far we have considered the critical conditions of buckling. If the external pressure exceeds the critical value given by Eq. (21), large deformations of the tube will occur—which are referred to as *post-buckling modes*. To determine these modes, Eqs. (1), (5), (8)–(10) must be integrated with the boundary conditions that the moment, shear, stress resultant, and curvature must be single-valued and continuous, so that when the arc length s becomes $2\pi R$,

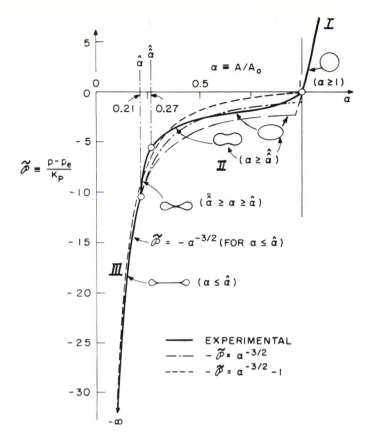

Figure 4.3:3 Behavior of a collapsible tube. Dimensionless transmural pressure difference, $\tilde{p}$, versus dimensionless area ratio, α. Solid curve shows a typical experimental curve for thin-walled latex tube, and adjacent to it, typical cross-sectional shapes for the different ranges of α. Dot–dash curve represents Eq. (8), coincides with solid curve for $\alpha < \hat{\alpha}$. Dashed curve represents Eq. (10). Curve with long dashes represents the theoretical result given by Flaherty *et al* for cylinders whose cross-sections are perfectly circular when $\tilde{p} = 0$. Point contact occurs at $\alpha = \overset{\approx}{\alpha}$, and line contact occurs at $\alpha = \hat{\alpha}$. From Shapiro (1977), by permission.

the values of M, Q, N, ξ at $s = 2\pi R$ must be equal to their values at $s = 0$. A condition of symmetry may be imposed so that $d\xi/ds$ and Q vanish at $s = 0$ and $2\pi R$.

It can be proved that these equations have a nontrivial solution (i.e., one with $\xi \not\equiv 0$) for every value of $p_e - p$ greater than the critical value given by Eq. (21), and for some $n \geq 2$. The solution obtained by Flaherty et al. (1972), by numerical integration on a computer, is shown by the dashed curve in Fig. 4.3:3. Of great interest is the relationship between the cross-sectional area of the tube in the post-buckling modes and the pressure difference $p - p_e$. Figure 4.3:3 shows this relationship expressed in nondimensional variables:

$$\tilde{p} = \frac{p - p_e}{(E'I/R^3)} \quad \text{and} \quad \alpha = \frac{A}{\pi R^2}. \tag{23}$$

The denominators in $\tilde{p}$ and α are also written as K_P and A_0 respectively. The dashed curve in this figure refers to initially perfectly circular cylinders. These cylinders will not buckle for $\tilde{p}$ above -3. Buckling starts at $\tilde{p} = -3$. For $\tilde{p} < -3$, post-buckling, the cross-sectional area decreases rapidly with decreasing $\tilde{p}$ until the opposite sides of the tube touch. The buckling patterns are illustrated in Fig. 4.3:4. Upon further increase in external pressure, the contact area increases and the open portion of the cross section is reduced in size but remains similar in shape. For this "self-similar" type of deformation Flaherty et al. obtained the relationship

$$-\tilde{p} = \alpha^{-3/2}. \tag{24}$$

The dashed curve shown in Fig. 4.3:3 is the relationship obtained for the mode $n = 2$. The mode $n = 3$ can occur when $\tilde{p} \leq -8$. At a sufficently large negative value of $\tilde{p}$ the opposite sides of the tube touch also in the $n = 3$ mode, and the same self-similar solution described by Eq. (24) holds. Without special precaution to prevent the $n = 2$ mode from occurring, however, the modes $n \geq 3$ cannot be realized.

The solid curve in Fig. 4.3:3 represents experimental results reported by Shapiro (1977). The other two curves in the figure represent two empirical formulas proposed by Shapiro (see Eqs. (8) and (10) of Sec. 4.4). These curves apply to cylinders whose cross sections are elliptical in the unloaded condition.

Effect of Lateral Support

In the analysis presented so far, the tube remains cylindrical (though not circular after buckling) because it is assumed that there is no lateral support. For a tube of finite length, the effect of lateral support on the stability can be very great. The critical pressure can be increased greatly by introducing reinforcing rings. Consider a tube *simple supported* at the ends, where the deflection and bending moments vanish. The analytical results in this case can be expressed in terms of two parameters, ϕ and λ:

$$\phi = \frac{Rp_{cr}(1 - v^2)}{Eh}, \quad \lambda = \frac{h^2}{12R^2}. \tag{25}$$

See Flügge (1960), or Timoshenko and Gere (1961). Figure 4.3:5 shows the relationship of ϕ to the ratio of the length L between supports and the tube

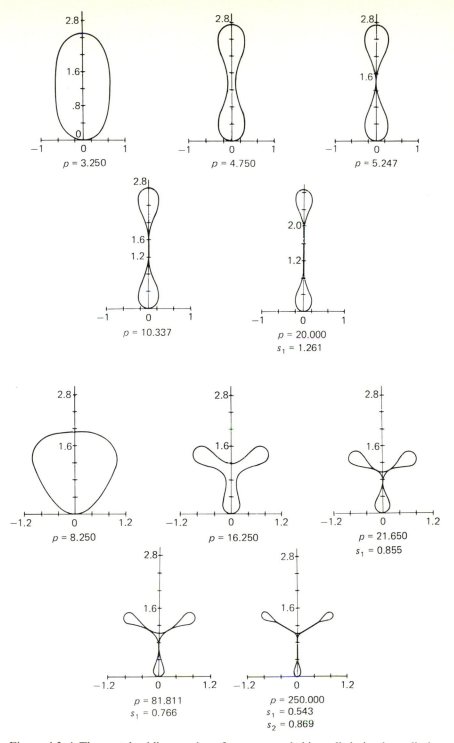

Figure 4.3:4 The post-buckling modes of unsupported thin-walled circular cylinder subjected to uniform external pressure as computed by Flaherty et al. (1972). The curves are the deformed cross-sectional shape of the cylinder. Reproduced by permission.

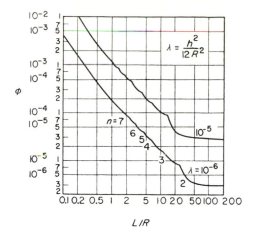

Figure 4.3:5 The critical buckling condition of a thin-walled circular cylinder of length L simply supported at both ends, and subjected to uniform external pressure. The critical pressure p_{cr} is contained in the parameter ϕ which is the ordinate. The abscissa is the ratio L/R. R is the cylinder radius. n is the number of waves around the circumference. From Timoshenko, S. (1936) *Theory of Elastic Stability*. McGraw–Hill, New York, by permission.

radius R, for two values of λ. The value of n in this figure is the number of circumferential waves similar to n in Eq. (18), resulting in a deformation described by Eq. (16).

Effects of Axial Thrust, Initial Imperfections, and Material Nonlinearity

Thin cylinder stability is also very sensitive to axial thrust and initial imperfections. These effects have been studied quite thoroughly because of their importance to engineering. For a critical review see Fung and Sechler (1960, 1974).

The application of these engineering studies to physiology may be questioned on the ground that biological tissues do not obey Hooke's law. For example, in Chapter 8 of *Biomechanics* (Fung, 1981), we have shown that the Young's modulus E of an artery increases with increasing stress level. A full analysis of cylindrical shell instability for a nonlinear pseudoelastic material is very complicated. For a rough estimation, it is reasonable to use the incremental modulus E at the prevailing state of stress in formulas such as Eq. (2) to obtain the critical pressure for buckling.

4.4 Vessels of Naturally Elliptic Cross Section

If the cross section of the tube is elliptical in the stress-free state, then under increasing external pressure the tube will be compressed and distorted in a sequence of shapes similar to those sketched in Fig. 4.4:1. At first, the eccentricity will be increased. Then the middle portion will be bent inward. Eventually, the opposite walls will touch, compressed flat in the middle, leaving only the corners open.

The basic equations governing the bending of noncircular tubes subjected to external pressure are similar to those of the preceding section. Equations (1) through (9) of Sec. 4.3 remain valid, but Eq. (10) of Sec. 4.3 is no longer true. The initial curvature, $\varkappa_o$, is not a constant, but varies around the circumference. An example is

$$\varkappa_o = \frac{1}{R}\left(1 + \varepsilon\cos\frac{s}{R}\right),\tag{1}$$

where s is the arc length measured on the middle surface of the vessel wall in the circumferential direction as it is in Sec. 4.3, Fig. 4.3:1, R is the radius of an equivalent circle which has the same circumference as the noncircular tube cross section, and ε ($\ll 1$) is a small parameter. If this is used in Eqs. (8) and (9) of Sec. 4.3, we obtain the basic equations

$$E'I\frac{d^2\xi}{ds^2} + N\left[\xi + \frac{1}{R}\left(1 + \varepsilon\cos\frac{s}{R}\right)\right] = p_e - p,\tag{2}$$

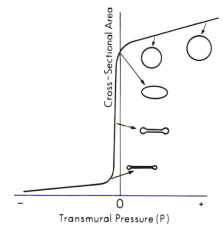

Figure 4.4:1 A sequence of cross-sectional shapes that occur as a naturally elliptic cylinder is subjected to gradually increasing external pressure. At first the eccentricity is increased. Then it buckles. The successive post-buckling modes become very similar to those of Fig. 4.3:4.

$$\frac{dN}{ds} + Q\left[\xi + \frac{1}{R}\left(1 + \varepsilon\cos\frac{s}{R}\right)\right] = 0, \tag{3}$$

whereas Eqs. (1) and (5) of Sec. 4.3 remain valid:

$$Q = -\frac{dM}{ds} = -E'I\frac{d\xi}{ds}. \tag{4}$$

Combining Eqs. (3) and (4) yields

$$\frac{dN}{ds} - E'I\left[\xi + \frac{1}{R}\left(1 + \varepsilon\cos\frac{s}{R}\right)\right]\frac{d\xi}{ds} = 0. \tag{5}$$

Equations (2)–(4), or (2) and (5) are sets of ordinary differential equations to be solved together with the boundary conditions that ξ, N, and Q are periodic:

$$\xi(2\pi R) = \xi(0), \qquad N(2\pi R) = N(0), \qquad Q(2\pi R) = Q(0), \tag{6}$$

and a condition of symmetry:

$$\frac{d\xi}{ds} = 0, \qquad Q = 0 \qquad \text{at } s = 0. \tag{7}$$

The analysis is more complex than that of the preceding section because ξ may not be considered infinitesimal in the present problem. There is no simple way to find analytic solutions, but a numerical solution is feasible.

Experimental results on a latex rubber tubing and a vein are shown in Fig. 4.3:3 and 4.4:2, respectively. In neither of these two examples was the geometry of the tubing in its natural, unstressed state accurately recorded. Hence, the data were not sufficient to check the theory. The effective Young's modulus in compression, and the bending rigidity $E'I$ of the vein are also unknown. The general trend, however, can be understood. When the internal pressure exceeds the external pressure, $p - p_e > 0$, the tube cross-sectional area increases with increasing $p - p_e$. When the external pressure exceeds the internal pressure, $p - p_e < 0$, the cross-sectional area decreases rapidly with increasing external pressure.

In Fig. 4.3:3, a chain–dot curve

$$-\tilde{p} = \alpha^{-n}, \qquad n = \tfrac{3}{2}, \tag{8}$$

is shown. This is an extension of Eq. (24) of Sec. 4.3 beyond the range $(\alpha \leq \hat{\alpha})$ in which the equation was originally derived. Here

$$\tilde{p} = (p - p_e)\frac{R^3}{E'I}, \qquad \alpha = \frac{A}{A_o}, \tag{9}$$

where A_o is the cross-sectional area in the unstressed state. Another curve indicated by short dashes is Shapiro's (1977) approximate formula

$$-\tilde{p} = \alpha^{-n} - 1; \qquad n = \tfrac{3}{2}. \tag{10}$$

It has the merit that it passes through the point $\tilde{p} = 0$, $\alpha = 1$.

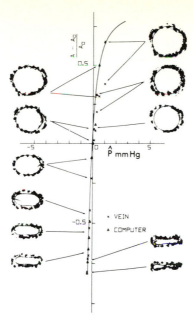

Figure 4.4:2 Relationship between transmural pressure and cross-sectional area of dog's vena cava. Experimental results from Moreno et al. (1970). Reproduced by permission.

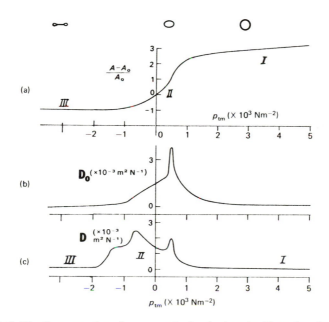

Figure 4.4:3 Elastic properties of a segment of a dog's vein. Here the abscissa is the transmural pressure measured in units of KPa (each KPa $\doteq$ 10 cm H_2O). The ordinate of (a) is $\alpha - 1$, i.e., the change of area $A - A_o$ divided by the area at zero transmural pressure. The ordinate of (b) is $D_o = (1/A_o)(dA/d(p - p_e))$, in units of KPa^{-1}. The ordinate of (c) is the distensibility D defined in Eq. (11). The difference between (b) and (c) shows that D_o is not a good approximation of D. Data from Moreno et al. (1970) and Attinger (1969). Adapted from Caro et al. (1978), by permission.

The most important feature of these curves relevant to the analysis of flow is the *distensibility* of the elastic tube defined by

$$D = \frac{1}{A} \frac{dA}{d(p - p_e)}. \tag{11}$$

Here, A is the cross-sectional area; $p - p_e$ is the transmural pressure. The variation of D with pressure $p - p_e$ for a vein is plotted in Fig. 4.4:3(c). The curve can be divided into three zones: in I and III, the distensibility is small; in II it is larger. It is expected that the interaction between a flowing fluid and the wall deformation will be most vigorous in zone II. That this is indeed the case will be seen in Secs. 4.6 and 4.8.

We could also mark the zones I, II, III on Figs. 4.4:2, and 4.3:3. With regard to the points of demarcation between the zones, there is a difference between those vessels that are naturally circular and those that are naturally elliptic or otherwise nonaxisymmetric. In all cases, there is no clearly definable point of demarcation between zone II and zone III, (in other words, the division is arbitrary). For the naturally elliptic or otherwise nonaxisymmetric vessels (as in Fig. 4.4:2, and also for the solid curve in Fig. 4.3:3), neither is there a definable point of demarcation between zone I and zone II. But, for a naturally circular cylindrical tube, as it is shown by the long-dashed curve in Fig. 4.3:3, there is a well-defined critical buckling point, and that point marks a sharp change of distensibility between zone I and zone II. This is clearly seen from the sudden change of the slope of the long-dashed curve for a circular cylinder at the critical buckling point in Fig. 4.3:3. For circular cylindrical tubes with very thin walls (with very small wall thickness to radius ratio, say, <0.01), the buckling load is so small that it is not too far wrong to take the point of demarcation between zone I and zone II at $p - p_e = 0$.

4.5 Steady Flow in Collapsible Tubes

Blood flow in veins is similar to that in the arteries except that (a) veins often have valves which prevent reversed flow, and (b) sometimes the transmural pressure in the vein is negative, i.e., the blood pressure in the vein is smaller than the pressure external to the vein. Transmural pressure in the arteries can be negative too, for example, in arteries in an arm under a pressure cuff in blood pressure measurement by means of Korotkow sound, but normally the arterial blood pressure is so high that this does not occur. In the vein, the blood pressure is low and the transmural pressure can become negative by hydraulic gradient, muscle action, or for other reasons. For example, the pressure in the vena cava is nearly atmospheric. If we raise our hands above our heads, the weight of blood in the vein will reduce the hydrostatic pressure in the veins of the hands by 60 or 70 cm

H_2O below that of the vena cava. If the tissue pressure outside the veins remains nearly atmospheric, then the transmural pressure would be negative 60 or 70 cm H_2O.

The feature introduced by the negative transmural pressure is the great distensibility of the vessel in a certain range of pressure. This is evident from Fig. 4.4:3 in region II. It is also seen in Figs. 4.4:2, and 4.3:3. Now the phase velocity of propagation of waves of small amplitude is (see Chap. 3, Sec. 3.8, Eq. (4))

$$c = \left(\frac{A}{\rho} \frac{dp}{dA} \right)^{1/2} = \left[\frac{A}{\rho} \frac{d(p - p_e)}{dA} \right]^{1/2} \tag{1}$$

If $Ad(p - p_e)/dA$ is low, c is small and the blood flow velocity u may be comparable with, or even larger than, c. This reminds us of transonic and supersonic flow in gas dynamics. Indeed, the analogy with gas dynamics and with channel flow of a liquid with a free surface is very close. To see this, consider a one-dimensional, unsteady, frictionless flow in a collapsible tube, a gas flow in a rigid tube, and a liquid flow in a uniform, horizontal open channel. The equation of motion is identical for each of the three cases:

$$\frac{\partial u}{\partial t} + u \frac{\partial u}{\partial x} = -\frac{1}{\rho} \frac{\partial p}{\partial x}, \tag{2}$$

where ρ is the mass density of the fluid, p is the pressure in the flowing fluid, u is the velocity, t is time, and x is longitudinal distance. The equations of continuity are

For a collapsible tube:
$$\frac{\partial A}{\partial t} + \frac{\partial}{\partial x} (Au) = 0; \tag{3a}$$

For the gas flow:
$$\frac{\partial \rho}{\partial t} + \frac{\partial}{\partial x} (\rho u) = 0; \tag{3b}$$

For the channel flow:
$$\frac{\partial h}{\partial t} + \frac{\partial}{\partial x} (hu) = 0. \tag{3c}$$

Here A is the cross-sectional area in the first case, ρ is the mass density in the second case, and h is the height of the free surface above the bottom in the third case. The phase velocity of propagation of small perturbations, c, is, in the three cases:

$$c^2 = \frac{A}{\rho} \frac{d(p - p_e)}{dA}; \tag{4a}$$

$$c^2 = \left(\frac{dp}{d\rho} \right) \quad \text{at constant entropy}; \tag{4b}$$

$$c^2 = \frac{h}{\rho} \frac{dp}{dh} = gh; \tag{4c}$$

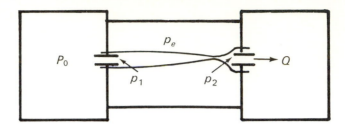

Figure 4.5:1 An experimental arrangement in which a collapsible tube is used as a "Starling resistor." The tube connects a reservoir at left which has a pressure p_0 to a reservoir at right at a lower pressure.

where g is the gravitational acceleration. Thus the analog is seen. Those readers who are familiar with gas dynamics may recall the shock waves, the supersonic wind tunnel, the Laval nozzle for steam turbine, the convergent section to accelerate the fluid in subsonic regime, the sonic throat, and the divergent section to accelerate the fluid in supersonic regime. Those familiar with the open channel flow may recall the flow over a dam, and the hydraulic jump. One could anticipate the existence of analogous phenomena in blood flow in collapsible vessels. One anticipates also, of course, that similar phenomena occur in air flow in the airways, Korotkov sound in arteries, urine flow in urethra, etc.

Flow Limitation

Consider a simple example of flow of a nonviscous liquid in a collapsible tube connected to two reservoirs (see Fig. 4.5:1). The tube is mounted by rigid connections to the reservoirs, and is enclosed in a chamber containing air or water at an adjustable pressure p_e. Such a tube is known as a "Starling resistor," which was first used by the English physiologist Starling (1866–1927) in his heart–lung machine.

Consider flow in such a tube. The flow depends on the inlet pressure p_1, the outlet pressure p_2, and the external pressure p_e, or, more precisely, on the pressure differences $p_1 - p_e, p_2 - p_e$, because the tube cross section depends only on the transmural pressure. If $p_1 - p_e$ were fixed and $p_2 - p_e$ were gradually decreased, the velocity of flow would increase, but in the meantime the tube cross-sectional area would decrease. The flow, being a product of velocity and cross-sectional area, would increase at first, but eventually may be limited.

What happens in such a tube may be illustrated by an example. Figure 4.5:2 shows the result of Conrad's (1969) experiment with the flow of water in a Starling resistor whose outlet was connected to a flow resistor and then exposed to the atmosphere. The chamber pressure p_e was fixed at 3.3 kPa

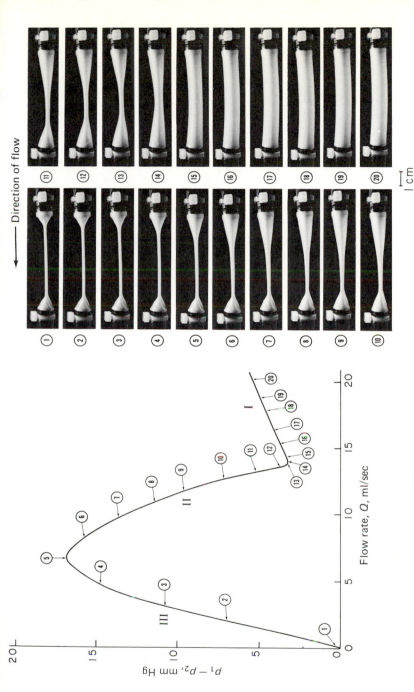

Figure 4.5:2 (a) Pressure–flow relationship in a Starling resistor. Ordinate: $p_1 - p_2$ or $(p_1 - p_e) - (p_2 - p_e)$. Abscissa: flow rate, Q. For this figure, $p_e = 3.3 \times 10^3 \text{ N m}^{-2}$ was kept fixed. The outlet of the tube was connected to a flow resistance and then exposed to the atmosphere. The resistance R was kept constant. The inlet transmural pressure $p_1 - p_e$ is equal to $Q \cdot R$ plus atmospheric pressure. The exit pressure p_2 is equal to $Q \cdot R$ plus atmospheric pressure. (b) Side views of the collapsible segment of tubing at different stages of experiment. Flow from right to left. Numbers correspond to the numbered positions on the graph in (a). From Conrad (1969). © 1969 IEEE. Reproduced by permission.

(~ 33 cm H_2O). The inlet pressure p_1 was varied. The pressure–flow relationship is shown in Fig. 4.5:2(a). If self-excited oscillations (flutter) occurred, the flow was averaged over time. The numbers indicated on the curve of Fig. 4.5:2(a) correspond to the photographs shown in Fig. 4.5:2(b), which are a sequence of side views of the tube at successive stages in the experiment. For these photographs, the flow was from right to left.

The pressure–flow relationship may be separated into three regimes, I, II, III, as marked on Fig. 4.5:2(a). (1) In regime I, both $p_1 - p_e$ and $p_2 - p_e$ are positive, there is no buckling of the tube, and the flow Q is essentially proportional to $p_1 - p_2$. (2) In regime II, $p_1 - p_e > 0$, $p_2 - p_e < 0$, buckling occurs towards the outlet, the tube cross section changes rapidly as the transmural pressure falls, and the tube may flutter (see Sec. 4.8). (3) In regime III, $p_1 - p_e < 0$, $p_2 - p_e < 0$, the tube is buckled, and the cross section becomes dumbbell shaped as described in Secs. 4.3 and 4.4. The flow rate is small, but again roughly proportional to the pressure drop $p_1 - p_2$.

The most fascinating part is regime II, in which the great distensibility of a collapsed tube takes effect. The tube starts to buckle at the downstream end at a condition corresponding to panel 14 in Fig. 4.5:2(b), or point 14 in Fig. 4.5:2(a). As flow is further reduced, the pressure p_2 decreases because, in Conrad's experimental set up, p_2 is equal to atmospheric pressure plus Q times the resistance, which is fixed, so that p_2 decreases if Q decreases. When $p_2 - p_e$ decreases, the buckle deepens, the resistance to flow increases, and the pressure drop required to maintain the rate of flow increases. The progressive collapse of the tube can be seen from panels 14 to 5 of Fig. 4.5:2(b). At point 5, virtually the whole tube is collapsed; and p_1 is approximately equal to p_e.

In a different experiment by Holt (1969), p_1 and p_e ($p_1 > p_e$) were fixed while the downstream pressure p_2 was varied. Then, as it can be seen from Fig. 4.5:3, the flow increased as $p_2 - p_e$ was decreased as long as $p_2 - p_e$ was

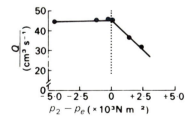

Figure 4.5:3 An illustration of flow limitation in a thin-walled rubber tube used as a Starling resistor. The upstream transmural pressure $p_1 - p_e$ was fixed, whereas the downstream transmural pressure $p_2 - p_e$ was continuously decreased. The mean flow rate was measured. In case of flutter, the flow was averaged over times. When $p_2 - p_e$ is negative, the flow rate is independent of $p_2 - p_e$. From Holt (1969), © 1969 IEEE. Reproduced by permission.

positive. But, when $p_2 - p_e$ was negative, the flow was practically independent of the values of $p_2 - p_e$: No increase of flow could be obtained by lowering the pressure at the exit end. A condition of *flow limitation* was reached.

The tube often flutters in regime II. The unsteady condition will be discussed in Sec. 4.8.

Figure 4.5:3 illustrates flow limitation in a collapsible tube. A simplified analysis of this situation is instructive. Consider laminar flow in an elastic tube at a large Reynolds number so that Bernoulli's equation holds:

$$p + \tfrac{1}{2}\rho u^2 = p_0, \tag{5}$$

where p_0 is the stagnation pressure, p is the static pressure, ρ is fluid mass density, and u is velocity. The volume flow rate, Q is

$$Q = Au = A\sqrt{\tfrac{2}{\rho}(p_0 - p)} = A\sqrt{\tfrac{2}{\rho}[(p_0 - p_e) - (p - p_e)]}. \tag{6}$$

A is the cross-sectional area which is a function of $p - p_e$. Although p varies with distance down the tube, Q remains constant, of course. Now if $p_0 - p_e$ is fixed and we change $p - p_e$, then the rate of change of Q is

$$\frac{dQ}{d(p - p_e)} = -\frac{A}{\rho}\left\{\frac{2}{\rho}\left[(p_0 - p_e) - (p - p_e)\right]\right\}^{-1/2} + \frac{dA}{d(p - p_e)}\left\{ \right\}^{1/2}$$

$$= -\frac{A}{\rho u} + \frac{dA}{d(p - p_e)}u = -\frac{A}{\rho u} + \left[\frac{\rho}{A}\frac{dA}{d(p - p_e)}\right]\frac{A}{\rho}u.$$

The factor in the bracket in the last term is $1/c^2$, according to Eq. (1). Hence we obtain

$$\frac{dQ}{d(p - p_e)} = \frac{A}{\rho u}\left(\frac{u^2}{c^2} - 1\right). \tag{7}$$

Thus the flow will increase with decreasing $p - p_e$ only if $u < c$. A maximum, i.e., a limitation, is reached when $u = c$. If $u > c$, then further decrease in $p - p_e$ decreases the flow! Thus $u = c$ signifies flow limitation, and the section where $u = c$ is analogous to the sonic section in the Laval nozzle or supersonic wind tunnel. It *chokes* the flow. The ratio

$$S = \frac{u}{c}, \tag{8}$$

is called the *speed index* by Shapiro (1977), and it plays a central role in liquid flow through a collapsible tube as the Mach number does in gas dynamics.

The maximum flow is given by Eq. (6) with $u = c$, and is $Q_{max} = Ac$. If the pressure–area relationship follows Eq. (8) or (10) of Sec. 4.4, then we have

$$c = \left[\frac{A}{\rho}\frac{d(p-p_e)}{dA}\right]^{1/2} = \left[\frac{A}{\rho}\frac{E'I}{R^3}\frac{d\tilde{p}}{d\alpha}\frac{1}{A_o}\right]^{1/2}$$

$$= \left[\frac{1}{\rho}\frac{E'I}{R^3}n\alpha^{-n}\right]^{1/2} = c_o\alpha^{-n/2}, \qquad \left(c_o = \sqrt{\frac{E'In}{\rho R^3}}\right), \tag{9}$$

where c_o is the value of c when $\alpha = 1$, i.e., when the tube is in the unstressed state, with $p - p_e = 0$. A_o is the cross sectional area at the unstressed state. Hence we have

$$\frac{Q_{\max}}{A_o c_o} = \frac{Ac}{A_o c_o} = \alpha^{1-n/2}. \tag{10}$$

If we use Eq. (8) or Eq. (10) of Sec. 4.4 as an approximation, we obtain, respectively,

$$\frac{Q_{\max}}{A_o c_o} = (-\tilde{p})^{(n-2)/2n} \qquad \text{or} \qquad (1 - \tilde{p})^{(n-2)/2n}. \tag{11}$$

In either case it is seen that the maximum flow rate depends solely upon the local transmural pressure difference at the "sonic" section, where $S = 1$, irrespective of the upstream driving pressure.

This analysis is based on the assumption that the frictional loss is negligible, and that the tube cross sectional area depends solely on the transmural pressure. Thus the viscosity of the fluid and longitudinal tension in the tube are neglected. If these assumptions do not apply, as in the lung, then the concludions are not valid. Flow limitation can still occur, however, by some other mechanisms which will be discussed in Sec. 4.10 and 6.13.

Problem

4.8 If the tube has a uniform cross section in the unstressed state, then $-\tilde{p}$ must be the largest at the outlet section. Show that if $n = 2$, the maximum possible flow rate does not depend on $-\tilde{p}$ at all. If $n = \frac{3}{2}$, determine $Q_{\max}/A_o c_o$ for $-\tilde{p} = 5$, 10, and 15.

General One-Dimensional Steady Flow

Shapiro (1977) presented a full analysis of one-dimensional steady flow through a collapsible tube, including considerations of friction, gravity, variations of external pressure, or of muscle tone. He considers the external pressure, p_e, the initial cross-sectional area of the tube, A_o, the radius R, and the bending rigidity $E'I$, as functions of x, the distance along the tube. He demonstrated the crucial role of the speed index S. For example, in a naturally uniform tube, when $S < 1$, friction causes the area and pressure to decrease in the downstream direction, and the velocity to increase. In contrast, when $S > 1$, the area and pressure will increase along the tube.

while the velocity decreases—exactly opposite to the former case. In general, whatever may be the effect of certain changes of A_o, p_e, etc., in a "sub-critical" flow ($S < 1$), the effect is of opposite sign in a "supercritical" flow ($S > 1$). As a consequence, a variety of unexpected and remarkable features can be found. Some of these may be counter to intuition. As an illustration, consider a small change of external pressure, p_e, while all other independent variables (A_o, friction, elasticity, etc.) are held constant. If p_e increases, both A and p decrease in subcritical flow, but they increase in supercritical flow!

The full analysis is intriguing, but quite complex. Let us quote here only Shapiro's examples (Fig. 4.5:4) of situations in which a continuous passage

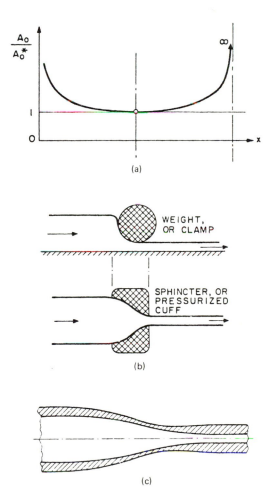

Figure 4.5:4 Several examples given by Shapiro (1977) in which a smooth transition through the critical condition $S = 1$ is possible. See text. Reproduced from Shapiro (1977), by permission.

of flow in regime $S < 1$ through $S = 1$ into $S > 1$ might occur. The pressure–area law given by Eq. (10) of Sec. 4.4 is assumed. Figure 4.5:4(a) shows the case with pure variation of initial cross sectional area, A_o, along the tube axis. A_o^* denotes the area at the location where $S = 1$. Assuming that the transition is from subcritical to supercritical flow, then the pressure decreases continuously in the axial direction, and the area of the actual, deformed cross section, A, would decrease continuously in the axial direction also (not shown in the figure). Figure 4.5:4(b) shows transition caused by a clamp, a cuff, or a sphinctor, through their effect on changing the external pressure, p_e. Both the fluid pressure and the area decrease continuously in the axial direction. $S = 1$ occurs at a point in the region where a sharp constriction exists. Figure 4.5:4(c) shows the case with a pure change in bending stiffness parameter $E'I/R^3$. This is physically realizable in a tube with variable wall thickness. Both the cross-sectional area and the pressure decrease continuously through the transition. Details can be found in Shapiro (1977).

In general it is not possible to have supercritical flow indefinitely along an originally uniform tube. Hence, one must consider transition from supercritical flow back to subcritical flow. In the analogous case of supersonic wind tunnel, this is done by a shock wave. Shapiro showed that in an elastic tube the shock wave may be very thick (several tube diameters), and that it is possible to have a transition from one supercritical flow to another supercritical flow through a shock wave (unlike the shock wave in gas dynamics). Later studies have shown that for the shock recovery problem the one-dimensional flow approximation is inadequate. For a realistic solution it is necessary to consider three-dimensional flow, taking the distortion of cross sections and nonaxisymmetric flow into consideration.

4.6 Unsteady Flow in Veins

Flow in veins is unsteady because of a variety of reasons, including the pulsatile action of the heart and the transient actions of the muscles. The heart affects the end conditions, the muscle affects the boundary conditions along the vessel, and a variety of other factors may affect the internal and external pressures in the vessel. As illustrated in Fig. 4.6:1, if the venous system is idealized as a system of pipes, then the right atrium controls the end condition at $x = L$, the capillaries control the pressure at $x = O$, while the muscles, body fluids, and neighboring organs control the pressure external to the veins. The muscle action may be indirect, as it happens when one uses abdominal muscles and the diaphragm to control the pressure surrounding the vena cava, or it may be direct, as it happens in the venules and veins in the muscles of the arms and legs. Other causes of transient changes could arise from breathing, exercise, change of posture, flying or diving, etc. In all cases, the valves in the vein act to stop reversed flow, but offer very little resistance to forward flow. These valves are very flexible,

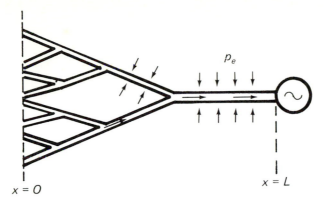

Figure 4.6:1 A schematic drawing of the venous system.

tenuous membranes. The hydrodynamic principles of valve action in the vein are the same as those in the heart, which are discussed in Sec. 2.5.

Pulsatile Flow into the Right Heart

The venous tree begins at the venules and ends at the right atrium. The periodic fluctuation of pressure in the right atrium is shown in Fig. 2.4:2 on p. 35, (the fifth curve from the top). In the right atrium of man, the mean pressure (averaged over time) is of the order of 3 cm H_2O, and the amplitude of pressure fluctuations is of the order of 7 cm H_2O. In the venules, the mean pressure is of the order of 25 cm H_2O, and the amplitude of fluctuations is of the order of 4 cm H_2O. The fluctuations in the pressure and flow waves in the venules are, however, not in phase with the pressure and flow waves at the right atrium, owing to wave propagation, reflection at branching points, and attenuation due to viscoelasticity of blood vessels. The situation is rather analogous to the flow of a river into an ocean. As the influence of the tide does not extend too far upstream, so the influence of the pressure fluctuations in the right atrium dies out gradually in the veins. This is illustrated in Fig. 4.6:2 which shows the pressure waves at four sites along the venous tree of a man. The big disturbance in trace (c) is almost certainly due to the presence of a valve in the vein as the catheter was gradually withdrawn through it. The wave form in the superior vena cava is almost identical to that in the right atrium. The wave in the sub-clavian vein shows a phase lag from that in the vena cava, consistent with the propagation of disturbances away from the source.

  The velocity waves in the venae cavae of man are presented in Fig. 4.6:3, which shows that in each cardiac cycle there are two main oscillations of flow velocity, which are out of phase with the pressure oscillations in the right atrium.

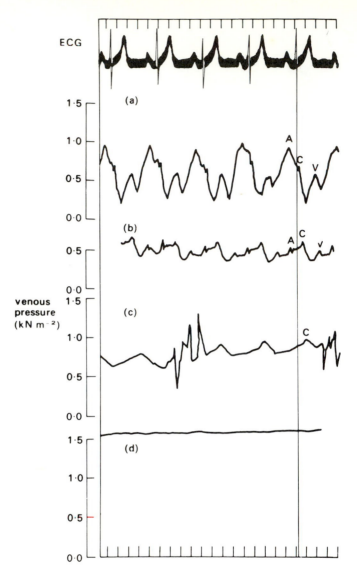

Figure 4.6:2 Pressure fluctuations in human venous system. From top to bottom: (a) the superior vena cava, (b) the subclavian vein, (c) the axillary vein, (d) the brachial vein. The pressures were measured sequentially with a single catheter. The values were relative to the atmosphere. The subject was supine so that all sites were at approximately the same level. The big disturbance in (c), the axillary vein is almost certain due to withdrawing the catheter through a valve. From Caro et al. (1978), and by courtesy of Dr. G. Miller, Brompton Hospital, London. Reproduced from Caro et al. (1978), by permission.

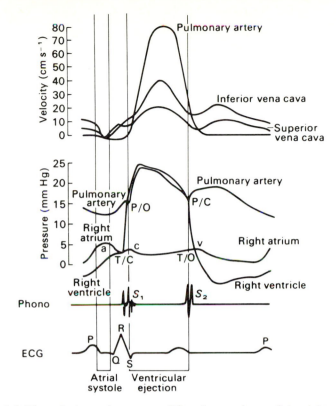

Figure 4.6:3 The velocity and pressure of flow into and out of the right atrium, co-ordinated with phonocardiogram and ECG. T/C indicates the closure of tricuspid valve; P/O: pulmonary valve open; P/C: pulmonary valve closed; T/O: tricuspid valve open. From Wexler et al. (1968). Reproduced by permission of the American Heart Association.

The pressure pulse in the jugular vein is presented in Fig. 2.4:2. The pulsation in the jugular vein is visible to the naked eye and palpable by the finger, and hence is used clinically to detect any abnormalities.

Propagation of Progressive Waves in Veins

Studies of propagation of progressive waves in veins are few. Some predictable features may be gathered from the principles discussed in Chap. 3, see Problems 4.9–11 at the end of this section.

Experiments done by Anliker et al. (1969) on anesthetized dogs reveal a number of interesting features of venous blood flow. They used high-frequency sinusoidal pressure waves of small amplitude generated either by a small sinusoidal pump introduced into the abdominal venae cavae, or by an electromagnetic wave generator attached to the vein's outer wall. A short train of high-frequency pressure waves was generated each time. Its propagation was detected by two pressure sensors mounted on catheter tips and placed in the vein at a known distance apart (from 4 to 8 cm). The high frequency and short wave train were used to avoid distortions due to wave reflection. The small amplitude was used to assure linearity of the system. Their results on the wave speed as a function of transmural pressure are shown in Fig. 4.6:4. The different symbols represent different frequencies of the waves. It is seen that the wave speed varies from 2 m sec^{-1} to 6 m sec^{-1} over the applied pressure range, and that the wave speed increases with increasing transmural pressure, reflecting the rapid increase in the incremental Young's modulus of the vessel wall as well as the change in the ratio of vessel wall thickness to diameter (see Eq. (2) *infra*). The wave speed at any given transmural pressure is essentially independent of the frequency of oscillation; i.e., the system is nondispersive in this frequency range.

The results of Anliker et al. on the attenuation of the wave amplitude with distance propagated along the vein are shown in Fig. 4.6:5. It is seen that the amplitude falls off exponentially with distance. The ratio x/λ is the distance (x) measured in units of wavelength (λ). The figure shows that the a/a_o vs x/λ relationship is almost unaffected by the frequency of the waves. In other words, the amount of attenuation *per wavelength* is almost independent of frequency in the frequency range tested. The experimental results may be expressed by the equation

$$a = a_o e^{-kx/\lambda},\tag{1}$$

in which a is the amplitude of the wave, a_o is the amplitude at $x = o$, x is the distance measured along the vessel, λ is the wavelength, and k is a constant. The value of k derived from the vena cava of the dog was found to lie in the range 1.0–2.5 (attenuation of 63–92% per wavelength), compared with the range 0.7–1.0 for the aorta.

There are at least three causes for the attenuation. One is the viscosity of the blood, but since both the Womersley number N_W and the Reynolds number N_R are quite large, the effect of blood viscosity is small. Another is the radiation or transmission to tissues or fluids surrounding the vessel, but since the experiment was performed on veins exposed to air (open chest and abdomen), this dissipation is minimal. The third cause, the viscoelasticity of the vessel wall, must be predominantly responsible for the attenuation.

The characteristic of the viscoelasticity of the vessel wall revealed by this experiment is that the attenuation per wavelength is almost independent of frequency. Translated into a statement about the energy dissipated by the vessel wall in executing sinusoidal motion, it says that the energy dissipated per cycle of oscillation is almost independent of the frequency. In other words, the energy dissipation mechanism is almost independent of strain rate. Although this was verified in this experiment only in the frequency range 20 to 100 Hz, it was found to be true also in wide frequency ranges

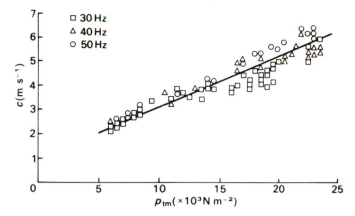

Figure 4.6:4 The speed of propagation c of short trains of sinusoidal waves of small amplitude imposed on the abdominal vena cava of a dog plotted against the transmural pressure p_{tm}. From Anliker et al. (1969). Reproduced by permission.

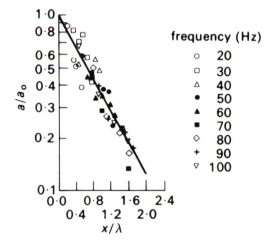

Figure 4.6:5 The attenuation of the amplitude of a short train of sinusoidal waves of small amplitude imposed on the abdominal vena cava of a dog with the distance of propagation. The ratio of the wave amplitude a, to the amplitude a_o at a fixed site is plotted against the ratio x/λ, the distance distal to the fixed site (x) divided by the wave length of the wave (λ). From Anliker et al. (1969). Reproduced by permission.

in a variety of experiments reported in *Biomechanics* (Fung, 1981). It is in keeping with a general observation that living tissues are *pseudo-elastic* (*Biomechanics*, p. 238).

Problems

4.9 Assume that a vein be circular cylindrical in the unstressed state, that its pressure–area relationship in the unbuckled state be derivable from the membrane theory, and that in the buckled state Eq. (8) or (10) of Sec. 4.4 holds. Derive an analytic expression for the distensibility of the vessel as defined by Eq. (11) of Sec. 4.4. It is well known that the Young's modulus E of a blood vessel wall varies with the stress in the wall, see Chap. 8 of *Biomechanics* (Fung, 1981). For states of the vein near buckling or post-buckling, one may use the value of E at zero stress, $p - p_e = 0$. For veins subjected to positive inflation, $p - p_e > 0$, show that the membrane theory gives the formula

$$\frac{1}{D} = \frac{Eh}{d}, \tag{2}$$

in which E is the incremental Young's modulus for circumferential stretch, h is the wall thickness, and d is the vessel diameter. Use the data given in Fig. 4.4:3, obtain an estimation of the incremental Young's modulus both for $p - p_e > 0$ and $p - p_e \leq 0$.

4.10 For progressive harmonic waves of small amplitude propagating in a cylindrical elastic tube, the wave speed c is given by the equation $c = (\rho D)^{-1/2}$, where ρ is the density of blood and D is the distensibility of the vessel. Using the values of D given in Fig. 4.4:3 and ρ about 1 g cm^{-3}, show that the wave speed in a vein varies from 5 m sec^{-1} or more at high transmural pressures, to a minimum of about 0.6 m sec^{-1} when the vein is collapsing.

4.11 If the average velocity of blood in the inferior vena cava of a dog is between 10 cm sec^{-1} and 20 cm sec^{-1}, and the diameter of the vessel is about 1 cm, what is the Reynolds number (N_R) of the flow? What is the frequency parameter or Womersley's number (N_W) at a heart rate of 2 Hz? What is the wavelength (λ) if the wave speed is 2 m sec^{-1} and frequency is 2 Hz?

Answer: N_R lies between 250 and 500. $N_W \doteq 8$. N_R and N_W are smaller in smaller veins. $\lambda \doteq 1$ m.

4.12 On the basis of N_R and N_W estimated in the preceding problem, would the flow be laminar or turbulent? How long is the entrance length for the mean flow? How thick is the oscillatory boundary layer on the vessel wall? How long is the entrance length for the unsteady flow?

Answer: Flow is laminar. Entrance length of the inferior vena cava is about 7.5–15 cm. Oscillatory boundary layer is thin. Unsteady flow entry length is about 4.5 cm.

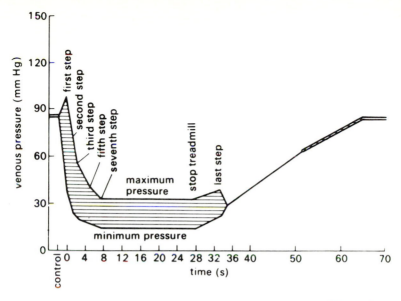

Figure 4.7:1 The change of pressure in an ankle vein of an erect subject as he stands and walks. The figure shows the maximum and minimum pressures. The subject is initially motionless, then walks, and finally again stands still. From Pollack and Wood (1949). Reproduced by permission.

4.7 Effect of Muscle Action on Venous Flow

If a vein is embedded in skeletal muscle, then the contraction of the muscle may squeeze the vein; this, in conjunction with the action of the valves in the vein, creates an interesting control of blood flow. If a man stands still, the veins in his leg are filled with blood, the hydrostatic pressure gradient must prevail, and the pressure in his ankle vein may reach, say, 85 mmHg. As he starts to walk, his muscles begin pumping the veins, which, because of their one-way valves, empty toward the heart. Segments of veins either empty or only partically fill, and the pressure drops. Measurements of ankle vein pressure were done a long time ago. Figure 4.7:1 shows the results of Pollack and Wood (1949). At first, the subject was motionless, and the pressure in the ankle was 85 mmHg. When the first step was taken, the pressure in the vein rose at first, then dropped as the muscle relaxed. With successive steps, the pressure continued to drop until it reached asymptotically a maximum of 30 mmHg and a minimum of 15 mmHg. When the walking stopped, the pressure in the vein gradually rose to its previous level.

These events can be explained easily by the squeezing and the valve actions. One may deduce that when the pressure in the vein decreased, the venous blood volume in the leg would decrease, and indeed this was verified by plethysmograph measurements. The squeezing action would be effective only if the leg motion is fast enough to keep the vein partially empty. The relevant time constant is the time it takes the microcirculation to refill the vein (about 50 sec at rest and 5 sec in exercise). If the valves were incompetent, the action would be somewhat less effective. But since the characteristic impedance of the vein closer to the heart is smaller than that closer to the microcirculation bed, squeezing of even valveless veins can produce the effect described above, that is, pumping blood into the heart.

Respiratory Maneuvers

Indirect action of muscle on venous blood flow may be illustrated by respiratory maneuvers. Any movement that reduces the thoracic pressure helps distend the thoracic vena cava. One that increases the abdominal pressure squeezes blood in the abdominal veins into the thorax and heart. Thus, in quite breathing, the enlargement of the thorax during inspiration reduces the intrathoracic pressure and causes blood to be drawn from the extrathoracic venis into the intrathoracic vessels and the heart. Expiration would have the opposite effect.

A *Mueller maneuver* refers to a deep, sustained inspiration against a closed glottis (usually used by patients taking X-ray photographs to examine blood filling in the thorax). In such a maneuver, the alveolar and the intrapleural pressures are reduced, as are the pressures in the right atrium and the thoracic vena cava. The diaphragm muscle contracts and the diaphragm is lowered, so the abdominal pressure and the pressure in the abdominal inferior vena cava is increased. Hence, upon the initiation of Mueller's maneuver, blood will be squeezed from the abdominal vena cava into the thorax, but the action will be transient. Afterwards, a steady-state limiting flow of the type discussed in Sec. 4.5 (waterfall phenomena, sluicing flow) will be established, and the flow will be independent of the downstream (right atrium) pressure.

A *Valsalva maneuver* refers to a deep, sustained expiration against a closed glottis. In this case both the thoracic and abdominal pressures are increased, and blood flow in the thoracic and abdominal vena cava may be shut off. The flow is restored when the microcirculation into these venae cavae has raised their pressures above the thoracic and abdominal pressures.

4.8 Flutter

A phenomenon that can be demonstrated easily in the laboratory is the flutter (a self-excited oscillation) of a collapsible tube conveying a fluid, operating in such a range that the transmural pressure is positive (distending)

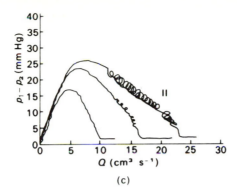

(c)

Figure 4.8:1 Flutter of a collapsible thin-walled rubber tube in certain range of flow. The tube was used as a Starling resistor, with the chamber pressure p_e kept fixed at 3.9 kPa. The outlet of the tube was connected to a flow resistance and then exposed to the atmosphere. The three curves were obtained by using three different resistors at the outlet. From Katz, Chen and Moreno (1969). Reproduced by permission.

at the inlet end and negative (collapsing) at the exit end. Since veins often operate in such a pressure range, it is often suggested that flutter occurs in veins, although direct *in vivo* evidence is lacking. On the other hand, the method commonly used to measure blood pressure, by inflating a cuff around an arm and listening to the Korotkov sound in an artery under the cuff, seems exactly analogous to such an experimental arrangement.

A Starling resistor, as shown in Fig. 4.5:1, is used by many to demonstrate flow limitation and flutter. As we have mentioned in Sec. 4.5, the tube often executes a self-excited oscillation in regime II, illustrated in Fig. 4.5:2(a). Further examples are given in Fig. 4.8:1, which shows three curves derived from three different values of downstream resistance, with the chamber pressure p_e kept constant. Each trace is a continuous recording made while the flow rate was gradually increased. The self-excited oscillations that occur in some cases can be seen.

The mechanism of flutter is not well understood. A detailed analysis of the stability of flow of a compressible or incompressible fluid in an elastic cylindrical tube with simply supported ends is given by Matsuzaki and Fung (1978). Limiting to the potential flow theory, but allowing full interplay of the inertial forces, hydrodynamic forces, and elastic forces, they show that the hydroelastic instability is in the nature of divergence (nonoscillatory), and not flutter (oscillatory). In this theory, the structural nonlinearity is included, but the hydrodynamic equations are linearized and viscosity is neglected. The failure of the theory suggests that the phenomenon is beyond the range of applicability of the linearized potential flow theory. Thus for future work the fluid mechanical analysis should be improved. In particular, the effect of viscosity should be considered, and the nonlinear effect of convective inertia should be included. It could be that flutter is a phenomenon of nonlinear oscillation that occurs only at finite amplitude.

A phenomenon associated with large deformation of the tube is the separation of streamlines from the wall as illustrated in Figs. 3.17:1 for a flow at a high Reynolds number of 20,000 and in Fig. 3.17:2 for flows at Reynolds numbers of 31, 70, and 185. Flow separation is usually associated with hysteresis in cyclic changes of flow and may lead to self-excited oscillations. It is caused by an adverse pressure gradient in the boundary layer in a divergent channel (i.e., one whose cross-sectional area increases in the direction of flow). Such a divergent section exists at the exit end of the Starling resistor shown in Figs. 4.5:1 and 4.5:2, for which flutter occurs under certain conditions. That the pressure gradient is adverse in a divergent channel can be seen from the Bernoulli's equation (Eq. (3) of Sec. 1.6), because in a divergent channel the velocity of flow decreases in the direction of flow and therefore the pressure increases in the same direction. The adverse pressure gradient makes the velocity profile in the boundary layer flatter, and eventually causes the boundary layer flow to be unstable, and the streamlines to separate from the wall.

Oscillatory Flow Due to Boundary Layer Separation

Since flutter and flow separation is important not only to the venous flow, but also to the generation of Korotkov sound in arteries, to post-stenotic dilatation, and to forced expiratory flow in the airways, coughing, etc., we would like to know as much about the hydrodynamics of these phenomena as possible. The full story is not yet available, but a review of the known facts is worthwhile.

One of the early experimental studies on a rigid pipe with a divergent boundary was made by Gibson (1910). Kline and his associates (1957, 1959) performed systematic experiments on two-dimensional divergent channels by means of a flow visualization technique in order to clarify the separation mechanism. They found four flow regimes:

1. No appreciable stall
2. Large transitory stall
3. Fully developed stall
4. Jet flow

Here the term "stall" means backflow at a wall. For a fixed inflow velocity, these regimes are influenced by total divergence angle, the ratio of the wall length to throat width, and the inflow turbulence. Their work, pertinent to diffuser designs, covers a Reynolds number range that is too large for physiological applications. For the moderate Reynolds number range of physiological interest, Young and Tsai (1973) measured pressure drop of flow through tubes with constrictions, and Matsuzaki and Fung (1976) studied

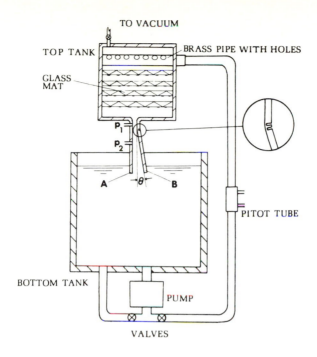

Figure 4.8:2 Schematic diagram of a "two-dimensional" test apparatus for the study of flow separation in a divergent channel. From Matsuzaki and Fung (1976). Reproduced by permission.

the separation phenomenon in two-dimensional channels. The model used by Matsuzaki and Fung is sketched in Fig. 4.8:2. It consists of a channel, one wall of which was movable to change the divergent angle. The inflow from the upper tank was very quiet (nonturbulent). The convergent segment of the channel was so designed that the flow had a uniform velocity profile at the throat. In each experiment the divergence angle θ was fixed, and the pressure differential between two points p_1, p_2 was measured. The length of the convergent segment, the throat, the divergent segment, and the distance between p_1 and p_2 were, respectively, 3.30, 2.54, 22.9, and 7.62 cm.

Figure 4.8:3 shows the experimental results on the pressure differential Δp (equal to the difference of pressures between p_1 and p_2 minus the hydrostatic head $\rho g z$, where z is the vertical distance between p_1 and p_2) as a function of the speed of flow expressed as the Reynolds number at the throat:

$$N_R = \frac{\bar{u} W}{\nu},$$

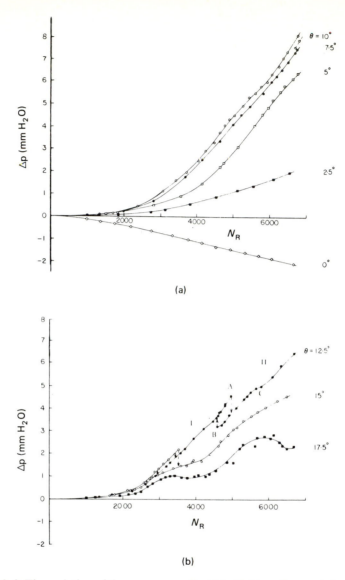

(a)

(b)

Figure 4.8:3 The variation of the pressure gradient ($\Delta p/\Delta x$) in a divergent channel with the speed of flow ($\bar{u}$) at several values of angle of divergence (θ). The speed of flow is expressed in terms of the Reynolds number $N_R = \bar{u}W/v$, where W is the width of the throat and v is the kinematic viscosity of the fluid. The pressure difference (Δp) was measured in a distance $\Delta x = 7.62$ cm. From Matsuzaki and Fung (1976), by permission.

where $\bar{u}$, W, and v are, respectively, the mean velocity at the throat, the throat width, and the kinematic viscosity of the fluid, water. Note that when the divergence angle $\theta = 0$, Δp is negative according to Poiseuille's formula. For the divergence angle $\theta = 2.5°$, Δp is positive and increases parabolically with N_R, in accordance with the Bernoulli equation. For $\theta = 5°$, $7.5°$, and $10°$, Δp increases with N_R, first parabolically, then more or less linearly. For $\theta = 10°$, fluctuating flow was observed at higher flow rates. For $\theta = 12.5°$, there is a sudden drop of Δp at a point A if the flow speed is increasing, and a sudden increase at B if the flow is decreasing. At flow speeds greater than those at A and B the amplitude of fluctuation is much greater. Beyond point C, the frequency of fluctuation decreases to a much lower value. If the free stream disturbances of the inflow are increased, points A, B, C would move to the left. This same type of hysteresis occurs at $\theta = 15°$. When $\theta = 17.5°$, the hysteresis loop becomes insignificant, but the Δp vs N_R relationship appears to be rather complex. Fluctuations in Δp were quite strong at all speeds when $\theta = 15°$ and $17.5°$.

If the curves of Fig. 4.8:3 were cross plotted for varying divergence angle, but a constant Reynolds number, the result would be that which is shown in Fig. 4.8:4. The divergence angle at which a discontinuous jump in Δp occurs is seen to vary with the Reynolds number.

Thus, the complex character of flow in divergent channels is seen. However, this information is still insufficient for the analysis of flutter because the boundary conditions are stationary in these experiments, whereas in flutter they are nonstationary. A full flutter analysis remains to be done.

Korotkov Sounds

We have mentioned that Korotkov sounds may be the physiological evidence of the flutter phenomenon. This is the sound used by physicians when they measure the patient's blood pressure by inflating a cuff on the arm. If a stethoscope bell is placed over the brachial artery, nothing can be heard at all in normal circumstances. However, when a wide cuff containing an inflatable bag is wrapped around the upper arm and the bag is inflated to pressures sufficient to collapse the artery and stop the flow and then the pressure is allowed to fall slowly, characteristic sounds are heard from the brachial artery (the Korotkov sounds). It has been shown by angiographic and ultrasound techniques that the first appearance of the sound coincides with the onset of blood flow through the collapsed artery segment. As the bag pressure falls, the sound becomes louder and more extended in time until it reaches a maximum intensity and begins to diminish, and then disappears. At a pressure just below that where the sound begins to diminish, there is a change in the character of the sound, known as "muffling." The sound loses its ringing, staccato quality and becomes a thumping. It is not certain which particular sounds are associated with the cuff pressure being

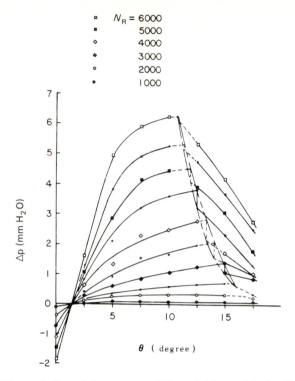

Figure 4.8:4 The variation of the pressure differential (Δp) with the divergence angle (θ) at several specific values of Reynolds number (N_R). The region in which a sharp change in pressure differential occurs is bounded by two chained curves. The interpolated portions of these curves are shown as dotted lines. From Matsuzaki and Fung (1976), by permission.

equal to the systolic and diastolic pressures in the heart, but by internationally agreed convention the cuff pressures at the appearance and the muffling of the Korotkov sounds are taken as the systolic and diastolic pressures, respectively. Burton (1965) says "the more one inquires into the basis of the Riva–Rocci indirect method of measuring arterial pressure, the less confidence one has in its accuracy, both for systolic and diastolic pressures. Yet it remains an invaluable aid to diagnostic medicine, in no way replaced in practice by the availability of methods involving direct arterial puncture."

McCutcheon and Rushmer (1967) and Ur and Gordon (1970) have provided basic experimental data on Korotkov sound. Anliker and Raman (1966), Pedley (1980), and Wild, Pedley, and Riley (1977) have made extensive mathematical analyses on the subject.

4.9 Patency of Pulmonary Veins When the Blood Pressure Is Exceeded by Airway Pressure

Not all veins collapse when the internal pressure is smaller than the external pressure. Such is the case with pulmonary veins. Although the pulmonary venous vessel wall is thin and flexible, it is tethered by the interalveolar septa, which lend support and stabilize the vessel wall. This fact is very important to the understanding of pulmonary blood flow. Historically, it was in the lung that the "waterfall" phenomenon was first discovered. But until the stability of the venous vessels was proven by Fung et al. (1983), one could only speculate on where the "falls" are on the vascular tree. With the proof, we know that the falls are not on the venous tree. They are certainly not on the arterial tree. So if they exist, they must be located on the capillary blood vessels.

To demonstrate the patency of pulmonary veins, Fung et al. (1983) perfused the pulmonary blood vessels of the cat with a low-viscosity (20 cp) silicone elastomer (with 3% stenous ethylhexoate and 1.5% ethyl silicate hardening agent freshly added). After perfusing at a pressure of 25 mmHg for 20 minutes, the flow was stopped and the perfusion pressure (p_v) was lowered to a desired level and held constant. At this selected static condition the silicone elastomer hardened. After hardening, the heart and lungs were removed and suspended in 10% KOH solution to corrode away the tissue. Then the arterial tree was gently separated from the venous tree, and casts of the two trees were obtained.

Patent Vessels

If a blood vessel is collapsed so that its internal cross-sectional area vanishes, then, after the process of tissue corrosion, that vessel will disappear from the tree. For the lungs prepared in the manner described above, the capillary blood vessels disappeared when the transmural pressure $p_v - p_A$ was sufficiently negative. Here p_v stands for blood pressure in the vein and p_A stands for airway pressure. Figure 4.9:1 shows a venous tree cast of a cat lung prepared with a perfusion pressure (measured at the level of the left atrium) that was 17 cm H_2O lower than the alveolar gas pressure. Casts made at other negative values of $p_v - p_A$ look similar. We conclude, therefore, that the pulmonary veins do not collapse at these negative transmural pressures.

The Smallest Open Veins, the Branching Pattern of the Venous Tree, and the Elasticity and Compliance Constants of the Venules

In our silicone rubber casts of the pulmonary venous tree, the smallest veins that remained open under negative transmural pressure are those smallest

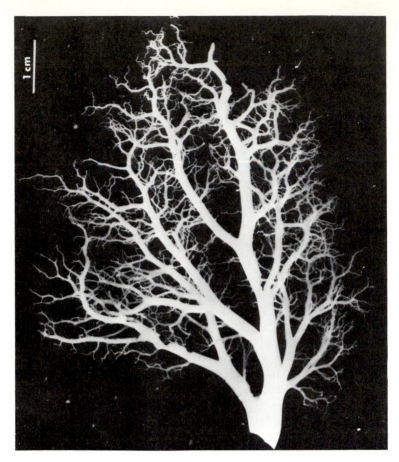

Figure 4.9:1 A silicone elastomer cast of the venous tree of a cat's lung whose veins are subjected to a pressure difference $p_v - p_A$ of -17 cm H_2O. Pleural pressure $= 0$ (atmospheric). Airway pressure $= 10$ cm H_2O. Blood vessel pressure was -7 cm H_2O.

twigs that remained on the tree and did not fall off. Hence, by measuring the dimensions of these smallest twigs, we can determine the dimensions of the smallest vessels that did not collapse.

There is, however, a logical possibility that under increasing negative transmural pressure the larger vessels became smaller while the smallest collapsed and disappeared. To make sure that this did not happen, we should verify that the branching pattern of the entire tree did not change; that the same number of generations remained as the negative transmural pressure was increased.

There are two ways to describe vascular trees. One uses *generations* in analogy with a familial tree, and counts the number of offspring in each generation. Difficulty arises in the lung because at each bifurcation of a vessel the two offspring are usually unequal in size (diameter, length). To systematize the counting, Weibel (1963) "symmetrizes" the offspring. The other way is to use the *Strahler system*, which is used in geography to describe rivers (see Cumming et al. (1968)). In the Strahler system, the smallest blood vessel is said to be of *order* 1. When two vessels of order 1 meet, the next larger vessel is called a vessel of *order* 2. Two order 2 vessels meet to form a larger vessel of order 3, etc. But if an order 1 vessel meets an order 2 vessel, the order number remains at 2. If a vessel of order 2 meets a vessel of order 3, the combined trunk's order remains at 3, and so on. If the branching pattern of the vascular tree were that of "symmetric" bifurcation, with every parent vessel yielding two equal offspring, then the ratio of the number of vessels of order n to that of $n + 1$, called the *branching ratio*, is 2. However, the pulmonary vascular tree does not bifurcate symmetrically, and the branching ratio is close to 3. In this situation the Strahler system gives a more accurate description of the branching pattern.

The results of our measurement are given in Tables 4.9:1 and 6.11:2 (p. 338). Table 4.9:1 (from Fung et al., 1983) presents the diameters and lengths of the small pulmonary veins. Table 6.11:2 (from Yen et al., 1983) presents the branching pattern of the entire venous tree of the right lung of the cat. It was found that there are 11 orders of pulmonary veins between pulmonary capillaries and the left atrium. The lungs of five cats were prepared at $p_v - p_A = -7$ cm H_2O, two cats were prepared at $p_v - p_A = -2$ cm H_2O, one was prepared at $p_v - p_A = -17$ cm H_2O. All were found to have 11 orders of veins. Hence the structure of the venous tree was not changed when $p_v - p_A$ was varied from -2 to -17 cm H_2O; and the meaningfulness of identifying the smallest vessels in all casts as order 1 is assured.

The data in Table 4.9:1 show that the diameters of the smallest open venules (vessels of order 1) are in the range of 22 to 27 μm. If the diameter is assumed to be a function of the pressure $p_v - p_A$ and a linear regression is assumed, then by least squares method we obtain the rate of decrease of the diameter (compliance constant) as approximately 0.32 μm per cm H_2O of pressure, or 1.24% per cm H_2O based on the average diameter at $p_v - p_A = -2$ for the vessels of order 1.

Earlier, Sobin et al. (1978) measured the diameters of the *smallest* non-capillary blood vessels in each photomicrograph of the cat's lung and found that these smallest vessels have mean diameters 14.5, 16.6, 17.0, 18.2, 21.0 μm when $p_v - p_A = $ (positive) $+ 0, 3, 10.25, 17, 23.75$ cm H_2O respectively. The compliance constant is 0.274 μm per cm H_2O, or 1.61% per cm H_2O, which is quite consistent with the mean value found above for the smallest venules. Hence, we conclude that the compliance constant of the venules does not change much as the transmural pressure $p_v - p_A$ changes from positive to negative values in the range -17 to 24 cm H_2O. Furthermore, since the smallest vessels must be smaller than the average order 1 vessels, we conclude that the smallest vessels listed in Table 4.9:1 are venules of order 1.

Table 4.9:1 lists also the *diameter ratio* (the ratio of the diameters of

TABLE 4.9:1 Diameters and Branching Ratios of the First Four Orders of Small-Pulmonary Veins of the Cat and the Lengths of Veins of Orders 3, 4, 5.[a]

		$p_v - p_A = -2$ cm H_2O		$p_v - p_A = -7$ cm H_2O	$p_v - p_A = -17$ cm H_2O
		Cat CFB (RLL)	Cat CFK (RLL)	Cat CET (LLL)	Cat CJG (RLL)
Diameter	Order 1	27.4 ± 10.1	24.2 ± 8.2	22.2 ± 4.1	23.6 ± 9.4
(μm)	Order 2	42.8 ± 10.0	41.0 ± 9.1	40.5 ± 7.3	37.0 ± 11.1
mean ± SD	Order 3	77.6 ± 19.8	73.9 ± 8.9	67.7 ± 11.5	71.0 ± 18.1
	Order 4	160.3 ± 39.5	142.0 ± 33.9	136.3 ± 44.7	126.1 ± 25.7
Diameter ratio		1.80	1.80	1.84	1.77
Length	Order 3	0.59 ± 0.27	0.56 ± 0.42	0.50 ± 0.21	0.58 ± 0.37
(mm)	Order 4	1.57 ± 0.60	1.47 ± 0.63	1.55 ± 1.11	1.48 ± 0.76
mean ± SD	Order 5	2.23 ± 1.58	2.44 ± 0.77	2.38 ± 1.74	2.69 ± 1.75
Length ratio		1.94	2.08	2.18	2.15
$\log \dfrac{N_i}{N_{i+1}} = B$		0.462	0.465	0.516	0.487
Average branching ratio		2.90	2.92	3.27	3.07

[a] $p_{PL} = 0$ (atmospheric), $p_A = 10$ cm H_2O, p_v = variable, measured at the level of the left atrium. N_i = the number of vessels of order i. p_v = blood pressure in vein, p_A = alveolar gas pressure, p_{PL} = pleural pressure.

successive orders of vessels), the average length of the vessels of successive orders, the *length ratio* (the ratio of the average length of successive orders of vessels), and the branching ratio. The last quantity is obtained by plotting the number of branches in successive orders on a semilog paper and finding the slope. The regression line yields

$$\log(N_i/N_{i+1}) = B,$$

where N_i is the number of vessels of order i, and B is a constant. The *branching ratio* is then given by 10^B. It is seen that the branching ratio is about 3.0.

These results tell us that all the pulmonary veins remain open when the blood pressure is less than the airway pressure by as much as -17 cm H_2O. In contrast, the capillaries would collapse completely when $p_v - p_A$ is -1 cm H_2O, (see Sec. 6.5). This difference in behavior between capillaries and venules is important for hemodynamics. It is the basis of our conclusion that the sluicing gates in the zone 2 condition are located at the junctions of the capillaries and venules, (Fung et al., 1972, p. 473).

Compliance of Pulmonary Veins Under Negative Transmural Pressure

To clarify the behavior of the pulmonary veins further, we measured the change of the diameters of these vessels with respect to blood pressure. The diameters were measured on the x-ray films of isolated lungs after perfusing them first with saline, and then with $BaSO_4$ suspension. The method is presented in Yen et al. (1980).

Our results are shown in Fig. 4.9:2 in which the distensibility of vessels in the diameter range of 100–200, 200–400, 400–800, 800–1200 μm and with pleural pressures of -20, -15, -10, and -5 cm H_2O is presented. On the ordinate is shown the percentage change in diameter normalized with respect to D_{10}, the diameter at a $\Delta p = p_v - p_{PL}$ of 10 cm H_2O. This Δp is the difference between the venous perfusion pressure (p_v) and the pleural pressure (p_{PL}). The ranges 100–200, etc., mean all vessels whose diameters fall in these ranges when $\Delta p = 10$ cm H_2O. At other Δp, the same vessels were followed. It appears from Fig. 4.9:2 that a linear relationship between pressure and diameter change exists for all these vessels in the ranges tested. In these figures, the vertical bars indicate the standard deviation (SD) of the D/D_{10} ratio of the vessels studied, whereas the horizontal bars indicate the S.D. of the pressure difference $p_v - p_A$ in these vessels. The scatter of $p_v - p_A$ was caused by the effect of gravity on the different heights of the branches, which resulted in different hydrostatic pressures in the vessels.

A linear regression line is assumed for each group of vessels (in a given diameter range), and slope and intercept of the regression line are determined by the method of least squares using the mean values of D/D_{10} and $p_v - p_A$. These regression lines are plotted in Fig. 4.9:2. Their slopes are called the

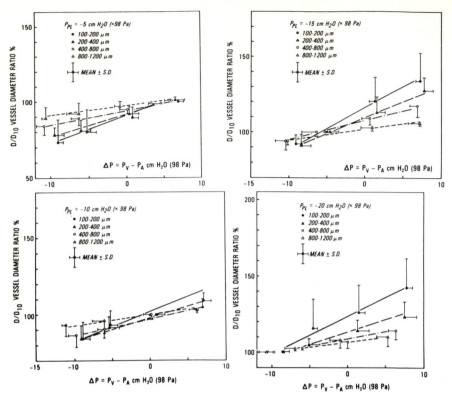

Figure 4.9:2 Percentage change in diameter of pulmonary veins of the cat as a function of the blood pressure. The airway pressure p_A, is zero. The values of the pleural pressure, p_{PL}, are noted in the figure. The vessel diameter is normalized against its value when $p_v - p_A$ is 10 cm H$_2$O at which the vessel cross section is circular. The nominal size of a vessel is its diameter at $p_v - p_A = 10$ cm H$_2$O. From Yen and Foppiano (1981). Reproduced by permission.

TABLE 4.9:2 The Compliance Coefficient
(% Change of Diameter per cm H_2O Change in
$p_V - p_A$) of a Cat's Pulmonary Veins When
$p_v - p_A$ Is Negative[a]

Vessel diameter range (μm)	p_{PL} (cm H_2O)	Compliance coefficient
100–200	−5	1.98
	−10	2.05
	−15	2.79
	−20	2.44
200–400	−5	1.83
	−10	1.44
	−15	2.01
	−20	1.60
400–800	−5	0.98
	−10	1.08
	−15	1.16
	−20	0.93
800–1200	−5	0.79
	−10	0.71
	−15	0.57
	−20	0.58

[a] The airway pressure is 0 (atmospheric). The pleural
pressure (p_{PL}) is listed. The compliance constant is the slope
of the linear regression line over a range $−10 < p_v - p_A <$
10 cm H_2O determined for each group of vessels.

compliance coefficients and are listed in Table 4.9:2. The unit of the compliance coefficient is the percent change in diameter per cm H_2O of pressure
change, or inverse Pascal. The table shows that smaller veins of the cat are
more compliant than larger veins. Furthermore, for smaller veins (100–
400 μm), inflation to a higher lung volume results in a higher compliance
coefficient initially until a pleural pressure of $−15$ cm H_2O is reached,
whereas further increase in lung volume decreases compliance. For larger
veins (400–1200 μm), the compliance coefficients are smaller and their variation with the degree of inflation is not as significant.

The difference between the mechanical properties of pulmonary veins and
the peripheral veins becomes evident if one compares the curves of Fig. 4.9:2
with those of Figs. 4.3:3, 4.4:2, and 4.4:3. Whereas the compliance of the
peripheral veins increases greatly when the transmural pressure becomes

negative, the compliance of the pulmonary veins changes hardly at all when the corresponding transmural pressure, $p_v - p_A$, changes from positive to negative.

Why Are the Pulmonary Veins so Stable?

The stability of the pulmonary veins against negative transmural pressure $p_v - p_A$ may be explained by the pull provided by the tension in the interalveolar septa on the veins. The relationship between the interalveolar septa and pulmonary venules is illustrated by a typical example shown in Fig. 4.9:3. Larger vessels may be pulled by four or more interalveolar septa. A few appear to be tethered by only two septa. We have never seen an isolated, untethered vessel in the lung.

For each blood vessel, there are tethering interalveolar septa either parallel to or intersecting it at various angles. Tensile stresses prevail in the interalveolar septa as long as the lung is inflated and the alveoli are open; and they tend to distend the blood vessel. Between the successive septa the vessel wall is subjected to the pressure of the blood, p_v, in the inside, and alveolar gas pressure, p_A, on the outside; the net pressure acting outward is $p_v - p_A$. When $p_v - p_A$ is negative, the transmural pressure acts inward.

As we have seen in Sec. 4.3, the stability of a circular cylindrical shell can be greatly improved by adding lateral and longitudinal supports. Figure 4.3:5 shows that the shorter the length of the cylinder L, and the larger the wave number n, the higher is the critical buckling pressure. Now, for a pulmonary vein, those interalveolar septa intersecting it perpendicular to its axis determine the length L (being the distance between successive septa, or approximately the alveolar diameter); whereas those tethering it parallel to its axis determine n (e.g., $n = 3$ for the vessel shown in Fig. 4.9:3). If there were no tethering interalveolar septa, the buckling mode of the veins would correspond to $n = 2$, and $L/R =$ vessel length/vessel radius which is very large. The great stabilizing influence of tethering is then very clear from Fig. 4.3:5.

Another factor that improves stability of pulmonary veins by tethering arises from the nonlinear mechanical behavior of the blood vessel wall material. As it is well-known, the vessel wall has an exponential stress–strain relationship (see *Biomechanics*, (Fung, 1981), Ch. 8), and the incremental Young's modulus increases with increasing stress. The tethering interalveolar septa stresses the blood vessel wall, and increases its elastic modulus. As we have seen in Secs 4.2–4.4, the critical buckling load is directly proportional to the elastic modulus; hence an increase of the elastic modulus improves the stability.

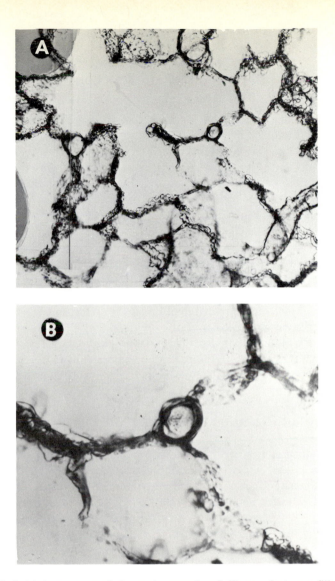

Figure 4.9:3 (a) A montage of photomicrographs of silicone elastomer filled cat lung showing two venules in the central portion of the figure each tethered by three interalveolar septa. Another venule which was cut lengthwise is seen at the lower right corner of the photograph. All noncapillary vessels in this figure are venous. Gelatinembedded preparation. Cresyl violet stain. 90-μm-thick sections. (b) An enlargement of a portion of (a), showing tethering of a venule by three interalveolar septa. These figures are enlargements of a small portion of the montage presented in Fig. 6.13:1, p. 348; located at the upper right corner of that figure, near the letter "a." The dark shadows at the left border of (a) are marks of the arterial regions as explained in Sec. 6.13. From Sobin et al. (1980). Reproduced by permission.

Conclusion

We conclude that in the normal range of airway, pleural, and blood pressures in the zone II condition, the pulmonary veins, including venules, will not collapse. The elasticity of the blood vessels is such that the slope of the diameter vs $p_v - p_A$ curve remains almost constant for $p_v - p_A$ in the range of $+10$ to -17 cm H_2O. There is no sudden change of pressure–diameter relationship as the transmural pressure changes from positive to negative values. This is in strong contrast to the curves shown in Fig. 4.4:2. The cause for this patency is the tension exerted on the vessels by the interalveolar septa which are attached to the outer walls of the vessels. Although this conclusion is based on cat lung, it should be applicable to other mammalian lungs because their basic structures are similar, as can be seen from the many illustrations in Krahl (1964), Miller (1947), von Hayek (1960), and Weibel (1963) listed at the end of chapter 6.

Pulmonary veins that remain patent under the condition $p_v - p_A < 0$ have been reported earlier by Glazier et al. (1969), Macklin (1946), Howell et al. (1961), and Permutt (1965). For larger veins (with diameter much larger than the diameter of alveoli), the patency has been fully explained by Mead and Whittenberger (1964), Permutt (1965), and Lai-Fook (1979).

4.10 Waterfall Condition in the Lung

In the preceding section we have shown that the pulmonary venules and veins remain patent when the blood pressure (p) is smaller than the gas pressure in the alveoli (p_A), provided that the lung is inflated. On the other hand, we know (see Chap. 6, Sec. 6.5) that the pulmonary capillary blood vessels can and will be collapsed if the transmural pressure $p - p_A$ is negative. It follows that the "waterfall" condition (Sec. 4.1), if it occurs in the lung, will occur in the capillary blood vessels. The principal fact about the capillaries is that they are very small. They are so small that the Reynolds number of flow and the Womersley number at the frequency of cardiac pulsation) are much less than one, (usually $< 10^{-3}$). Hence, the inertial force in the blood vessel due to transient and convective accelerations is very small compared with the gradients of viscous stresses and pressure. In this condition, the phenomena of collapsing, choking, flow limitation, etc., discussed in Secs. 4.2–4.7 can occur, but the vessel will not flutter (Fung and Sobin, 1972). Flutter (Sec. 4.8) is a phenomenon caused by a competition between the inertial, pressure, and elastic forces. For flow in capillary blood vessels the inertial force is almost absent, and the balance of the elastic and pressure forces results in a static deformation. Thus, waterfall occurs, but statically.

In the lung, the waterfall phenomenon is a common occurrence, and the discussion presented here is necessary for its understanding. Further analysis is given in Chapter 6.

Problem

4.13 Show that if a circle is deformed into an ellipse of the same circumferential length, then the ratio of the mean diameter of the ellipse, defined as the average of the major and minor axes, to the diameter of the circle, is 0.998 when a/b = 1.25, 0.976 when a/b = 1.75, and 0.965 when a/b = 2.0, a being the major diameter, b being the minor diameter. In other words, if an inextensible circle is deformed into an ellipse with the major axis twice as large as the minor axes, the mean diameter of the ellipse is only 3.5% smaller than that of the circle. Therefore, if the blood vessel cross sections were circular originally and were deformed into elliptical shapes under a negative transmural pressure, then a collection of random samples of the projected widths will yield a mean diameter quite close to the mean diameter of the original circular vessels. The standard deviation will reflect the degree of deformation as well as the variation in the original diameter.

References

Alexander, R. S. (1963). The peripheral venous system. Chapter 31 of *Handbook of Physiology*, Sec. 2, Vol. 2. *Circulation*. American Physiological Society, Bethesda, MD, pp. 1075–1098.

Anliker, M. and Raman, K. R. (1966). Korotkoff sounds at diastole—a phenomenon of dynamic instability of fluid-filled shells. *Inst. J. Solids & Struct.* **2**: 467–491.

Anliker. M., Wells, M. K. and Ogden, E. (1969). The transmission characteristics of large and small pressure waves in the abdominal vena cava. *IEEE Trans. Biomedical Eng.* **BME-16**: 262–273.

Attinger, E. O. (1969). Wall properties of veins. *IEEE Trans. Biomedical Eng.* **BME-16**: 253–261.

Banister, J. and Torrance, R. W. (1960). The effects of the tracheal pressure upon flow: Pressure relations in the vascular bed of isolated lungs. *Quart. J. Exp. Physiol.* **45**: 353–367.

Brown, E., Greenfield, A. D. M., Goei, J. S., and Plassaras, G. (1966). Filling and emptying of the low-pressure blood vessels of the human forearm. *J. Appl. Physiol.* **21**(2): 573–582.

Burton, A. C. (1965). *Physiology and Biophysics of the Circulation*. Year Book Medical Pub., Chicago, Ill.

Caro, C. G. and Harrison, G. K. (1962). Observations on pulse wave velocity and pulsatile blood pressure in the human pulmonary circulation. *Clin. Sci.* **23**: 271–329.

Caro. C. G., Pedley, T. J., Schroter, R. C. and Seed, W. A. (1978). *The Mechanics of the Circulation*, Oxford Univ. Press, Oxford.

Conrad, W. A. (1969). Pressure flow relationship in collapsible tubes. *IEEE Trans. Biomedical Eng.* **BME-16**: 284–295.

Cumming, G., Henderson, R. Horsfield, K. and Singhal, S. S. (1968). The functional morphology of the pulmonary circulation. In *The Pulmonary Circulation and Interstitial Space*. (A. Fishman and H. Hecht, eds.) Univ. Chicago Press, Chicago, pp. 327–338.

Dawson, S. V. and Elliott, E. A. Wave-speed limitation on expiratory flow—a unifying concept. *J. Appl. Physiol.* **43**(3): 498–515.

Downey, J. M. and Kirk, E. S. (1975). Inhibition of coronary blood flow by vascular waterfall phenomenon. *Circ. Res.* **36**: 753–760.

Duomarco. J. L. and Rimini, R. (1954). Energy and hydraulic gradients along systemic veins. *Am. J. Physiol.* **178**: 215–220.

Elliott, E. A. and Dawson, S. V. (1977). Test of wave-speed theory of flow limitation in elastic tubes. *J. Appl. Physiol.* **43**: 516–522.

Flaherty, J. E., Keller, J. B. and Rubinow, S. I. (1972). Post buckling behavior of elastic tubes and rings with opposite sides in contact. *SIAM J. Applied Mathematics* **23**(4): 446–455.

Flügge, W. (1960). *Stresses in Shells*. Springer-Verlag, Heidelberg.

Fry, D. L., Thomas, L. J. and Greenfield, J. C. (1980). Flow in collapsible tubes. In *Basic Hemodynamics and Its Role in Disease Processes*, (Patel, D. J., and Vaishnav, R. N, eds.) University Park, Baltimore, Ch. 9, pp. 407–424.

Fung, Y. C. (1977). *A First Course in Continuum Mechanics*. 2nd ed. Prentice-Hall, Englewood Cliffs, N. J.

Fung, Y. C. (1981). *Biomechanics: Mechanical Properties of Living Tissues*. Springer-Verlag, New York.

Fung, Y. C. and Sechler, E. E. (1960). Instability of thin elastic shells. In *Structural Mechanics*. Proc. of Symp. on Naval Structure Mechanics, (Goodier, J. N. and Hoff, N., eds.) Pergamon Press.

Fung, Y. C. and Sobin, S. S. (1972a). Elasticity of the pulmonary alveolar sheet. *Circulation Res.* **30**: 451–469.

Fung, Y. C. and Sobin, S. S. (1972b). Pulmonary alveolar blood flow. *Circulation Res.* **30**: 470–490.

Fung, Y. C., Perrone, N. and Anliker, M. (1972). *Biomechanics: Its Foundations and Objectives*. Prentice-Hall, Englewood Cliffs, N. J.

Fung, Y. C. and Sechler, E. E. (eds.) (1974). *Thin Shell Structures: Theory, Experiment and Design*. Prentice-Hall, Englewood Cliffs, N. J..

Fung, Y. C., Sobin, S. S., Tremer, H., Yen, M. R. T. and Ho, H. H. (1983). Patency and compliance of pulmonary veins when airway pressure exceeds blood pressure. *J. Appl. Physiol: Respir., Exercise, and Environ. Physiol.* **54**: 1538–1549.

Gibson, A. H. (1910). On the flow of water through pipes and passages having converging or diverging boundaries. *Proc. Roy. Soc. London*, A, **83**: 366–378.

Glazier, J. B., Hughes, J. M. B., Maloney, J. E. and West, J. B. (1969). Measurements of capillary dimensions and blood volume in rapidly frozen lungs. *J. Appl. Physiol.* **26**: 65–76.

Greenfield, J. C., Jr., and Tindall, G. T. (1965). Effect of acute increase in intracranicl pressure on blood flow in the internal carotid artery of man. *J. Clin. Invest.* **44**: 1343–1351.

Griffiths, D. J. (1969). Urethral elasticity and micturition hydrodynamics in females. *Medical and Biological Engineering* **7**: 201–215.

Griffiths, D. J. (1971). Hydrodynamics of male micturition—I. Theory of steady flow through elastic-walled tubes. *Medical & Biol. Engineering* **9**: 581–588. II. Measurements of stream parameters and urethral elasticity. *ibid.* **9**: 589–596.

Griffiths, D. J. (1973). The mechanics of the urethra and of micturition. *British J. of Urology* **45**: 497–507.

Guntheroth, W. G. (1969). In vivo measurement of dimensions of veins with implications regarding control of venous return. *IEEE Trans. Biomededical Eng.* **BME-16**(4): 247–253.

Henderson. Y. and Johnson, F. E. (1912). Two modes of closure of the heart valve. *Heart*, **4**: 69–82.

Holt, J. P. (1941). The collapse factor in the measurement of venous pressure: The flow of fluid through collapsible tubes. *Am. J. Physiol.* **134**: 292–299.

Holt, J. P. (1953). Flow of liquids through collapsible tubes. *Amer. Heart J.* **46**: 715–725.

Holt, J. P. (1969). Flow through collapsible tubes and through in situ veins. *IEEE Trans. Biomedical Eng.* **BME-16**: 274–283.

Howell, J. B. L., Permutt, S., Proctor, D. F. and Riley, R. L. (1961). Effect of inflation of the lung on different parts of pulmonary vascular bed. *J. Appl. Physiol.* **16**: 71–76.

Hyatt, R. E., Schilder, D. P. and Fry, D. L. (1958). Relationship between maximum expiratory flow and degree of lung inflation. *J. Appl. Physiol.* **13**: 331–336.

Kamm, R. D. and Shapiro, A. H. (1970). Unsteady flow in collapsible tube subjected to external pressure or body forces. *J. Fluid Mechanics* **95**: Part 1, 1–78.

Katz, A. I., Chen, Y. and Moreno, A. H. (1969). Flow through a collapsible tube: Experimental analysis and mathematical model. *Biophysical J.* **9**: 1261–1279.

Kececioglu, I., Kamm, R. D. and Shapiro, A. H. (1978). Structure of shock waves in collapsible tube flow (Abstract) *Proc. 31st Ann. Conf. Engng. in Medicine & Biol.*, Atlanta, Ga.

Kety, S. S., Shenkin, H. A. and Schmidt, C. F. (1948). The effects of increased intracranial pressure on cerebral circulatory functions in man. *J. Clin. Invest.* **27**: 493–499.

Kline, S. J. (1959). On the nature of stall. *J. of Basic Eng., Trans. ASME* **81**, Ser. D: 305–320. See also Kline et al., *loc. cit.*: 321–331.

Kline, S. J., Moore, C. A. and Cochran, D. L. (1957). Wide-angle diffusers of high performance and diffuser flow mechanisms. *J. Aeronautical Sci.* **24**: 469–471.

Knowlton, F. P. and Starling, E. H. (1912). The influence of variations in temperature and blood pressure on the performance of the isolated mammalian heart. *J. Physiol.* (London) **44**: 206–219.

Kresch, E. (1979). Compliance of flexible tubes. *J. Biomechanics.* **12**: 825–839.

Kresch, E. and Noordergraaf, A. (1969). A mathematical model for the pressure-flow relationship in segment of vein. *IEEE Trans. Biomedical Eng.* **BME-16**: 296–307.

Lai-Fook, S. J. (1979). A continuum mechanics analysis of pulmonary vascular interdependence in isolated dog lobes. *J. Appl. Physiol.* **45**: 419–429.

Lyon, C. K., Scott, J. B., and Wang, C. Y. (1980). Flow through collapsible tubes at low Reynolds numbers: Applicability of the waterfall model. *Circulation Res.* **47**: 68–73.

Macklin, C. C. (1946). Evidences of increase in the capacity of the pulmonary arteries and veins of dogs, cats and rabbits during inflation of the freshly excised lung. *Revue canadienne de Biol.* **5**: 199–232.

Matsuzaki, Y. and Fung, Y. C. (1976). On separation of a divergent flow at moderate Reynolds numbers. *J. Appl. Mech., Trans. ASME* **98**: 227–231.

Matsuzaki, Y. and Fung, Y. C. (1977). Unsteady fluid dynamic forces on a simply-supported circular cylinder of finite length conveying a flow, with applications to stability analysis. *J. of Sound and Vibration*, **54**(3): 317–330.

McCutcheon, E. P. and Rushmer, R. F. (1967). Korotkoff sounds: an experimental critique. *Circulation Res.* **20**: 149–169.

Mead, J. and Whittenberger, J. L. (1964). Lung inflation and hemodynamics. In *Handbook of Physiology* Sec. 3, *Respiration*, (W. O. Fenn and H. Rahn, eds.) Vol 1, Amer. Physiol. Soc., Washington, D.C. pp. 477–486.

Moreno, A. H., Katz, A. I., Gold, L. D. and Reddy, R. V. (1970). Mechanics of distension of dog veins and other very thin-walled tubular structures. *Circulation Res.* **27**: 1069–1079.

Morkin, E., Collins, J. A., Goldman, H. S. and Fishman, A. P. (1965). Pattern of blood flow in the pulmonary veins of the dog. *J. Appl. Physiol.* **20**: 1118–1128.

Moses, R. A. (1963). Hydrodynamic model cyc. *Ophthalmologica* **146**: 137–142.

Olsen, J. H. and Shapiro, A. H. (1967). Large amplitude unsteady flow in liquid-filled elastic tubes. *J. Fluid Mechanics* **29**: 513–538.

Pedley, T. J. (1980). *The Fluid Mechanics of Large Blood Vessels*. Cambridge Univ. Press, Cambridge & New York, Ch. 6, Flow in collapsible tubes. pp. 301–368.

Permutt, S., Bromberger-Barnea, B. and Bane, H. N. (1962). Alveolar pressure, pulmonary venous pressure, and the vascular waterfall. *Med. Thorac.* **19**: 239–260.

Permutt, S. and Riley, R. L. (1963). Hemodynamics of collapsible vessels with tone: vascular waterfall. *J. Appl. Physiol.* **18**: 924–932.

Pollack, A. A. and Wood, E. H. (1949). Venous pressure in the saphenous vein at the ankle in man during exercise and changes in posture. *J. Appl. Physiol.* **1**: 649–662.

Prescott, J. (1924). *Applied Elasticity*. 1st ed. 1924. Reprint, Dover Publications, New York.

Ribreau, C. and Bonis, M. (1978). Propagation et écoulement dans les tubes collabables. Contribution à l'étude des vaisseaux sanguins. *J. Fr. Biophy. & Med. Nucl.* **2**: 153–158.

Rodbard, S. (1955). Flow through collapsible tubes: augmented flow resistance produced by resistance at the outlet. *Circulation* **11**: 280–287.

Rodbard, S. and Saiki, H. (1953). Flow through collapsible tubes. *Amer. Heart J.* **46**: 715–725.

Rubinow, S. I. and Keller, J. B. (1972). Flow of a viscous fluid through an elastic tube with application to blood flow. *J. Theor. Biology*. **35**: 299–313.

Shapiro. A. H. (1977). Steady flow in collapsible tubes, *J. Biomech. Engng. Trans. ASME* **99**(K): 126–147.

Shepherd, J. T., and Vanhoutte, P. M. (1975). *Veins and their Control*. Saunders, London, Philadephia.

Singhal, S., Henderson, R., Horsfield, K., Harding, K. and Cumming, G. (1973). Morphometry of the human pulmonary arterial tree. *Circulation Res.* **33**: 190–197.

Smith, F. T. (1977). Upstream interactions in channel flows. *J. Fluid Mechanics*. **79**: 631–655.

Sobin, S. S., Fung, Y. C., Tremer, H. and Rosenquist, T. H. (1972). Elasticity of the pulmonary interalveolar microvascular sheet in the cat. *Circulation Res.* **30**: 440–450.

Sobin, S. S., Lindal, R. G., Fung, Y. C. and Tremer, H. M. (1978). Elasticity of the smallest noncapillary pulmonary blood vessels in the cat. *Microvas. Res.* **15**: 57–68.

Sobin, S. S., Fung, Y. C., Lindal, R. G., Tremer, H. M. and Clark, L. (1980). Topology of pulmonary arterioles, capillaries and venules in the cat. *Microvas. Res.* **19**: 217–233.

Strahler, A. N. (1964). Quantitative geomorphology of drainage basin and channel networks. In *Handbook of Applied Hydrology: Compedium of Water Resources Technology* (Chow, V. T., ed.) McGraw-Hill, New York.

Szidon, J. P., Ingram, R. H. and Fishman, A. P. (1968). Origin of the pulmonary venous flow pulse. *Amer. J. Physiol.* **214**: 10–14.

Timoshenko, S. and Gere, J. M. (1961). *Theory of Elastic Stability*. McGraw–Hill, New York, 1st ed. 1936., 2nd ed. 1961.

Ur. A. and Gordon, M. (1970). Origin of Korotkoff sounds. *Am. J. Physiol.* **218**: 524–529.

Weibel, E. R. (1963). *Morphometry of the Human Lung*. Springer-Verlag, Berlin.

Wexler, L., Bergel, D. H., Gabe, I. T., Makin, G. S., and Mills, C. J. (1968). Velocity of blood flow in normal human venae cavae. *Circulation Res.* **23**: 349–359.

Wild, R., Pedley, T. J. and Riley, D. S. (1977). Viscous flow in collapsible tubes of slowly-varying elliptical cross-section. *J. Fluid Mech.* **81**: 273–294.

Wood, J. E. (1965). *The Veins: normal and abnormal functions*. Little, Brown, Boston, 224 pp.

Yen, R. T. and Foppiano, L. (1981). Elasticity of small pulmonary veins in the cat. *J. Biomech. Engng. Trans. ASME* **103**: 38–42.

Yen, R. T., Fung, Y. C. and Bingham, N. (1980). Elasticity of small pulmonary arteries in the cat. *J. Biomech. Engng. Trans. ASME* **102**: 170–177.

Yen, R. T., Zhuang, F. Y., Fung, Y. C., Ho, H. H., Tremer, H. and Sobin, S. S. (1983). Morphometry of cat's pulmonary venous tree. *J. Appl. Physiol.* In press.

Young, D. F. and Tsai, F. Y. (1973). Flow characteristics in models of arterial stenosis. I. Steady flow. *J. Biomechanics.* **6**: 395–410.

Young, D. F., Cholvin, N. R., and Roth, A. C. (1975). Pressure drop across artificially induced stenoses in the femoral arteries of dogs. *Circ. Res.* **36**: 735–743.

CHAPTER 5

Microcirculation

5.1 Introduction

In the preceding chapters we studied the flow of blood in large blood vessels in which the main feature is a balance between the pressure forces and inertial forces (due to transient acceleration and convective acceleration). Only in the boundary layer are the viscous friction forces important. The boundary layer thickness grows with increasing distance from the entry section, and in a long tube the boundary layer on the wall eventually becomes so thick as to fill the entire tube. The flow is then said to be *fully developed*. In a fully developed flow, there is an interplay of inertial forces, pressure forces, and viscous forces. In the aorta of man, the length is not sufficient to allow full development of boundary layer; hence the whole aorta may be considered an entrance region, and the pulse wave can be analyzed approximately by neglecting the viscous stresses. However, arteries divide and divide again. The vessel diameter decreases with each division, and soon the Reynolds number becomes quite small, the entry length becomes only a small multiple of the vessel diameter, and the flow becomes fully developed over most of the length of the vessel. At the same time, the frequency parameter, or the Womersley number, also decreases, so the transient boundary layer also becomes as thick as the tube radius, and the flow becomes in phase with the pressure gradient. Hence, in the smaller arteries the anslysis given in Sec. 3.2 is applicable.

The Reynolds number and Womersley number tend to 1 at the level of the terminal arteries. Further downstream, in the arterioles, capillaries, and venules, both the Reynolds number and the Womersley number become less than 1. In these vessels, the inertial force becomes less important; and the flow is determined by the balance of viscous stresses and pressure gradient. This is the realm of microcirculation.

Small Reynolds numbers ($\ll 1$) are not the only characteristics of micro-circulation. At least three other features are unique:

(a) The individuality of blood cells must be recognized.
(b) Exchange of fluid and other matters between blood and tissue sur-rounding the blood vessel occurs.
(c) The smooth muscle of the microvasculature operates to regulate the flow locally.

We have already discussed the role of red blood cells in the rheology of blood in microvessels in Chapter 5 of *Biomechanics* (Fung, 1981); and more will be said in the present chapter. Fluid exchange will be discussed in Chapter 2 of the companion volume, *Biodynamics: Flow, Motion, and Stress* (Fung, 1984). The regulation of blood flow locally by arterioles will be discussed in Sec. 5.12.

A striking characteristic of the capillary circulation is the continuous variation of the blood flow. Changes are seen in the velocity, direction of movement, and number of capillaries with an active circulation. During the ebb and tide of flow, a continuous circulation persists in certain channels, whereas in the majority of capillaries the circulation is intermittent. At one time, the blood stream courses from arteriole to venule through two or three pathways. At a subsequent phase, the blood spills over into numerous side branches so that as many as 15–20 capillary vessels contain an active circula-tion originating from a single arteriole.

These features can be explained on the basis of mechanics: with the active contraction of smooth muscle on the one hand, and the basic laws of continum mechanics on the other.

As usual, we shall start with anatomy, then proceed to the mechanical properties of tissues, and finally, system dynamics. The importance of the subject is unquestionable, because the whole purpose of the heart and the arteries is to carry blood to the capillaries to nourish the cells in the body.

5.2 Anatomy of Microvascular Beds

There are infinite variations in the detailed geometry of microvascular beds, just as there are infinite varieties of irrigation fields in agriculture. Figure 5.2:1 shows threee major models. In (a) an artery supplies a number of parallel microvessels which drain into a vein. In (b) an arterial network and a venous network are nearly parallel. Many microvessels connect various points of the arterial network to points of the venous network. In (c), an artery supplies a region which is drained by veins and lymph vessels. Three different things are sketched in (c). One is a *glomerulus*, whose capillaries have a large caliber and many local dilatations. The second is a *sinusoid*, which has a dense network and dilates easily. The third is a *sinus*, which is a wide capillary without forming any meshes or networks. To help visualize the differences between these models, the analogous agricultural irrigation

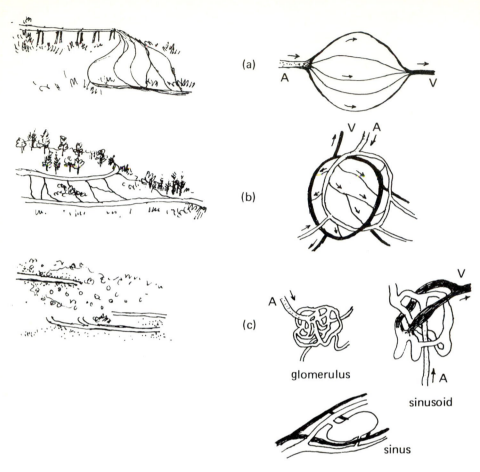

Figure 5.2:1 Sketch of four topological models of microvascular beds and their irrigation analogs.

channels are sketched on the side. The analog of the blood pressure is the elevation of the irrigation channels.

   With the topology illustrated in these sketches, it is not surprising that the flow in all microvessels is not the same: some carry stronger currents, some less. The ones in which flow is more robust than their neighbors are called *thoroughfares*. Some microvessels, especially in cases (a) and (c), are so short that they appear to connect an artery to a vein directly, to form shortcuts that bypass the capillary network: these are called *anastomosis*. Thoroughfares and anastomoses are important flow control gates.

   The draining of fluid is assisted by lymph vessels, which are analogous to subterrainean drainage in agriculture.

   These conceptual models can help us understand the structure of various organs. Figure 5.2:2 shows a photomicrograph of rat cremaster muscle

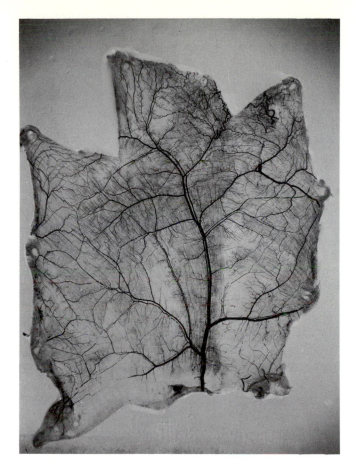

Figure 5.2:2 Photomicrograph of rat cremaster muscle after intravenous injection of carbon to visualize the vascular pattern. Note parallel course of small arteries and veins, and interarcading pattern of terminal arterioles and venules ($\times 20$). From Smaje, et al. (1970). Reproduced by permission.

after intravenous injection of carbon to visualize the vascular pattern. The small arteries and veins run parallel to each other, the arterioles branch off at right angles, and the capillary networks are arranged so that the capillaries run parallel to the muscle fibers. The photograph shows two layers of muscle fibers which lie approximately at right angles to each other. Figure 5.2:3 is a schematic abstraction of the vascular structure.

Figure 5.2:4 shows a schematic drawing of the microvascular bed of the human skin. Here vessel networks of all three types (a), (b), and (c), can be clearly seen. The sweat gland is surrounded by vessels of the type (c).

Readers interested in seeing pictures of many different kinds of microvascular beds in various organs may consult Wiedeman et al. (1981), Johnson (1978), Kaley and Altura (1977).

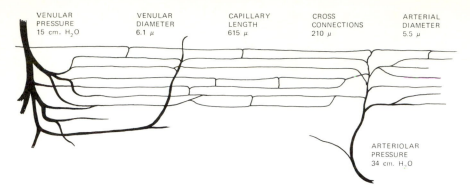

Figure 5.2:3 An abstraction of the cremaster muscle capillary blood vessel network, showing the type of arrangement of the vessels and mean values obtained in the experiments. From Smaje, et al. (1970). Reproduced by permission. *Additional data:* capillary density = 1300/mm², distance between capillaries = 34 μm, capillary surface area = 244 cm²/cm³ muscle, red cell velocity = 700 μ/sec, capillary filtration coefficient = 0.001 $\mu^3/\mu^2 \cdot$ sec $\cdot$ cm $\cdot$ H$_2$O difference.

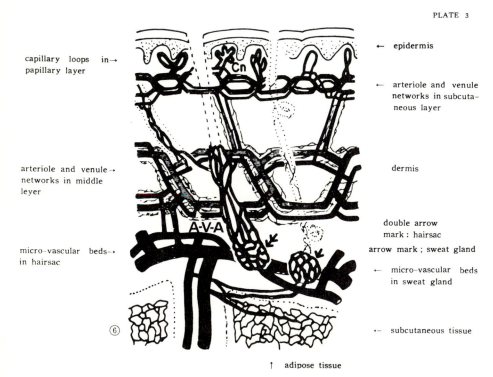

Figure 5.2:4 Schematic drawing of micro-blood-vessel distribution in the skin of an adult human. From Ogawa (1976). Reproduced by permission.

Arterioles and Venules

Most authors base the terminology of arterioles and venules on histological characteristics. Thus a *terminal arteriole* is a final arterial ramification of 10–50 μm diameter endowed with a continuous single layer of smooth muscle cells and scant supporting connective tissue. A *metarteriole* is one with discontinuous smooth muscle cells in the wall. The *precapillary sphincter* is the last smooth muscle cell along any branch of a terminal arteriole. An *arteriole* is a small artery ranging approximately between 10–125 μm in diameter, and having more than one smooth muscle layer, and nerve association in the outermost muscle layer. The inner wall of these vessels is lined with endothelial cells which are flat in shape and abut a basement membrane and an elastic layer. Fine elastic fibers are interspersed among the muscle cells.

Analogously, a *postcapillary venule* is a vessel with a diameter of 8–30 μm formed by, and is a continuation of, two to four confluencing venous capillaries, with an increasing number of pericytes as the lumen increases. A *collecting venule* is one of 10–50 μm diameter, with one complete layer of pericytes and a complete layer of veil cells, and occasional smooth muscle cells. A *muscular venule* is one of 50–100 μm diameter, with a thick wall of smooth muscle cells that sometimes overlap to form two layers. The confluence of muscular venules forms larger, 100–300 μm diameter, *small collecting veins*, with a prominent media of continuous layers of smooth muscle cells.

These descriptive definitions lack precision, and their use is not universally adhered to by all authors. Furthermore, not all organs have all these vessels. For example, neither metarteriole, nor precapillary sphinctor have been found in skeletal muscle. Also, the precapillary arteries (i.e., arterioles) in the lung do not have layers of smooth muscles, and thus do not fit the definition of an arteriole named above. In these cases, counting generations from capillaries is the simplest way to identify the hierarchy of the vascular tree, as it is illustrated in Sec. 4.9 in Chapter 4.

Perhaps the most important thing for us to remember is that the microvascular bed of different organs are different. To study the function of an organ, we must familiarize ourselves with the special structure of the vasculature of that organ.

The Capillaries

The wall of a capillary blood vessel consists of a single layer of endothelial cells surrounded by a basement membrane which splits to enclose occasional cells called *pericytes*. The pericytes are thought to have the potential to become smooth muscle cells. There is a large number of vesicles in the endothelial cells. These vesicles are believed to be transporters of materials.

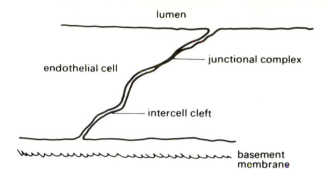

Figure 5.2:5 A schematic view of the endothelial layer showing the intercell cleft and junctional complex between adjacent cells viewed in cross-section. From Caro et al. (1978, p. 369). Reproduced by permission.

The endothelial cells of the capillary wall have their edges closely apposed to one another. In electron microscopy, apposing cell membranes appear very close, with a gap of 10–20 nm. At certain points, these membranes and the adjacent cytoplasm appear darker. At these points, the intercellular clefts are also sealed by tight junctions or *maculae occludens*, which are formed by the close apposition or fusion of the external leaflets of the plasmalemma, completely obliterating the intercellular space. In certain areas (e.g., in the brain) these junctions form an uninterrupted seal, i.e., *zonulae occludens*, preventing the passage of molecules with radius of 2.5 nm or above. These tight junctions are like spot welding (maculae) and seam welding (zonula) in industrial metal construction. They connect the endothelial cells together to form a continuous barrier. They play an important role in determining the permeability of the endothelium to water and other molecules. A schematic drawing is given in Fig. 5.2:5.

The appearance of the endothelial cell lining of blood vessels may be different in different organs, as is illustrated in Fig. 5.2:6. In the first, *continuous* type, the endothelial cells are joined tightly together. In the vessels of striated muscle, the cells may be quite flat and thin. In postcapillary venules, they may be cuboidal and form a thick layer. In the second, *fenestrated type* the endothelial cells are so thin that the opposite surfaces of their membrane are very close together, and form small circular areas known as *diaphragms of fenestrate* approximately 25 nm thick, and of the order of 100 nm across. Adjacent endothelial cells are still tightly joined. This type of vessel has been described in three groups or organs: (1) endocrine gland, (2) structures engaged in the production or absorption of fluids (e.g., renal glomerulus, choroid plexus of the brain, ciliary body of the eye, intestinal villus), and (3) retia mirabilia (e.g., renal medulla, fish swim bladder).

The third type of endothelium is the *discontinuous* type in which there are distinct intercellular gaps and discontinuous basement membrane. These

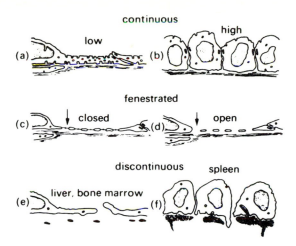

Figure 5.2:6 Schematic view of different types of endothelial lining, classified according to the degree of continuity. From Majno (1965). Reproduced by permission.

occur in those vessels commonly called *sinusoids*. They are common in organs whose primary functions are to add or to extract from the blood whole cells as well as large molecules and extraneous particles, e.g., liver, spleen, and bone marrow.

The Lymphatics

A lymphatic capillary has a single layer of endothelium surrounded by a basement membrane, and lacks smooth muscle in its walls. The lymphatic endothelial cells contain more microfilaments than the systemic capillary cells. The basement membrane of the lymphatic capillaries is incomplete, and there are filaments running through it to the endothelial cell membrane from the collagen and elastin fibers of the interstitial space. The intercellular junction of adjoining lymphatic endothelial cells is similar to that of blood capillaries, except that open junctions are seen in all lymphatic capillaries. The gap of the open junction may be some microns across, but is usually about 0.1 μm. These open gaps play an important role in the uptake of material and its retention in the lymphatics.

The lymphatic capillaries are blind sacs. They merge to form *collecting lymphatics* which transport material to the vein. Collecting lymphatics have an endothelium, a basement membrane, and a layer of smooth muscle cells. They have valves which are either truncated cones or paired leaflets originating from opposite sides of the lymphatic wall. These valves assure unidirectional movement of lymph.

The Interstitial Space

The complement to the space occupied by the blood vessels, lymphatics, and cells of a tissue is called the interstitial space of that tissue. It is mainly connective tissue, containing collagen, elastin, hyaluronic acid, and other substances, either bathed in some kind of fluid, or embedded in a gel. See Chapter 2 of the author's companion volume, *Biodynamics: Flow, Motion, and Stress.*

Nerves

Sympathetic fibers invest the aorta, large and small arteries and veins, and to a variable degree the networks of the arteriolar vessels and muscular venules in each organ. There appears to be no direct innervation of the capillary blood vessels and collecting venules, although fibers may be found in the capillary region. Sympathetic fibers are usually superimposed on the smooth muscle layer of the blood vessel wall, but do not make direct synaptic contact with the vascular smooth muscle cells. See Norberg and Hamberger (1964).

Stimulation of sympathetic nerves generally constricts the blood vessel. The blood vessels in most organs show a maintained constriction during tonic sympathetic stimulation. However, the contribution of sympathetic nerves to resting or basal vascular tone varies greatly among different organs. Acute denervation has no effect on cerebral blood flow, whereas denervation in skin increases flow 5- to 10-fold. In intestine, liver, spleen, and lymph nodal tissue the response to a continued stimulus is transient and the vascular bed "escapes" from the constrictor influence within a few minutes.

If the effect of the sympathetic transmitter norepinephrine is blocked by an α-adrenergic blocking agent, a vasodilator influence acting through β-receptors is unmasked. When the β-receptor is also blocked, the catecholamine is without effect. Sympathetic activity may cause vasodilation also through effects on tissue metabolism, as seen in cardiac muscle and liver.

The parasympathetic system produces vasodilation in those tissues that are innervated by it. The vasodilation action involves either an alteration in metabolism or (in salivary and sweat glands) release of an enzyme that diffuses into the tissue spaces.

The central nervous system has various sites where neural control mechanisms of vasomotor tone are located. See Folkow and Neil (1971), and Sagawa et al. (1974). On the aortic arch and carotid sinus there are baroreceptors which inhibit the medullary vasomotor activity when stimulated. The effect of the reflex mechanisms differs considerably from organ to organ. Reduction of pressure in the carotid sinus causes strong constriction in muscle and has a lesser effect on the kidney, liver and intestine. Brain apparently is not significantly affected. Distention of pulmonary veins and artial junction also inhibit sympathetic tone arising from the medullary neurons. There are similar receptors in the atria, ventricles, and the lung.

The chemoreceptors in carotid sinus and aortic arch affects the peripheral blood vessels in a complex way. If other factors are held constant, stimulation of either the aortic or carotid bodies causes reflex vasoconstriction. However, the normal increase in ventilation that accompanies chemoreceptor activity overrides this reflex response and causes vasodilation.

In addition to control by central nervous system, the vascular smooth muscle cells respond to changes in tension, stretch, and metabolities. These responses are responsible for the moment-to-moment regulation of vascular tone in individual organs. This local control mechanism will be discussed in Sec. 5.12.

5.3 Pressure Distribution in Microvessels

Systematic measurement of pressure distribution in small blood vessels is usually done by a probe originally designed by Wiederhielm et al. (1964). Zweifach and his associates have made extensive measurements of pressure distribution in microvessels. In a typical microvascular bed of the cat mesentery, the arterial to venous distribution of intravascular pressure and velocity is shown in Fig. 5.3:1. The pressure decreases rapidly in arterioles of diameters in the range of 10–35 μm. The decline in pressure within the true capillaries and postcapillaries is much more gradual.

The pressure gradient, dp/dL, can be measured by using two pressure probes inserted into two side branches of a given vessel and occluding flow in these side branches. The two pressure readings divided by the distance between the stations gives the pressure gradient. As is shown in Fig. 5.3:2, the pressure gradient increases as vessel size decreases.

Figures 5.3:1 and 5.3:2 show the data obtained from cats whose central arterial pressures were in the normal range of 101–142 mmHg. Data were also obtained in hypertensive cats with arterial pressures in the range 142–194 mmHg, and hypotensive cats with pressures of 60–100 mmHg. These are shown in Fig. 5.3:3. The pressure drop in arterioles in the hypertensive cats was larger than in the normals, whereas that in the hypotensive cats was smaller. Pressures in the capillaries and postcapillary vessels were similar in the two groups, the difference between the mean pressures being only 3–5 mmHg. Thus it appears that the arterioles control the blood pressure in such a way that the capillary pressure is maintained in the normal range while the central arterial pressure may fluctuate.

In the skeletal muscle of the cat, the pressure drop in the arterioles is even stronger. See Fig. 5.3:4.

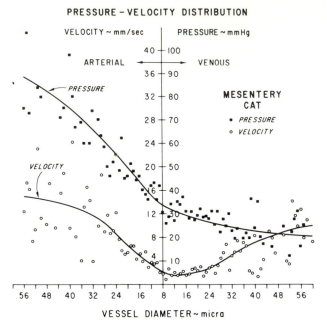

Figure 5.3:1 Arterial to venous distribution of intravascular pressure and velocity in the mesentery of the cat. Vessel diameter (abscissa) is taken to be representative of the functional position of each vessel in the microvascular network. Each data point represents the average value of three to five individual measurements at the abscissa (diameter) value. The solid curves are piece-wise cubic spline fits of the data and are statistically representative of the arterial to venous trends. From Zweifach and Lipowsky (1977, p. 386). Reproduced by permission of the American Heart Association, Inc.

Shunts

It was observed that in the skin pressures in about 10% of the venules were sometimes higher than expected (approximately 70 mmHg compared with the usual value of 30 mmHg). This is taken to be an evidence of the existence of shunts (such as thoroughfare channels) in the microvascular bed. These shunts are more direct low-resistance pathways connecting arterioles to venules.

Temporal Variation

The pressure wave forms in the microvessels are illustrated in Fig. 5.3:5. One sees the cardiac oscillations with an amplitude of 1–2 mmHg normally, and 2–4 mmHg if the precapillary sphincter were dilated. One sees also a

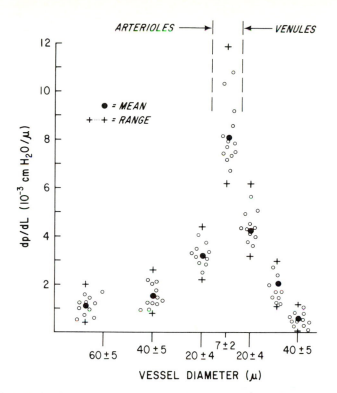

Figure 5.3:2 Reduction in pressure measured by two microprobes separated by the maximum distance possible between branches. In arterioles, dP/dL was measured along a 1500–2500 μ interval; in venules, longer segments were usually available, 2000–3000 μ. In the capillary region, the interprobe separation was usually 200–350 μ. Values indicated cover a diameter range of $\pm 5\mu$ for each of the categories listed, except for capillaries, in which the range is $\pm 2\mu$. Cat's mesentery. From Zweifach (1974, p. 850). Reproduced by permission of the American Heart Association, Inc.

random-fluctuation of a period in the order of 15 to 20 sec, with an amplitude of 3–5 mmHg. A third type of pressure variation is not shown in the figure, it is more substantial and lasts longer, in the order of 10 mmHg and 5–8 min, followed by a return to the steady-state condition in about 2–3 min.

That cardiac pulses must leave ripples in the capillaries is not surprising. The records shown in Fig. 5.3:5 show them clearly. These waves are attenuated in the direction of propagation, reflecting the fact that in the capillaries the viscous stress dissipates the pressure fluctuations. By measuring the phase shift of a wave from the arterial end to the venular end of a capillary, the wave speed is estimated to be about 7.2 cm/sec^{-1}.

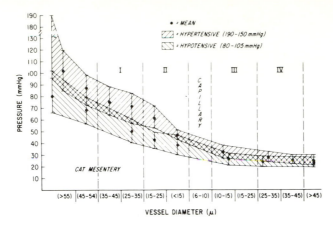

Figure 5.3:3 Pressure profiles for cats with extreme pressures (hypertension and hypotension). Note the trend for pressure to converge in the precapillary (15–20 μ) region. Postcapillary pressures were essentially the same for all groups (12 hypertensive, 8 hypotensive cats). From Zweifach (1974, p. 849). Reproduced by permission of the American Heart Association, Inc.

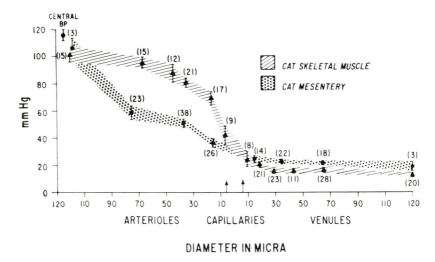

Figure 5.3:4 Micropressure distribution in two different tissues in relation to average diameter of given vessels. Vertical bars express $\pm$SEM and number of measurement is given in parentheses. Central BP—central arterial pressure—an average from all experiments. From Fronek and Zweifach (1974). Reproduced by permission of the American Heart Association, Inc.

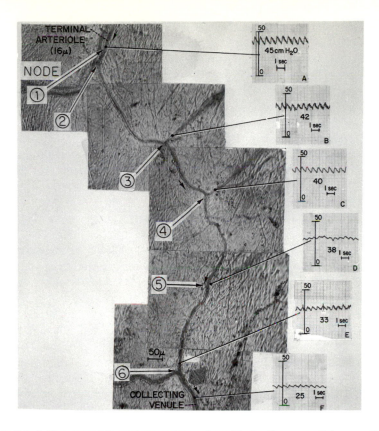

Figure 5.3:5 Photographic reconstruction of capillaries from arteriole to collecting venule with direct recordings of pressure taken at the points indicated. The capillaries ranged from 7.5 μm to 9 μm in width. Note the persistence of the pulse pressure throughout. Each reading was taken at a side branch so as not to interrupt the flow through the feeding capillary. From Zweifach (1974, p. 858). Reproduced by permission.

5.4 Pressure in the Interstitial Space

The pressure in the interstitial space is of great importance in the study of fluid movement in the tissue. If we treat the capillary blood vessel wall as a semi-permeable membrane, the rate of movement of water across the wall (from blood into the interstitium) may be assumed to obey Starling's hypothesis:

$$\dot{m} = K(p_b - p_t - \pi_b + \pi_t), \qquad (1)$$

where p stands for hydrostatic pressure, π stands for osmotic pressure, the subscript b stands for blood, t stands for tissue, $\dot{m}$ represents the volume flow rate per unit area of the membrane, and K is the *permeability constant*.

In order to calculate the fluid transfer rate $\dot{m}$, we must know all five quantities, p_b, p_t, π_b, π_t, and K; they are equally important. Since fluid movement in the tissue space is very important to health (too much or too little fluid in the tissue means edema or dehydration), the measurement of p_t and π_t has engaged attention of physiologists for a long time.

Methods of measuring the interstitial pressure in the tissues of various organs are discussed in Chap. 2 of the companion volume, *Biodynamics: Flow, Motion, and Stress.* (Fung, 1984). These methods are ingenious. The results are, however, controversial, yielding values of p_t ranging from a few mmHg below atmospheric to slightly above atmospheric pressure.

5.5 Velocity Distribution in Microvessels

In large blood vessels the velocity of red blood cells can be measured by an electromagnetic flow meter, based on the fact that the red cells are charged particles. For microvessels, such a small electromagnetic flow meter is not available. For capillary blood vessels in a suitable preparation, it is possible to measure red cell velocity by optical means because red cells are optically dense in mercury arc emission light. By observing a red cell in a capillary blood vessel at two stations of known distance apart, and measuring the time of travel between the stations, the velocity of the red cell can be calculated. This is called the *two-slit method.* In practice, the transmitted light at any station fluctuates with time because red cells are nonuniformly distributed. By recording the transmitted light intensity at two stations, one can calculate the cross-correlation of the two signals. Now, if the signal of the first station is delayed by a time period τ and then correlated with the signal from the second station, we can obtain a cross-correlation function as a function of τ. The value of delay time τ at which the correlation is the maximum is then taken to be the time required for the red cells to move from the first station to the second. A division of the known distance between stations by the lapse time τ yields the average red cell velocity.

This method can be used with confidence in narrow capillaries in which the red cells move in single file. For larger vessels, the velocity of red cells in any cross section vary from a maximum at the center to near zero at the wall. Hence, if we measure red cell velocity, we have to explain carefully where it is measured, whether it is centerline velocity, or is an average over the entire cross section. Since the diameters of the red cells of most mammals are in the range of 6–9 μm, it is possible to select a microscope objective so that the red cells in a focal plane are clearly seen, while others not in focus are blurred. Thus, if the vessel is several cell diameters large, you can focus up and down and get an impression of the velocity profile. Now, for quantitative work you will probably use a photoelectric multiplier to record the optical signals. The question then arises as to what is seen by the photoelectric tube. Wayland (1982) emphasized the fact that if a photomultiplier is used to "observe" the cells, the tube integrates the signals both from those cells sharply in focus and some cells not so sharply in focus. If then you focus up and down, the photomultiplier will give you a velocity profile which is *blunter* than the real one. This is an important factor to remember. For example, if a laminar flow of blood in a glass tube is observed, Baker and Wayland (1974) found that the photoelectric tube yields a maximum velocity of red cells on the centerline of the tube equal to 1.6 times the mean velocity of flow, instead of the theoretical factor of 2.0. Lipowsky and Zweifach (1978) confirmed the result for tubes of diameter from 80 to 17 μm, and erythrocytes of diameter about 6 μm, but the scatter of the data was large. Lee et al. (1983) have shown that this ratio depends on light intensity and tube diameter.

Usually we wish to know the flow rate of whole blood. Thus, if red cell velocity is measured, we should know the ratio of the average red cell velocity to the mean velocity of whole blood. In a large blood vessel this ratio approaches 1, since the cells, small compared to the tube, will be convected with the plasma. In a microvessel, the ratio will be larger than 1 because the cells tend to concentrate in the center of the tube where the velocity is higher than the average. If the vessel is so very narrow that the red cells effectively plug up the tube, then the particle velocity and the whole blood velocity tend to be equal again, because the "leak back" (see *Biomechanics* (Fung, 1981, p. 168) of the plasma in the narrow gap between the red cell and the tube wall is small.

To clarify this ratio, a model experiment was done by Yen and Fung (1978) with gelatin pellets simulating red cells, and silicone fluid simulating plasma. (See Sec. 5.6). The results are shown in Fig. 5.5:1 and Table 5.5:1. The velocity ratio $v/\overline{V}$ (average particle velocity v divided by mean velocity of whole blood $\overline{V}$) is seen to be independent of flow velocity, but depends strongly on the ratio of the diameter of the cell, D_c, to that of the tube, D_t. When the hematocrit is 10% the velocity ratio is about 1.21 when the diameter of the tube is equal to that of the cell, ($D_c/D_t = 1.0$). It increases to 1.47 when D_c/D_t is 0.67, and to 1.49 when D_c/D_t is 0.5. Each point in Fig. 5.5:1 represents an experimental measurement. The scatter of the data is seen to be very large, reflecting the fact that the exact value of the velocity ratio $v/\overline{V}$ depends on the incidental factor of particle configuration relative to the tube. The red cells deform severely in such a flow, and can assume all kinds of configurations: with their axes parallel to the cylinder axis, or perpendicular to it, or at some angles in between. For larger tubes Lee et al. (1983) have obtained a good empirical formula for $v/\overline{V}$.

From measurements on red cell velocity, one can compute the mean flow velocity using the velocity ratio named above. A multiplication with the measured cross-sectional area of the vessel then yields the flow.

Zweifach and Lipowsky's (1977) results on the average values of the velocity of flow in the microvessels in cat's mesentery is shown in Fig. 5.3:1.

Using two pressure probes of the type discussed in Section 5.3 to measure

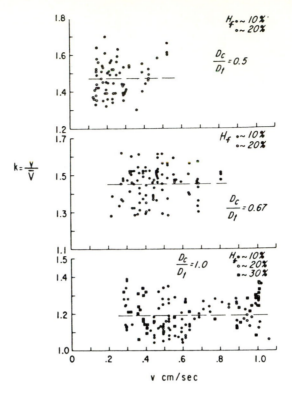

Figure 5.5:1 Experimental results of test model for $D_c/D_t = 0.5$, 0.67, and 1.0, where D_c is the diameter of the simulated red cells, D_t is the diameter of the tube. The ratio k between the average particle velocity v and the mean flow velocity $\bar{V}$ of the whole blood (simulated plasma and cells) is plotted against v for different feed-tube hematocrit H_f. Dotted lines are mean values of k computed for combined values of H_f for each value of D_c/D_t. From Yen and Fung (1978). Reproduced by permission.

TABLE 5.5:1 Ratio of Particle Velocity to Mean Flow Velocity[a]

D_c/D_t	Hematocrit			Combined Data
	10%	20%	30%	
1.0	1.21 ± 0.012	1.17 ± 0.012	1.20 ± 0.016	1.19 ± 0.008
0.67	1.47 ± 0.010	1.42 ± 0.014		1.45 ± 0.008
0.5	1.49 ± 0.014	1.45 ± 0.014		1.48 ± 0.011

[a] Experimental results of test model for $D_c/D_t = 1.0$, 0.67, and 0.5. Means $\pm$ SE of the ratio between particle velocity and mean flow velocity are listed corresponding to feed-tube hematocrit and combined for each value of D_c/D_t. D_c is the diameter of the simulated red blood cell. D_t is the diameter of the tube. Data from Yen and Fung (1978).

TABLE 5.5:2 Rheological Parameter[a] for Several Microvessels of the Cat's Mesentery. From Lipowsky and Zweifach (1977). Reproduced by permission.

Vessel type	Diameter (μm)	Length (μm)	$\langle V_{RBC}\rangle$[b] (mm/sec)	$\langle\Delta P\rangle$[c] (cm H$_2$O)	$\bar{V}$ (mm/sec)	μ (cP)	τ_w (dyn/cm^2)
Arteriole	45.0	632.0	20.8	4.3	13.0	3.25	75.0
Arteriole	23.0	429.0	23.2	6.7	14.5	1.75	88.0
Capillary	7.0	481.0	0.67	11.1	—[b]	5.17	39.6
Venule	17.0	667.0	2.00	2.10	1.25	2.23	13.1
Venule	54.0	403.0	7.50	0.71	4.69	3.36	23.3

[a] Based on time-averaged red cell velocities and pressure drops for the first 2 sec of each record.
[b] Baker and Wayland correction factor not applied. Flow is based on $\langle V_{RBC}\rangle$.
[c] ΔP is the pressure difference measured in a blood vessel at two points separated by a distance equal to the "length" listed in the table. $\bar{V}$ is equal to $\langle V_{RBC}\rangle/1.6$ according to Baker and Wayland (1974). μ is the apparent viscosity of blood. τ_w is the shear stress acting on the vessel wall calculated according to Eqs. (19)–(21) of Sec. 3.2.

the difference in pressure Δp at a distance ΔL apart, a dimensional analyzer to measure vessel diameter, and an aforementioned velocity diode, Zweifach and Lipowsky (1977) obtained data on volume-flow rate $\dot{Q}$ and pressure gradient $\Delta p/\Delta L$ in microvessels. From these data one can calculate the specific resistance R according to the formula

$$-\frac{\Delta p}{\Delta L} = \dot{Q}R. \tag{1}$$

According to Poiseuille formula (Eq (17) of Sec. 3.2), we have

$$R = \frac{8\mu}{\pi a^4}. \tag{2}$$

Hence, one can calculate the apparent viscosity of the blood, μ, in these vessels. Table 5.5:2 shows the rheological parameters culculated from data from several microvessels of the cat's mesentery.

The hematocrit distribution in microvasculature can be measured by optical means (Lipowsky et al., 1979). Figure 5.5:2 shows the hematocrit in mesenteric microvasculature of the cat. The very significant decrease in hematocrit in microvessels is noteworthy.

5.6 The Velocity–Hematocrit Relationship

If one observes capillary blood flow *in vivo*, one sees that the flow is non-homogeneous and unsteady. The major part of the unsteadiness is not due to the heartbeat, to which it is not synchronous. It changes much more slowly, and without a definite period. In one period, we see red cells rush by; in another period, we do not see any red cells at all. Since the volume

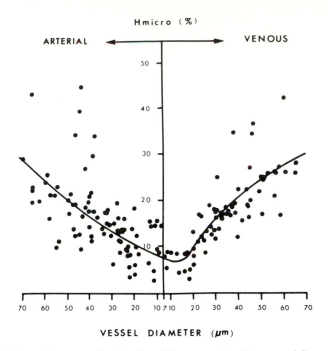

Figure 5.5:2 Arteriovenous distribution of hematocrit in the normal flow state of the mesenteric microvasculature (cat). Each point represents hematocrit in a single un-branched microvessel of the indicated luminal diameter (abscissa). Hematocrit was obtained by *in situ* measurement of optical density and *in vitro* correlation with hemato-crit following the technique of Jendrucko and Lee (1973). Hematocrits of microvessels smaller than 20 μm diameter were obtained by rapid occlusion of the vessel and cell counting. The solid curve is a piece-wise cubic spline smoothing of the 150 individual measurements taken in 15 animals. Arteriolar hematocrits averaged 15.9% and venular hematocrits averaged 17.3%. In contrast, systemic hematocrit averaged 33.8% ± 8.4% (SD). From Lipowsky et al. (1980). Reproduced by permission.

fraction of red cells in whole blood is called hematocrit, we say that the hematocrit in capillary blood vessels is unsteady. One of the reasons for the unsteadiness of hematocrit in capillary blood vessels is the unsteadiness of velocity in these vessels. In *Biomechanics* (Fung, 1981 Chap. 5, p. 161), we have explained that if a narrow capillary bifurcates into two equal daughters, the faster branch will get more red cells, thus having a higher hematocrit. Since any microcirculation circuit is derived from bifurcating blood vessels, there must exist a relationship between the distributions of blood flow velocity and hematocrit. Too many factors influence this rela-tionship, however, and only in the simplest case can a definitive mathematical relationship be stated. This is the case of one vessel bifurcating into two equal daughters. This case has been studied by Fung (1973) theoretically, by Yen and Fung (1978) using a simulated model, by Gaehtgens (1980)

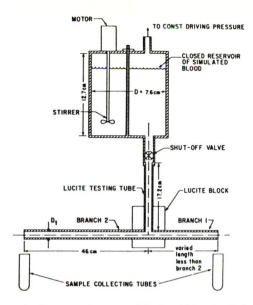

Figure 5.6:1 Schematic diagram of test model of red blood cell flow in a bifurcating capillary blood vessel. Three cylindrical tubes meet to form an inverted T joint. Flow in branch 1 is faster than that in branch 2. Inner diameters of test tubes, D_t, are 0.32, 0.48, and 0.64 cm. From Yen and Fung (1978). Reproduced by permission.

using blood in micropipette and *in vivo* observations, and by G. W. Schmid-Schoenbein et al. (1980a) in rabbit ear-chamber with particular attention to leucocytes. *In vivo* observations are necessary, but accurate measurements are difficult, especially because a method to determine the capillary blood vessel diameter to a desired level of accuracy is still unavailable. Model experiments are simpler. By fixing a number of parameters they yield precise mathematical relations more readily, and can be understood and analyzed more easily. In the following, we shall discuss a model approach.

In Yen and Fung's (1978) model, the plasma is simulated by a silicone fluid, the red blood cells are simulated by gelatin pellets, and the blood vessel is simulated by lucite tubes. The model was designed according to the principle of kinematic and dynamic similarity, at Reynolds number in the range 10^{-2}–10^{-3}. At such a low Reynolds number, the angle of branching is umimportant, and therefore 90° was used. A schematic diagram of the apparatus is shown in Fig. 5.6:1. It consists of a closed reservoir of simulated blood with an inverted T tube of lucite attached as shown. All branches are circular cylinders and of the same diameter.

The hematocrit and velocity relationship in bifurcation branches was determined by allowing a gelatin-pellet suspension to flow through the T tube. The experiment consisted of collecting quantities of fluid from the two branches in a steady-state condition. Flow can be stopped by closing

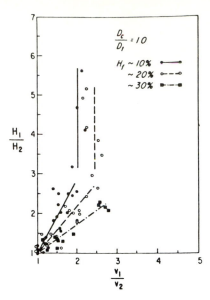

Figure 5.6:2 Experimental results of test model for $D_c/D_t = 1.0$. H_1/H_2 is plotted against v_1/v_2 for three different feed-tube hematocrits H_f. From Yen and Fung (1978). Reproduced by permission.

the shut-off valve after each test. Velocities in the two branches were varied by changing the lengths of the branches by cutting off a segment of one branch at a time. The pellet velocities were obtained by measuring the time required for a pellet to travel a known distance. The mean velocity of flow in each tube was computed from the volume discharge rate. The discharge hematocrit was measured by centrifuging the collected sample, and obtaining the ratio of the volume of the packed particles to the total volume. The tube hematocrit is computed according to the following consideration: In each tube the volume of the pellets that crossed a given cross section in unit time is equal to the product of (mean speed of tube flow) · (tube cross section) · (discharge hematocrit). It is also equal to the product (mean speed of pellets) · (tube cross section) · (tube hematocrit). Hence

$$\frac{\text{discharge hematocrit}}{\text{tube hematocrit}} = \frac{\text{mean speed of pellets}}{\text{mean speed of tube flow}}. \tag{1}$$

Hematocrit of the feeding tube (H_f) was calculated as follows. Let $\bar{V}_f$ be the mean volume-flow rate in the feeding tube, $\bar{V}_1$ be that in branch 1, $\bar{V}_2$ be that in branch 2; and let v_f be the average particle velocity in the feeding tube, v_1 be that in branch 1, v_2 be that in branch 2. Without loss of generality, we may let $v_1 \geq v_2$, and $\bar{V}_1 \geq \bar{V}_2$. Then, by the principle of conservation of mass of the mixture and of the pellets, we have, since the cross-sectional area of all branches is the same,

$$\bar{V}_f = \bar{V}_1 + \bar{V}_2, \tag{2}$$

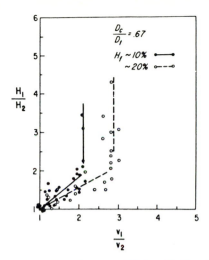

Figure 5.6:3 Experimental results of test model for $D_c/D_t = 0.67$. H_1/H_2 is plotted against v_1/v_2 for two different feed-tube hematocrits H_f. From Yen and Fung (1978). Reproduced by permission.

$$H_f v_f = H_1 v_1 + H_2 v_2. \qquad (3)$$

The mean flow velocities $\bar{V}_f$, $\bar{V}_1$, $\bar{V}_2$ are related to the particle velocities v_f, v_1, v_2 as is discussed in Sec. 5.5 and illustrated in Fig. 5.5:1 and Table 5.5:1. It is seen that the ratio of particle velocity to mean flow velocity depends strongly on the ratio of cell to tube diameters, D_c/D_t, but does not vary significantly with hematocrit. Nor does it vary with flow rate. Hence, for each value of D_c/D_t, we can replace Eq. (2) by

$$v_f = v_1 + v_2. \qquad (4)$$

On substituting Eq. (4) into Eq. (3), we obtain the feed tube hematocrit H_f

$$H_f = \frac{H_1 v_1 + H_2 v_2}{v_1 + v_2}. \qquad (5)$$

Figures 5.6:2–4 show the experimental results. In these figures, the ratio H_1/H_2 is plotted against the ratio v_1/v_2 for different feed-tube hematocrit H_f. The symbols v_1, v_2, H_1, H_2 are the particle velocities and tube hematocrits in the branches 1 and 2, respectively. It is seen that for narrow capillaries (with the cell diameter/tube diameter $= D_c/D_t = 1.0$, 0.67, and 0.5), the branch with faster flow (branch 1) will have more cells. In general, for velocity ratios sufficiently smaller than a critical value, the hematocrit ratio can be expressed by a linear relationship given by

$$\frac{H_1}{H_2} - 1 = a\left(\frac{v_1}{v_2} - 1\right). \qquad (6)$$

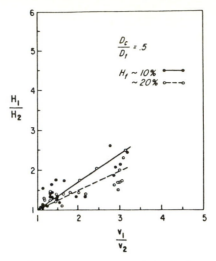

Figure 5.6:4 Experimental results of test model for $D_c/D_t = 0.5$. H_1/H_2 is plotted against v_1/v_2 for two different feed-tube hematocrits H_f. From Yen and Fung (1978). Reproduced by permission.

In Eq. (6), the dimensionless constant, a, depends on a number of factors, the most important of which are (i) the ratio of cell diameter to tube diameter, (ii) the shape and rigidity of the pellets, and (iii) the hematocrit in the feeding tube.

Figures 5.6:2 and 3 also show that for velocity ratios beyond a critical value nearly all the cells flow into the faster branch. The smaller the feeding tube hematocrit is, the smaller is the critical velocity ratio at which this phenomenon occurred. The critical velocity ratio lies in the range of 2–3.0 when $D_c/D_t = 1.0$, with exact value depending on the feed hematocrit. The critical velocity ratio becomes higher when D_c/D_t decreases.

Theoretical Analysis of the Experiment

An approximate analysis of the forces that act on a particle at a bifurcation point will clarify the theme of this article. We shall show that if the mean velocities of flow in the two daughter branches are $\bar{V}_1$ and $\bar{V}_2$, with $\bar{V}_1 > \bar{V}_2$, then the resultant forces due to pressure and shear stress are both proportional to $\bar{V}_1 - \bar{V}_2$, and act in the direction of the daughter tube with higher velocity, $\bar{V}_1$.

First, consider disk-shaped flexible pellets. Such a pellet can assume all kinds of orientation in the tube. Let us consider two configurations, one in which the plane of the disk is perpendicular to the axis of the tube, and

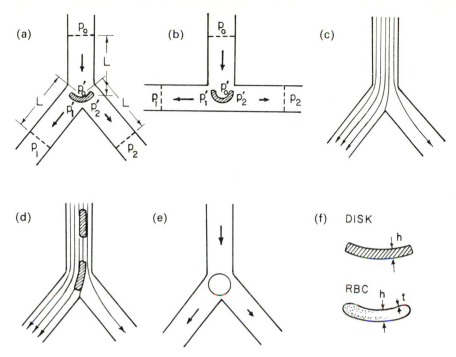

Figure 5.6:5 Illustration of the features of modeling. Flow is directed downward. Velocity in left branch (tube 1) is faster than that in right branch (tube 2). (a) A plugging pellet at the fork. (b) Similar to (a), but with branching angle equal to 90°. (c) Stream-line pattern in the case $\bar{V}_1 = 2\bar{V}_2$, as seen in the middle section. (d) pellets flowing edge-on, and astride of the dividing stream surface. (e) Flow of a rigid spherical particle at the fork. (f) Cross sections of a pellet in the model and a red blood cell. Pellet is a solid disk of homogeneous elastic material. Red blood cell is considered to be a thin shell filled with a liquid. From Yen and Fung (1978). Reproduced by permission.

another in which the plane of the disk is parallel to the axis of the tube. For conciseness, we say that the first case is plugging, the second is edge-on.

Consider the plugging case. Since the local velocity of flow must vanish on the wall of the tube and is maximal at the center, the flexible pellet must deform. Consistent with the principle of minimum potential energy, the deformation of a thin disk will be planar, i.e., its midplane will deform into a developable cylindrical surface, which requires no membrane strain in the midplane of the disk. Most of the energy of deformation will be used in bending, very little in stretching the midplane. (If h represents the thickness of the disk, then the bending rigidity is proportional to h^3, whereas stretching rigidity is proportional to h. When $h \to 0$, it becomes much easier to bend than to stretch.) Let us sketch such a deformed pellet in a branching tube as shown in Fig. 5.6:5 (a) or (b). Let us consider three sections of the tubes as indicated by dotted lines in the figure: one in the mother tube and two in the daughter tubes, all at a distance L from the point of bifurcation. In a flow of a homogeneous viscous fluid before the arrival of the pellet, let the pressures at these sections be P_0, P_1, P_2, respectively. Obviously $P_0 > P_2 > P_1$ on account of the assumption $\bar{V}_1 > \bar{V}_2$. When the pellet arrives at the junction, let the pressures acting on the pellet surface facing the three branches be denoted by P_0', P_1', P_2', respectively, as indicated in the figure. Now, the values of P_0', P_1', P_2' depend on how tightly the pellet plugs up the flow. If the flow is momentarilly plugged completely, then we have

$$P_0' = P_0, \qquad P_1' = P_1, \qquad P_2' = P_2. \tag{7}$$

If the flow can leak past the pellet then $P_0' < P_0$, $P_1' > P_1$, $P_2' > P_2$. But they are releated, $P_1' < P_2' < P_0'$; and $P_0' = P_1' = P_2'$ only in the limiting case of no pellet. The force that acts on the pellet that pulls the pellet into branch 1 is equal to the difference of pressures acting on the two sides of the pellet multiplied by the projected area in branch 1; i.e., $(P_0' - P_1')\pi D_c^2/8$. The pressure difference that pulls the pellet into the branch 2 is $(P_0' - P_2')\pi D_c^2/8$. Here D_c is the diameter of the pellet. The resultant force due to the pressure difference is F_p. In the case shown in Fig. 5.6:5(b),

$$F_p = (P_0' - P_1')\frac{\pi D_c^2}{8} - (P_0' - P_2')\frac{\pi D_c^2}{8} = (P_2' - P_1')\frac{\pi D_c^2}{8}, \tag{8}$$

and is directed into branch 1 because $P_1' < P_2'$. We can convert this expression into the mean velocities of flow as follows. Assuming Poiseuille flow, we have, from Eq. (18) of Sec. 3.2.,

$$\bar{V} = \frac{D_t^2}{32\mu}\frac{(P_0' - P_0)}{L}, \qquad \bar{V}_1 = \frac{D_t^2}{32\mu}\frac{(P_0' - P_1)}{L}, \qquad \bar{V}_2 = \frac{D_t^2}{32\mu}\frac{(P_0' - P_2)}{L}, \tag{9}$$

where μ is the apparent viscosity of the fluid. If the flow is momentarily plugged so that Eq. (7) applies, then by using Eq. (7) in (9) and (8) we obtain

$$F_p = 4\mu L\pi\frac{D_c^2}{D_t^2}(\bar{V}_1 - \bar{V}_2). \tag{10}$$

This shows that the resultant force is proportional to the velocity difference of the two branches, and to the square of the particle-to-tube diameter ratio.

Next, consider the edge-on case. Here it is necessary to consider the shear stress and velocity gradient, and hence the velocity distribution. The easiest way to understand the velocity distribution in a branching flow is to look at the streamline pattern. A sketch of the streamline of a flow of a homogeneous fluid in a branching tube is shown in Fig. 5.6:5(c). A streamline is a curve whose tangent is parallel to the velocity of a particle of the fluid lying at the point of tangency. A stream tube is a tube whose wall is composed of streamlines. Fluid contained in a stream tube will not leave the tube in a steady flow. Hence, the rate of volume flow is a constant in each stream tube. This consideration tells us how to quantitize the flow field by stream-lines. Let the cross section of the mother tube be divided into N equal areas. Let N stream tubes enclose these areas. The walls of these tubes are uniformly spaced far away from the bifurcation point. As the fluid velocity becomes nonuniform, the spacing of the stream tubes will vary. The higher the velocity, the more crowded the tubes will be. Figure 5.6:5(c) shows the distribution of the stream tubes of a flow of a homogeneous fluid in the case in which $\bar{V}_1 = 2\bar{V}_2$. Note that there is a dividing stream surface: All fluid on its left goes into tube 1, all on its right goes into tube 2.

Now, let there be an edge-on pellet in the tube. If it lies entirely to the left of the dividing stream surface it will flow into tube 1. If it lies to the right, it flows into tube 2. The borderline cases, in which the pellet lies astride the dividing stream surface, as shown in Fig. 5.6:5(d), is the one that needs attention. In this case the streamlines are crowded on the left hand side of the pellet, indicating that the flow velocity is high there. On the right the streamlines are rarified. This feature is accentuated especially in the neighborhood of the bifurcation point. The velocity gradients on the two sides can be assumed to be proportional to $\bar{V}_1/D_t$ and $\bar{V}_2/D_t$. The resultant shear force is therefore

$$F_s = \text{const} \cdot \frac{D_c^2}{D_t}(\bar{V}_1 - \bar{V}_2), \tag{11}$$

and is directed toward tube 1.

Pellets in other configurations and of other shapes will be acted on by stress resultants similar to those given by Eqs. (10) and (11), though different in magnitude. Thus, it is seen that the net pressure and shear forces tend to pull pellets to the faster side.

The analysis presented above is simple because many details are left in a qualitative state. A more refined analysis must be based on the solution of Stokes equation with appropriate boundary conditions. The question of simulating the flexibility of the red blood cells by pellets is discussed in Yen and Fung (1978). A more compact method of presentation with additional results is given by Schmid-Shönbein et al. (1980a & b).

5.7 Mechanics of Flow at Very Low Reynolds Numbers

As we have said before, blood flow in micro-blood-vessels is characterized by small Reynolds and Womersley numbers. If we assume a velocity of flow of 1 mm/sec, a vessel diameter of 10 μm, a viscosity of blood of 0.02 poise, a density of 1 g/cm^3, and a heart rate of 2 Hz, then the Reynolds number is 0.005 and the Womersley number is also 0.005, both much smaller than 1. The smallness is typical in microcirculation. At such small Reynolds and Womersley numbers, the viscosity effect becomes predominant. By compairson, the inertial forces due to transient and convective accelerations become negligible. Thus the Navier–Stokes equations (see Appendix, Eq. (A.3:2)) are simplified into

$$\mu\nabla^2 u = \frac{\partial p}{\partial x}, \qquad \mu\nabla^2 v = \frac{\partial p}{\partial y}, \qquad \mu\nabla^2 w = \frac{\partial p}{\partial z}, \tag{1}$$

where u, v, w are the velocity components in Cartesian coordinates x, y, z, and

$$\nabla^2 = \frac{\partial^2}{\partial x^2} + \frac{\partial^2}{\partial y^2} + \frac{\partial^2}{\partial z^2}.$$

If we differentiate the first of Eq. (1) with respect to y, the second of Eq. (1) with respect to x, and subtract, we obtain

$$\mu\nabla^2\left(\frac{\partial v}{\partial x} - \frac{\partial u}{\partial y}\right) = 0. \tag{2}$$

The quantities

$$\xi = \frac{\partial v}{\partial z} - \frac{\partial w}{\partial y}, \qquad \eta = \frac{\partial w}{\partial x} - \frac{\partial u}{\partial z}, \qquad \zeta = \frac{\partial u}{\partial y} - \frac{\partial v}{\partial x}, \tag{3}$$

are the Cartesian components of the vorticity. Hence

$$\nabla^2\xi = 0, \qquad \nabla^2\eta = 0, \qquad \nabla^2\zeta = 0. \tag{4}$$

The equation of continuity of an incompressible fluid is

$$\frac{\partial u}{\partial x} + \frac{\partial v}{\partial y} + \frac{\partial w}{\partial z} = 0. \tag{5}$$

Differentiating the three Eqs. (1) with respect to x, y, z, adding, and using Eq. (5), we obtain

$$\nabla^2 p = 0. \tag{6}$$

Applying the Laplacian operator ∇^2 to Eqs. (1) and using Eq. (6), we have

$$\nabla^4 u = 0, \qquad \nabla^4 v = 0, \qquad \nabla^4 w = 0. \tag{7}$$

Thus, when the Reynolds and Womersley numbers are very small, the pressure p satisfies the Laplace Eq. (6), and the components of velocity satisfy the biharmonic Eq. (7). Equation (1) is known as *Stokes equation*, and a flow obeying this equation is called a *Stokes flow*.

Stokes' Solution for a Falling Sphere

Consider a sphere of radius a falling in a fluid of viscosity μ. It is convenient to consider the sphere to be stationary, and the velocity of the flow relative to the sphere to be U at infinite distance from the sphere. The flow field is

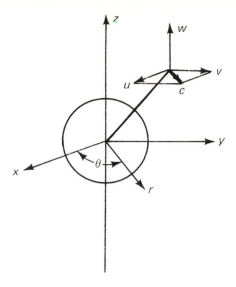

Figure 5.7:1 Use of cylindrical–polar coordinates for the falling sphere problem.

obviously axisymmetric. If cylindrical coordinates (r, θ, z) are used, with the z axis vertical, (see Fig. 5.7:1), then

$$u = c \cos \theta, \qquad v = c \sin \theta, \qquad w = w, \tag{8}$$

in which c is the velocity component in the r direction. c and w are functions of r and z only. It follows from Eqs. (8) and (3) that

$$\xi = -2\omega \sin \theta, \qquad \eta = 2\omega \cos \theta, \qquad \zeta = 0, \tag{9}$$

in which 2ω is the *resultant vorticity* given by

$$2\omega = \frac{\partial c}{\partial z} - \frac{\partial w}{\partial r}. \tag{10}$$

From Eq. (9) one obtains

$$\frac{1}{2}\nabla^2 \xi = -\left(\frac{\partial^2}{\partial z^2} + \frac{\partial^2}{\partial r^2} + \frac{1}{r}\frac{\partial}{\partial r} + \frac{1}{r^2}\frac{\partial^2}{\partial \theta^2}\right)\omega \sin \theta$$

$$= -\sin \theta \left(\frac{\partial^2}{\partial z^2} + \frac{\partial^2}{\partial r^2} + \frac{1}{r}\frac{\partial}{\partial r} - \frac{1}{r^2}\right)\omega \tag{11}$$

$$= -\frac{\sin \theta}{r}\left(\frac{\partial^2}{\partial z^2} + \frac{\partial^2}{\partial r^2} - \frac{1}{r}\frac{\partial}{\partial r}\right)r\omega = -\frac{\sin \theta}{r}L(r\omega)$$

if

$$L = \frac{\partial^2}{\partial z^2} + \frac{\partial^2}{\partial r^2} - \frac{1}{r}\frac{\partial}{\partial r}. \tag{12}$$

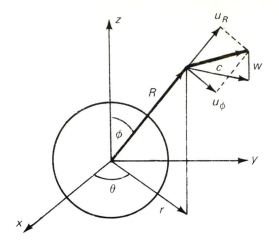

Figure 5.7:2 Spherical–polar coordinates.

Similarly,

$$\frac{1}{2}\nabla^2\eta = \frac{\cos\theta}{r}L(r\omega). \tag{13}$$

Thus, the three Eqs. (4) can be represented by the single equation (since $\zeta = 0$):

$$L(r\omega) = 0. \tag{14}$$

If we now introduce the *stream function* ψ so that

$$w = \frac{1}{r}\frac{\partial\psi}{\partial r}, \qquad c = -\frac{1}{r}\frac{\partial\psi}{\partial z}, \tag{15}$$

we have

$$-\omega = \frac{1}{2}\frac{1}{r}\left(\frac{\partial^2}{\partial z^2} + \frac{\partial^2}{\partial r^2} - \frac{1}{r}\frac{\partial}{\partial r}\right)\psi = \frac{1}{2r}L\psi. \tag{16}$$

Thus Eq. (14) becomes

$$L^2\psi = 0. \tag{17}$$

Now, let us introduce spherical coordinates (R, ϕ, θ) with the polar axis pointing to the direction opposite to the direction of motion of the sphere, Fig 5.7:2. Then

$$z = R\cos\phi, \qquad r = R\sin\phi, \tag{18}$$

and Eq. (17) becomes

$$\left[\frac{\partial^2}{\partial R^2} + \frac{\sin\phi}{R^2}\frac{\partial}{\partial\phi}\left(\frac{1}{\sin\phi}\frac{\partial}{\partial\phi}\right)\right]^2\psi = 0. \tag{19}$$

This is satisfied by

$$\psi = \sin^2 \phi f(R), \tag{20}$$

if

$$\left(\frac{d^2}{dR^2} - \frac{2}{R^2}\right)^2 f(R) = 0. \tag{21}$$

The solution of Eq. (21) is

$$f(R) = \frac{A}{R} + BR + CR^2 + DR^4. \tag{22}$$

The boundary conditions are undisturbed flow at infinity and no-slip on the surface of the sphere, i.e.,

at $R = \infty$: $\quad w = U$, $\quad c = 0$, $\quad$ or $\quad v_R = U\cos\phi$, $\quad v_\phi = U\sin\phi$,

at $R = a$: $\quad w = 0$, $\quad c = 0$, $\quad$ or $\quad v_R = v_\phi = 0$, $\tag{23}$

where v_R, v_ϕ are velocity components in the directions of increasing R and ϕ, respectively. It can be shown that

$$v_R = \frac{1}{R^2 \sin\phi} \frac{\partial\psi}{\partial\phi}, \qquad v_\phi = -\frac{1}{R\sin\phi} \frac{\partial\psi}{\partial R}. \tag{24}$$

From Eqs. (20), (22), and (24), it is seen that the boundary conditions are satisfied by choosing

$$C = \tfrac{1}{2}U, \qquad D = 0,$$
$$A = \tfrac{1}{4}Ua^3, \qquad B = -\tfrac{3}{4}Ua. \tag{25}$$

Thus

$$v_R = U\cos\theta - 2\left(\frac{A}{R^3} + \frac{B}{R}\right)\cos\theta,$$

$$v_\phi = -U\sin\theta - \left(\frac{A}{R^3} - \frac{B}{R}\right)\sin\theta. \tag{26}$$

The problem is now solved. The streamlines $\psi = $ constant can be plotted, and are as shown in Fig. 5.7:3.

A quantity of interest is the total hydrodynamic resistance encountered by the sphere. To evaluate this force, we must compute the stress tensor τ_{ij} from the constitutive equation

$$\tau_{ij} = -p\delta_{ij} + 2\mu\dot{e}_{ij} = -p + \mu\left(\frac{\partial v_i}{\partial x_j} + \frac{\partial v_j}{\partial x_i}\right),$$

and the stress vector acting on the surface of the sphere at radius $R = a$:

$$\overset{v}{T}_i = v_j\tau_{ij},$$

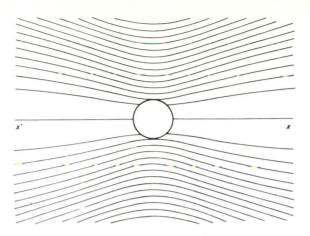

Figure 5.7:3 Streamlines in the flow caused by a sphere moving with a small constant velocity: Stoke's solution. From Lamb (1932), p. 599. By permission of Cambridge Univ. Press.

where $v = (v_1, v_2, v_3)$ unit vector normal to the surface. Clearly, v is the radius vector

$$(v_1, v_2, v_3) = \left(\frac{x}{R}, \frac{y}{R}, \frac{z}{R} \right).$$

By consideration of the axisymmetry of the flow field it is evident that the resultant forces in the x and y directions are zero, and that the resultant force in the z direction is given by

$$F = \oint \overset{v}{T_z} dS = 2\pi a^2 \int_0^\pi \overset{v}{T_z} \sin \phi \, d\phi. \tag{27}$$

It turns out that on the surface of the sphere, $R = a$,

$$\overset{v}{T_z} = -\frac{z}{a} p_o + \frac{3}{2} \mu \frac{U}{a}, \qquad \overset{v}{T_x} = -\frac{x}{a} p_o, \qquad \overset{v}{T_y} = -\frac{y}{a} p_o, \tag{28}$$

and the resultant force is

$$F = 6\pi \mu a U. \tag{29}$$

This solution, due to Stokes (1851), has been well verified experimentally, as shown in Fig. 5.7:4, where the ordinate is the so-called *drag coefficient* C_D defined by

$$C_D = \frac{F}{\frac{1}{2}\rho U^2 A}, \tag{30}$$

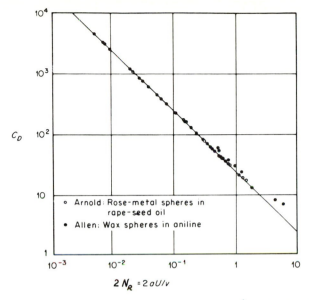

$$2\,N_R = 2\,aU/v$$

Figure 5.7:4 Experimental verification of the Stoke's law, $\dot{C}_D = 12/N_R$ which is repre-sented by the straight line. By permission from Rouse (1959, p. 240).

A being the projected area πa^2 in this case. From Eq. (29) we have

$$C_D = \frac{12}{N_R}, \tag{31}$$

where N_R is the Reynolds number, $aU\rho/\mu$. Equation (31) is plotted as the solid line in Fig. 5.7:4.

A note may be added with regard to the actual calculations leading to Eqs. (28) and (29). Instead of finding the full tensor τ_{ij} and then proceeding as outlined above, the following steps will greatly lessen the labor. We note that

$$\overset{v}{T_z} = \frac{z}{R}\tau_{zz} + \frac{y}{R}\tau_{zy} + \frac{x}{R}\tau_{zx}$$

$$= \cos\phi\left(-p + 2\mu\frac{\partial w}{\partial z}\right) + \mu\frac{y}{R}\left(\frac{\partial w}{\partial y} + \frac{\partial v}{\partial z}\right) + \mu\frac{x}{R}\left(\frac{\partial u}{\partial x} + \frac{\partial u}{\partial z}\right)$$

$$= -p\cos\phi + \mu\frac{\partial w}{\partial R} - \frac{\mu w}{R} + \frac{\mu}{R}\frac{\partial}{\partial z}(xu + yv + zw)$$

$$= -p\cos\phi + \mu\frac{\partial w}{\partial R} - \frac{\mu w}{R} + \frac{\mu}{R}\frac{\partial}{\partial z}Rv_R.$$

But

$$w = v_R \cos\phi - v_\phi \sin\phi, \qquad \frac{\partial v_R}{\partial z} = \frac{\partial v_R}{\partial R}\cos\phi - \frac{\partial v_R}{\partial\phi}\frac{\sin\phi}{R}.$$

Hence

$$\overset{v}{T_z} = -p\cos\phi + 2\mu\cos\phi\frac{\partial v_R}{\partial R} - \mu\sin\phi\frac{\partial v_\phi}{\partial R} + \frac{1}{R}\frac{\partial v_R}{\partial\phi} - \frac{v_\phi}{R}.$$

Equation (28) is then obtained by substituting $R = a$ into the equation above.

A further alternative is to note that in spherical coordinates,

$$\overset{v}{T_R} = \tau_{RR}\cos\phi - \tau_{R\phi}\sin\phi = (-p + 2\mu\dot{e}_{RR})\cos\phi - \mu\dot{e}_{R\phi}\sin\phi.$$

The strain rate components $\dot{e}_{RR}$ and $\dot{e}_{R\phi}$ are given by

$$\dot{e}_{RR} = \frac{\partial v_R}{\partial R}, \qquad \dot{e}_{R\phi} = R\frac{\partial}{\partial R}\frac{v_\phi}{R} + \frac{1}{R}\frac{\partial v_R}{\partial\phi}.$$

This classical work illustrates the method of formulation and analysis of a flow of very low Reynolds number. It is presented here not only for its beauty, but also for its importance. The slow motion of small particles in a fluid is a common occurrence in the biological world. Equation (29) is used very frequently in connection with flow of fluid containing particles, sedimentation of particles, centrifugation or ultracentrifugation of suspensions, colloids, and blood, isolation of tumor antigens, etc. The fluid does not have to be liquid, the particle does not have to be solid. The formula is useful in the analysis of natural fog or smog formation, the atomization of liquids, etc., with milliards of medical and industrial applications.

An analogous problem of a long circular cylinder slowly falling in a liquid in the direction perpendicular to the cylinder axis, i.e., the two-dimensional version of Eqs. (1) and (23), has no solution. The lack of a solution of Eq. (1) for two-dimensional flow is called the *Whitehead paradox*. It illustrates the delicate nature of mathematical idealization of physical problems.

Problems

5.1 Consider a very slow falling of a sphere in a viscous fluid. Let $\Delta\gamma$ be the difference in specific weight of the sphere and the fluid. Use dimensional analysis, show that the only dimensionless parameter is another Stokes number $S = U\mu/(a^2\Delta\gamma)$, which must therefore be a constant if inertial forces are neglected.

5.2 Apply Stokes' solution to the problem above. If the sphere is not accelerating, the hydrodynamic drag force is balanced by the weight of the sphere minus the buoyancy. Show that when the Reynolds number tends to zero, the Stokes number is

$$S = \frac{U\mu}{a^2\Delta\gamma} = \frac{2}{9}.$$

5.8 Oseen's Approximation and Other Developments

In Stokes' solution for the moving sphere, the inertial terms are entirely neglected. It is a limiting solution when the Reynolds number tends to zero. For small but finite Reynolds number, say, with N_R of the order of 0.1, some correction of the inertial terms is needed. Oseen (1910) proposed the following method to treat problems in which the flow field consists of a small perturbation of a constant mean flow, U. He made the substitution

$$v_1 = U + v_1', \qquad v_2 = v_2', \qquad v_3 = v_3', \tag{1}$$

in the Navier–Stokes equations, and neglected the quadratic terms in the primed quantities. This leads to the following equation:

$$U\frac{\partial v_i'}{\partial x_1} = -\frac{1}{\rho}\frac{\partial p}{\partial x_i} + \nu\nabla^2 v_i', \qquad (i = 1, 2, 3) \tag{2}$$

which is known as *Oseen's equation*. The approximation which Eq. (2) stands for is called *Oseen's approximation*.

When the moving sphere problem of the preceeding section is solved on the basis of Eq. (2), Oseen found that the resultant hydrodynamic force (drag) is

$$F = 6\pi\mu aU(1 + \tfrac{3}{8}N_R), \tag{3}$$

where N_R is the Reynolds number Ua/ν. The streamline pattern in this case is shown in Fig. 5.8:1.

The difference between Eq. (3) above and Eq. (29) of Sec. 5.7 lies in the factor $(3/8)N_R$. One may question, however, whether the correction term is not fortuitous, because in a frame of reference moving with the sphere, the fluid near the sphere is almost at rest, and in that region inertial force is negligible and Stokes equation is well justified. Far away from the sphere,

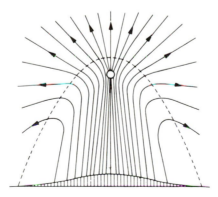

Figure 5.8:1 Streamlines in the flow caused by a sphere moving with a small constant velocity: Oseen's solution. From Schlichting (1962). Reproduced by permission.

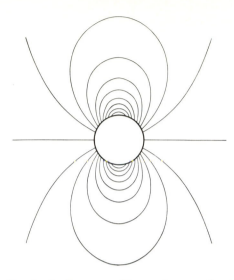

Figure 5.8:2 Streamlines in the flow caused by a sphere moving in a nonviscous fluid. Potential flow solution. From Lamb (1932, p. 128). Reproduced by permission.

the flow velocity approaches U and Oseen's approximation is more accurate. But Eq. (3) was obtained by using Oseen's equation for the entire flow field. This question was answered by Proudman and Pearson (1957), who solved the Navier–Stokes equations and gave an improved Stokes solution in the neighborhood of the sphere and an improved Oseen solution at infinity, and matched the two solutions in a supposed common region of their validity. They obtained

$$F = 6\pi\mu a U[1 + \tfrac{3}{8}N_R + \tfrac{9}{40}N_R^2 \ln N_R + O(N_R^2)]. \tag{4}$$

To the order N_R, Eqs. (3) and (4) agree. Equation (4) is valid for Reynolds numbers which is so small that the square of N_R is negligible compared with 1.

The details of the solution of the falling sphere problem based on Oseen's equation, and other developments concerning forces acting on an oscillating sphere, forces acting on a sphere moving with arbitrary speed in a straight line, motion of a sphere released from rest, etc., can be found in the excellent textbook by C. S. Yih, *Fluid Mechanics* (1969).

It is instructive to compare the solutions to the problem of moving sphere in an incompressible fluid by neglecting one term or another in the Navier–Stokes equation:

$$\rho\left(\frac{\partial u_i}{\partial t} + u_j\frac{\partial u_i}{\partial x_j}\right) = -\frac{\partial p}{\partial x_i} + \mu\nabla^2 u_i.$$

When the inertial force terms on the left-hand side are neglected, the streamlines are shown in Fig. 5.7:3. When the fluid is nonviscous, $\mu = 0$, then the last term $\mu\nabla^2 u_i$ can be dropped, the solution is well known from the potential flow theory, and the streamline pattern is shown in Fig. 5.8:2. Comparison of Figs. 5.7:3, 5.8:1, and 5.8:2 shows the tremendous differences implied by these assumptions.

The streamline pattern of the solution based on Oseen equation shows already the development of a wake behind the sphere. The wake becomes more pronounced as the Reynolds number of flow increases. Separation of streamlines from the solid surface of the sphere seems to begin in the neighborhood of the rear stagnation point at a Reynolds number of about 5. As the Reynolds number increases the separation region increases, and standing vortices develop. The point of separation depends on the flow condition in the boundary layer, whether it is laminar or turbulent. These fascinating and important features of flow and drag variation are discussed in several books, e.g., Yih (1969).

5.9 Entry Flow, Bolus Flow, and Other Examples

Features of entry flow have already been discussed in Sec. 3.14. With the background presented in Sec. 5.7 et seq., we can now discuss the mathematical side of the problem.

Entry Flow into a Circular Cylindrical Tube at a Very Low Reynolds Number

For a steady flow of an incompressible flow at a low Reynolds number, the Stokes approximation prevails and the equation of momemtum becomes the Stokes equation (Eq. (1) of Sec. 5.7)

$$-\nabla p + \mu \nabla^2 \mathbf{v} = 0. \tag{1}$$

Here, and in the rest of this section, letters printed in boldface denote vectors. The equation of continuity of an incompressible fluid is

$$\nabla \cdot \mathbf{v} = 0. \tag{2}$$

The boundary conditions are:

(a) The adherence of the fluid to the wall of the tube,

$$\mathbf{v} = 0 \qquad \text{on the wall of the tube.} \tag{3}$$

(b) $\mathbf{v} = $ a specified distribution at the inlet cross section of the tube.
(c) $\mathbf{v}$ and p are given by the Poiseuille formulas far downstream of the tube.

The mathematical problem is fully specified by these equations. To solve them, Lew and Fung (1969a) split $\mathbf{v}$ and p into two parts,

$$\mathbf{v} = \mathbf{v}' + \mathbf{v}_\infty, \qquad p = p' + p_\infty, \tag{4}$$

where $\mathbf{v}_\infty$ and p_∞ correspond to Poiseuille flow. $\mathbf{v}'$ and p' satisfy eqs. (1) and (2) because $\mathbf{v}_\infty$ and p_∞ satisfy them. Equation (2) is satisfied if $\mathbf{v}'$ is derived from an arbitrary function $f(x, r)$ as follows:

$$\mathbf{v}' = \nabla \times \nabla \times [\hat{x} f(x, r)], \tag{5}$$

where $\hat{x}$ designates the unit base vector of x-axis and r, θ, x are a system of cylindrical polar coordinates with the x-axis coinciding with the axis of the tube, and the origin of the coordinate system located at the entrance section. Since $f(x, r)$ is independent of θ, Eq. (5) can be expanded as

$$\mathbf{v}' = \hat{r} \frac{\partial^2 f}{\partial r \partial x} - \hat{x} \frac{1}{r} \frac{\partial}{\partial r}\left(r \frac{\partial f}{\partial r}\right). \tag{6}$$

Substitution of Eq. (5) into Eq. (1) yields the equation

$$-\nabla\left(p' - \mu\nabla^2 \frac{\partial f}{\partial x}\right) - \hat{x}\mu\nabla^4 f = 0, \tag{7}$$

which is satisfied if

$$p' = \mu\nabla^2 \frac{\partial f}{\partial x}, \tag{8}$$

$$\nabla^4 f = 0. \tag{9}$$

A general solution of Eq. (9), which has bounded values in the whole region of consideration, is

$$f(x, r) = \left(A + B\lambda\frac{x}{a}\right)e^{-\lambda x/a} J_0\left(\lambda\frac{r}{a}\right)$$
$$+ \left[C\cos\left(\eta\frac{x}{a}\right) + D\sin\left(\eta\frac{x}{a}\right)\right]\left[I_0\left(\eta\frac{r}{a}\right) + E\frac{r}{a}I_1\left(\eta\frac{r}{a}\right)\right], \tag{10}$$

where A, B, C, D, E, λ, and η are arbitrary constants; a is the radius of the tube, J_0 is the Bessel function of the first kind of order zero, and I_0, I_1 are the modified Bessel functions of the first kind of order zero and one, respectively.

Since the governing differential equations and boundary conditions are linear, we can superpose solutions of the type Eq. (10) to construct a general solution. In particular, we construct terms like

$$\sum_{n=1}^{\infty} A_n \left\{\left(1 + k_n\frac{x}{a}\right)e^{-k_n x/a} J_0\left(k_n\frac{r}{a}\right) + \int_0^\infty C_n(\eta)\cos\left(\eta\frac{x}{a}\right)\right.$$
$$\left.\left[I_0\left(\eta\frac{r}{a}\right) - \frac{I_0(\eta)}{\frac{2}{\eta}I_0(\eta) + I_1(\eta)}\frac{r}{a}I_1\left(\eta\frac{r}{a}\right)\right] d\eta\right\} \tag{11}$$

as part of the general solution, in which k_n is the nth zero of the Bessel function, $J_0(k_n) = 0$. With such superposition, one obtains a solution that is sufficiently general to satisfy all the boundary conditions if the velocity distribution at the inlet is axisymmetric. The full details are given in Lew and Fung (1969a). The velocity distribution is sketched in Fig. 3.14:2.

Entry Flow into Circular Cylinder at an Arbitrary Reynolds Number

Entry flow at a high Reynolds number (say $N_R > 100$, with Reynolds number $N_R = \rho a U / \mu$ defined on the basis of the mean flow velocity U and the tube radius (a) can be analyzed by the boundary layer theory, from which Targ (1951) obtained the result that the entry length L is

$$L = 0.16 a N_R, \tag{12}$$

where a is the tube radius, and L is defined as the distance of transition from a uniform inflow at the inlet to a section where the velocity profile differs from the Poiseuille profile by less than 1%. Entry flow at zero Reynolds number is discussed in the preceding paragraph, and we obtained the entry length

$$L = 1.3a. \tag{13}$$

For flow with Reynolds number between 0 and 100, Lew and Fung (1970b) used the Oseen approximation (Sec. 5.8):

$$\rho U \frac{\partial \mathbf{v}}{\partial x} = -\nabla p + \mu \nabla^2 \mathbf{v}, \tag{14}$$

where U is the average speed of flow over the cross section of the tube, and $\mathbf{v}$ is the velocity. The equation of continuity and boundary conditions are the same as Eqs. (2), (3) above. To solve these equations, Eqs. (4), (5), and (6) remain valid, while Eq. (7) becomes

$$-\nabla\left[p' - \mu\left(\nabla^2 - \frac{N_R}{a}\frac{\partial}{\partial x}\right)\frac{\partial f}{\partial x}\right] - \hat{x}\mu\left(\nabla^2 - \frac{N_R}{a}\frac{\partial}{\partial x}\right)\nabla^2 f = 0, \tag{15}$$

where N_R is the Reynolds number $\rho a U / \mu$. This equation is satisfied if

$$p' = \mu\left(\nabla^2 - \frac{N_R}{a}\frac{\partial}{\partial x}\right)\frac{\partial f}{\partial x}, \tag{16}$$

$$\left(\nabla^2 - \frac{N_R}{a}\frac{\partial}{\partial x}\right)\nabla^2 f = 0. \tag{17}$$

A solution of Eq. (17), which is bounded in the region of the tube is

$$
f(x, r) = \left[Ae^{-\lambda x/a} + Be^{-(\sqrt{4\lambda^2 + N_R^2} - N_R)x/2a} \right] J_0\left(\lambda \frac{r}{a} \right)
$$

$$
+ \left[C\cos\left(\eta \frac{x}{a} \right) + D\sin\left(\eta \frac{x}{a} \right) \right] I_0\left(\eta \frac{r}{a} \right)
$$

$$
+ E\left\{ \cos\left(\eta \frac{x}{a} \right) I_0\left[e^{i\alpha/2}\left(1 + \frac{N_R^2}{\eta^2} \right)^{1/4} \eta \frac{r}{a} \right] \Bigg|_R \right.
$$

$$
\left. - \sin\left(\eta \frac{x}{a} \right) I_0\left[e^{i\alpha/2}\left(1 + \frac{N_R^2}{\eta^2} \right)^{1/4} \eta \frac{r}{a} \right] \Bigg|_I \right\}
$$

$$
+ F\left\{ \cos\left(\eta \frac{x}{a} \right) I_0\left[e^{i\alpha/2}\left(1 + \frac{N_R^2}{\eta^2} \right)^{1/4} \eta \frac{r}{a} \right] \Bigg|_I \right.
$$

$$
\left. + \sin\left(\eta \frac{x}{a} \right) I_0\left[e^{i\alpha/2}\left(1 + \frac{N_R^2}{\eta^2} \right)^{1/4} \eta \frac{r}{a} \right] \Bigg|_R \right\},
$$

(18)

where A, B, C, D, E, F, λ, and η are constants, J_0 is a Bessel function, I_0 is a modified Bessel function, both of the first kind and zeroth order. $I_0|_R$ and $I_0|_I$ denote the real and imaginary part of I_0, respectively, and

$$
\alpha = \tan^{-1}\frac{N_R}{\eta}.
$$

(19)

Equation (18) corresponds to Eq. (10) of the case $N_R = 0$. By a superposition of terms of the type given in Eq. (18), we can construct a full solution analogous to Eq. (11) of the zero-N_R case. The details are given by Lew and Fung (1970b) and the results are sketched in Fig. 3.14:2.

The Motion of the Plasma Between the Red Cells in a Bolus Flow

A photograph of blood flow in a capillary blood vessel in the mesentery of a dog is given on p. 103 of *Biomechanics* (Fung, 1981). The red blood cells are seen to be severely deformed. In such a flow, the red cells seem to plug the capillary blood vessel. The motion of the plasma in the capillary between successive red cells is called *bolus flow*. The significance of bolus flow was pointed out by Prothero and Burton (1961). If streamlines are drawn relative to a frame of reference moving with the red cells, the streamlines will be seen to form eddies, thus creating a stirring mechanism which brings material on the centerline to the tube wall by convection. One might suspect that this action will help mass transfer. It was looked into and concluded that the influence of this on oxygenation and CO_2 removal is minor, but its effect on macromolecules may be significant (Aroesty and Gross, 1970).

The mathematical theory can be based on Stokes Eq. (1) and the con-

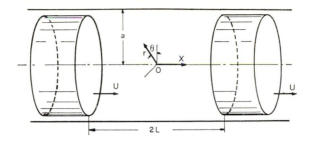

Figure 5.9:1 Idealized geometry of bolus flow. From Lew and Fung (1969b).

tinuity Eq. (2). Consider plug flow and an idealized geometry shown in Fig. 5.9:1. We have the boundary conditions:

$$u(x, r) = -U \quad \text{for } r = a \quad \text{and } -L \leq x \leq L,$$

$$v(x, r) = 0 \quad \text{for } r = a \quad \text{and } -L \leq x \leq L,$$

$$u(x, r) = 0 \quad \text{for } x = \pm L \text{ and } 0 \leq r \leq a,$$

$$v(x, r) = 0 \quad \text{for } x = \pm L \text{ and } 0 \leq r \leq 0,$$

where a is the radius of the capillary, U is the velocity of the red cells, and $2L$ is the distance between the two consecutive red blood cells.

A solution given by Lew and Fung (1969b) is quite similar to that of the entry flow problem mentioned earlier. In fact, the results can be easily understood in the light of the entry flow solution. We have seen that at a very low Reynolds number the entry length is about $1.3a$. Hence, if $L = 1.3a$, the velocity profile at midway between the cells will be almost parabolic, differing from it by less than 1%. For smaller L, the velocity profile would not have enough space to be readjusted to the parabolic profile; the u, v distributions are shown in Fig. 5.9:2, and are quite similar to those shown in Fig. 3.14:2.

5.10 Interaction between Particles and Tube Wall

As a mathematical model of blood flow in capillaries (Fig. 5.9:1), Skalak and his associates have published a series of papers on the motion of particles in a circular cylindrical tube. The governing equations are Eqs. (1) and (2) of Sec. 5.9, because plasma is an incompressible Newtonian fluid. The boundary conditions are: (a) zero velocity at the tube wall, (b) matching particle velocity and traction on the surface of the suspended particles, (c) a specification of either the total discharge or the pressure drop over some appropriate length of the capillary, and (d) on neutrally bouyant particles the net force on any particle and the net moment must be equal to

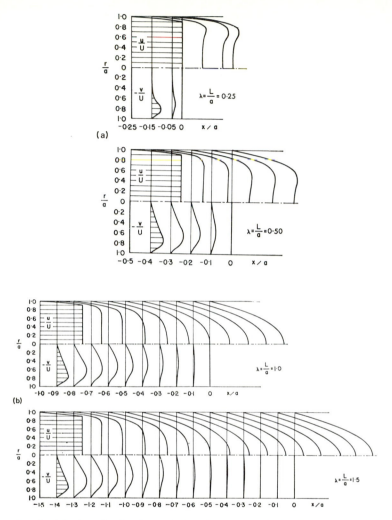

(a)

(b)

Figure 5.9:2 Velocity distribution of the plasma in a bolus flow induced by two adjacent red cells. Tube fixed. Figure shows in each cross section the axial component of velocity u above the centerline, and the radial component of velocity v below the centerline. The velocity specified at the red cell is $u = U$ in $0 \leq r/a \leq 0.9$, where U is a constant. In the gap between, the red cell and the tube wall, u decreases from U to 0 in $0.9 \leq r/a \leq 1$. On the red cell, $x = \pm L$, the vertical velocity $v = 0$ in $0 \leq r/a \leq 1$. The parameter λ is L/a, i.e., (distance between cells)/(tube diameter). From Lew and Fung (1969b). Reproduced by permission.

zero. The condition (d) is called the *zero-drag condition*. For deformable particles, the equations of motion and appropriate constitutive equations of the particles must be satisfied, and the internal velocity and stress fields must match the fluid stresses on the boundary of the particles.

Rigid Particles

In a steady axisymmetric flow, solutions have been developed for a line of spheres (Wang and Skalak 1969, Hochmuth and Sutera 1970, Bungay and Brenner 1973), spheroids (Chen and Skalak, 1970), disks (Bugliarello and Hsiao, 1967, Lew and Fung, 1969b, 1970a, Tong and Fung, 1971, Aroesty and Gross 1970), and biconcave rigid disk shapes (Skalak et al. 1972). The general features of the solutions are the same for all these shapes: (1) A particle on the axis of the capillary travels faster than the mean flow. (2) The pressure drop depends most strongly on the ratio of the maximum diameter of the particle to the tube diameter, (3) The pressure drop due to a given particle is independent of the presence of other particles if the spacing is greater than about one tube diameter. The last point is easily understood if one recalls the results of the entry length analysis presented in Sec. 5.9. There it is shown that at very low Reynolds number the entry length L is equal to 1.3 times the radius of the tube (Lew and Fung 1969a, 1970b). In other words, in a distance equal to 1.3 times the radius of the tube, the flow velocity profile will be able to change from a flat one to one that deviates from the Poiseuille (parabolic) profile by less than 1%. Analogously, in the case of suspended particles in a tube the velocity profile approaches the parabolic one between two particles if they are about 1 tube diameter apart. It follows that at low hematocrit the apparent viscosity of blood in a capillary vessel is proportional to the hematocrit.

When the particle spacing becomes small, the plasma trapped between neighboring particles will move almost as a rigid body with the particles. Hence, at high hematocrit the apparent viscosity of blood in a capillary is relatively independent of hematocrit.

The methods used to obtain these solutions are of four kinds. Skalak et al. (1972) and Tong and Fung (1971) used finite element method. Wang and Skalak (1969), Chen and Skalak (1970), Hyman and Skalak (1972), Lew and Fung (1969b, 1970a) used infinite series. Bungay and Brenner (1973) used asymptotic expansions. Skalak et al. (1972) used M. J. Lighthill's (1968) lubrication layer method (see *Biomechanics* (Fung, 1981, p. 168)). All authors treated axisymmetric flow, except Bungay and Brenner (1973) who treated an eccentrically located sphere, in which case the sphere rotates as it translates down the capillary along a line parallel to the axis of the tube.

Elastic Spheres

Tözeren and Skalak (1978, 1979) analyzed the steady flow of elastic spheres in a circular cylindrical tube, using a series expansion for the particle displacements and lubrication theory for the fluid motion. The results show that the apparent viscosity depends on the shear modulus of elasticity of the particle. In the later paper (1979), the authors extended the calculation to tapered tubes.

Flexible Red Cell Models

Zarda et al. (1977) analyzed the steady flow of a row of flexible red blood cells in a circular cylindrical tube in axisymmetric configuration. The membrane of the red cell is assumed to be elastic in shear and in bending, but its area is assumed to remain constant during any deformation. The tensile stress resultants T_1, T_2 (dyn/cm) in principal directions are adopted from Skalak et al. (1973) in the form:

$$T_1 = B(\lambda_1^2 - 1)\lambda_1/2\lambda_2 + T_0,$$
$$T_2 = B(\lambda_2^2 - 1)\lambda_2/2\lambda_1 + T_0,$$

where λ_1 and λ_2 are the principal extension ratios, and T_0 is an isotropic stress, analogous to the pressure in an incompressible fluid, introduced in response to the hypothesis that the cell membrane area is unchangeable. The coefficient B is an elastic modulus which is taken to be 0.0005 dyn/cm in the computations.

The principal bending moments, M_1, M_2, are assumed to depend on the change of curvature, K_1, K_2, according to the formulas

$$M_1 = D(K_1 + \nu K_2)/\lambda_2,$$
$$M_2 = D(K_2 + \nu K_1)/\lambda_1,$$

where D is a bending stiffness coefficient taken to be equal to 10^{-12} dyn/cm in the computations. The interior of the red cell is assumed to be a fluid, so that in static condition the internal pressure is uniform. The exterior fluid is the blood plasma which is assumed to be a Newtonian fluid with a viscosity of 1.2 cp. The pressure drop over a typical length of the capillary containing one blood cell is assumed to be given, and the computations seek the shape and velocity of the red blood cells.

Finite element method is used in conjunction with a variational principle. The nodal variables are the radial and axial velocities, and the pressure at each node of the finite element network. The numerical work proceeds in two stages. For any assumed positions of the red cells it is possible to solve for all of the fluid velocities and pressures, including the velocities at the nodes on the membrane. The solution which is sought for steady flow is one

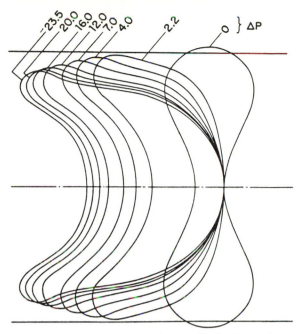

Figure 5.10:1 Shapes computed for red blood cells flowing axisymmetrically in a capillary. The unstressed radius of the red cell is 3.91 μm, and is 5% larger than the radius of the tube. From Zarda et al. (1977). Reproduced by permission.

in which all nodal points on the cell membrane move at the same velocity. If this condition is not satisfied, the position of the membrane is adjusted until it is satisfied. At the same time, the zero-drag condition is incorporated into the computation.

Some of their results for a line of cells in a tube with a hematocrit close to 26% are given in Fig. 5.10:1. The assumed unstressed shape of the cell is the one given on pp. 106, 107 of *Biomechanics* (Fung, 1981) at a tonicity of 300 mosmol. The figure shows the successive shapes of a cell for increasing dimensionless pressure drop, Δp, as indicated in the figure. From the pressure drop and velocity of flow the apparent viscosity of blood in the tube can be calculated. The results show that the apparent viscosity for a given initial cell/tube diameter ratio will generally decrease as the pressure drop increases. This is because at higher pressure drop the cells are deformed more and thereby pull away further from the tube wall.

All the literature cited above is concerned with axisymmetric flow in circular cylinders. In reality, the non-axisymmetric cases are of great importance, and should be investigated in the future. As it is discussed in Chapter 5 of the author's *Biomechanics* (Fung, 1981), experiments have shown that the most common configuration for a red cell to enter a capillary blood vessel is edge on—with the axis of symmetry of the cell perpendicular

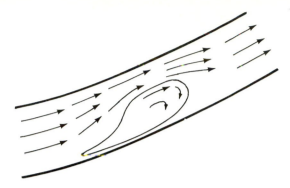

Figure 5.10:2 An illustration that tank treading of a red cell eccentrically placed in a tube will reduce viscous drag.

to the axis of the cylinder. Furthermore, the "tank-treading" mechanism, first pointed out by Holger Schmid–Schoenbein and Roe Wells (1969) and Fischer et al. (1978), offers an elegant mechanism for reducing friction between a red cell and the blood vessel wall. An illustration is shown in Fig. 5.10:2. The red cell is deformed into the shape of a slipper. The cell membrane rotates around, i.e., tank-treads. The cell is asymmetrically placed in the tube. The part of the cell membrane that is very close to the tube wall has small relative motion with respect to the wall. The part of the cell membrane closer to the center of the tube moves forward, thus reducing its effect on the motion of the plasma. If we compare this situation with the condition shown in Fig. 5.10:1, we can expect that the resistance to the movement of the cell in the tube is much reduced in the asymmetric, tank-treading case. The more the cell can be deformed to one side of the tube, the more effective is the mechanism. Only a thorough analysis of the cell deformation and fluid mechanics can put the mechanism on a quantitative basis. Secomb and Skalak (1982) have made an initial approach.

Such an analysis of a non-axisymmetric flow of particles in a tube will have applications also to the problem of leucocytes sticking to the wall of the blood vessel. The mathematical problem is admittedly difficult to solve. In the section to follow, we shall present a solution on the basis of model experiments.

5.11 Force of Interaction of Leucocytes and Vascular Endothelium

As an example of using model testing to study the mechanics of micro-circulation, let us consider the interaction of white blood cells and the endothelium of the blood vessel. Red blood cells do not stick to the endothelium unless the latter is damaged. White blood cells, however, are

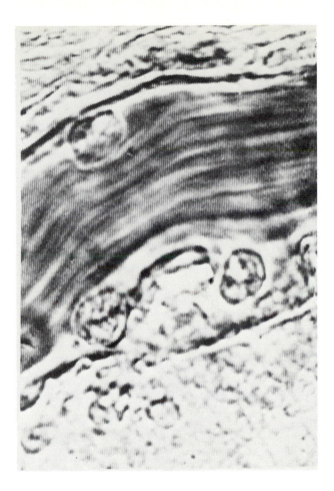

Figure 5.11:1 A 23-μm postcapillary blood vessel with a leukocyte adhering to the endothelium. Rabbit omemtum. The red cells move in a stream whose streamlines are seen but individual cells are not recognizable. Photographed from television screen by Dr. Geert Schmid–Schönbein.

often seen sticking to the endothelial wall or rolling slowly on it, while the plasma and the red cells whiz by around them. The biochemical details of this endothelium–leukocyte interaction are yet unknown, but they are certainly very important to both physiology and pathology. As a first step in an investigation of this phenomenon, one could ask how large is the force of interaction between the endothelial wall and a white blood cell that is sticking or rolling on it.

The sticking phenomenon is illustrated in Fig. 5.11:1, which is a view taken from the omentum of an anesthetized rabbit. In similar views taken from a high-speed cinemicrograph, the individual red blood cells can be identified. The motion of the red cells, plasma, and leucocytes was measured from successive frames of such a cinemicrograph by Schmid–Schoenbein, Fung and Zweifach (1975). From the kinematics data they proceeded to determine the shear force acting on a leukocyte sticking to the wall of a venule. They replaced the mathematical problem of calculating the force of interaction by testing a physical model. A kinematically and dynamically similar model of the venule–leukocyte system was made. By the principle of dynamic similarity, the dimensionless shear force coefficient is the same for the blood vessel and the model. Thus, the experimental shear force coefficient can be used to calculate the force acting on the leukocyte.

Analysis

Two flow systems are said to be *kinematically similar* if their geometric shapes are similar, although their linear dimensions can be different. Two systems are said to be *dynamically similar* if the systems of differential equations describing their motion, written in dimensionless form, are the same. If two systems are both kinematically and dynamically similar, then the dimensionless variables (expressing stresses, velocities, displacements, etc. nondimensionally by forming ratios to characteric values of these variables) will have exactly the same values at corresponding points in the two systems. This is the basic *principle of similarity*.

In the blood flow problem, the principal variables describing the geometry

TABLE 5.11:1 List of Variables[a]

Symbol	Definition	Dimensions
d_c	Diameter of the leukocyte considered as a sphere	L
d_t	Diameter of the blood vessel	L
V_M	Maximum velocity of undisturbed flow in the blood vessel	LT^{-1}
V_c	Linear velocity of the centroid of the white blood cell	LT^{-1}
μ	Coefficient of viscosity of plasma	$ML^{-1}T^{-1}$
ρ	Density of plasma ($\bar{\rho}$ is that of the silicone oil)	ML^{-3}
H	Hematocrit of the blood, i.e., the volume fraction of the cellcular content in the blood	—

[a] All symbols with an overbar refer to the model. For example, μ signifies the viscosity of plasma and $\bar{\mu}$ denotes the viscosity of the silicone oil in the model experiment.

and motion of our system are listed in Table 5.11:1. In this table, the hematocrit H is dimensionless. From the remaining six variables, three independent *dimensionless parameters* can be formed. The following is a convenient set:

$$d_c/d_t, \qquad V_c/V_M, \qquad V_M d_c \rho/\mu. \tag{1}$$

All other dimensionless parameters are functions of these basic variables. For example, if we are interested in the resultant shear force, S (dynes), imparted to the white blood cell by the blood flow, we note that the ratio $S/(V_M \mu d_c)$ is dimensionless, and we can express this ratio as a function of the three dimensionless parameters listed in Eq. (1) and the hematocrit H:

$$\frac{S}{V_M \mu d_c} = f\left(\frac{d_c}{d_t}, \frac{V_c}{V_M}, \frac{V_M d_c \rho}{\mu}, H\right), \tag{2}$$

where $f(\cdots)$ denotes a functional relationship that can be determined either by solving the differential equations or by using a model experiment. We notice that the parameter $V_M d_c \rho/\mu$ is a *Reynolds number* (N_R). The other parameter $S/(V_M \mu d_c)$ will be called the *shear coefficient* and is denoted by C_S; thus,

$$C_S = \frac{S}{V_M \mu d_c}, \tag{3}$$

$$N_R = \frac{\rho V_M d_c}{\mu}, \tag{4}$$

and Eq. (2) can be written as

$$C_S = f(N_R, d_c/d_t, V_c/V_M, H). \tag{5}$$

If we use a bar over a variable to indicate that it belongs to a geometrically similar model, then

$$\overline{C_S} = f(\overline{N_R}, \overline{d_c/d_t}, \overline{V_c/V_M}, \overline{H}). \tag{6}$$

Our basic approach is to determine Eq. (6) by model experiments, then to identify $\overline{C_S}$ with C_S in Eq. (5), and to use Eq. (3) to compute the shear force S:

$$S = C_S \mu V_M d_c. \tag{7}$$

It turns out that the shear coefficient C_S is strongly dependent on the hematocrit. Since the hematocrit is stochastic in vivo, the shear force must fluctuate as time passes. The fluctuation is quasi-static, because the Reynolds number of flow is very small.

Figure 5.11:2 shows a free-body diagram of a white blood cell adhering to a blood vessel wall. It is subjected to shear stresses imparted on its surface by a number of factors: by the plasma and the red blood cells, by pressure variations in the flowing blood, by a shear stress at the interface of the white

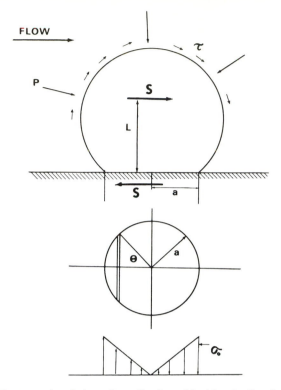

Figure 5.11:2 Cross-sectional view of an adhering white blood cell. P is the hydrostatic pressure, τ is the shear stress exerted on the surface of the white blood cell, and S is the resultant shear force. The two lower diagrams show the assumed contact area and the normal stress distribution on that contact area. A uniform normal stress acting on the contact area due to pressure over the cell is omitted from the lowest diagram: only the part needed to resist rolling of the cell is shown. See text for other abbreviations. From Schmid–Schöenbein et al. (1975). Reproduced by permission of the American Heart Association, Inc.

blood cell and the endothelium, by a variable normal stress σ on the interface, and by a body force due to acceleration and gravity. To examine the magnitude of these forces, it is necessary to remember that the Reynolds number of flow in the small venular vessels is very small, on the order of 10^{-2}. Hence, the inertial force due to fluid acceleration is negligible. The motion of the white blood cell is slow compared with that of the red cells. Furthermore, because its body is so small and because it is suspended in a fluid of almost equal density, the body force is insignificant. The resultant pressure force in the axial direction can also be neglected for the following reason. The pressure drop in a venule with an average length of 2000 μm is at most on the order of 5 mmHg. A sphere with a radius of 5 μm situated in such a pressure field will be subjected to a resultant force on the order of 3×10^{-8} dyn. The resultant of the pressure changes due to local disturbances in the flow caused by the presence of the body has a comparable magnitude. Thus, the resultant force in the axial direction due to pressure variation is on the order of 10^{-7} dyn. As will be seen later, the resultant of the shear forces acting on the free surface of the white blood cell is on the order of 10^{-4} dyn. Hence, in the axial direction, the resultant of the pressure forces is small in comparison with the resultant of the shear forces. Thus, the total drag force is approximately equal to the resultant of the shear force acting on the white blood cell.

The normal stress σ acting on the interface between the endothelium and the white blood cell must balance the forces and moments of the pressure and shear acting on the cell. Since the surface traction acting on the white blood cell has a resultant torque SL which does not vanish, where L represents the moment arm as shown in Fig. 5.11:2, the normal stress σ on the interface cannot be uniform and must have a resultant moment equal to SL.

The preceding analysis is applicable both when the white blood cell rolls at a constant speed and when it remains stationary. If the torque SL exceeds the torque of the normal stresses acting on the interface, then the rolling of the white blood cell will be accelerated. The normal stress of interaction between the endothelium and a stationary white blood cell will be maximum when the cell is on the verge of rolling down the wall. Experimentally, it was found that the average rolling velocity of the white blood cell is only about 4% of the mean blood flow velocity in the venule. With such a small rolling velocity, the flow pattern around the rolling white blood cell should be almost the same as that around a stationary cell.

The Model

The model is sketched in Fig. 5.11:3. The plasma was modeled by a silicone oil with a coefficient of viscosity of 47 poise. The red blood cells were modeled by gelatin pellets. The white blood cells were modeled by rigid spheres of certain diameters $(\overline{d_c} = 0.63$ cm, 0.55 cm, and 0.4 cm) mounted on a lever and introduced into a tube through a boring 0.65 cm in diameter. The blood vessel was modeled by a circular cylindrical tube $(\overline{d_t} = 2.25$ cm) connected to a container filled with a silicone oil-gelatin pellet suspension. The fluid was allowed to flow under gravity, using a valve to regulate the velocity.

As a tracer for the velocity measurement, tiny air bubbles were introduced into the silicone oil simply by pouring the oil into the container. A camera with a lens of short depth of field (3 mm) was focused on the plane of symmetry of the sphere and the tube. The velocity, V_M, was measured from 16-mm film recordings.

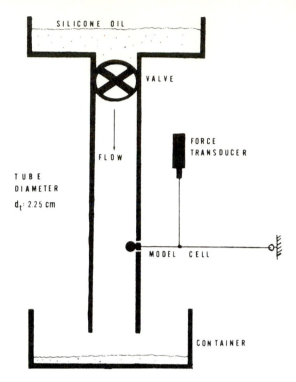

Figure 5.11:3 Cross-sectional view of the experimental model. The camera was focused precisely on the midplane of the tube in which the velocity of flow was determined. From Schmid–Schöenbein, et al. (1975). Reproduced by permission of the American Heart Association, Inc.

Results

At zero hematocrit, the model experiment was performed with spheres of several diameters. Figure 5.11:4 shows that $\overline{C_S}$ calculated according to Eq. (3) increases with increasing Reynolds number and increasing $\overline{d_c/d_t}$:

$$\overline{d_c/d_t} = 0.17: \qquad \overline{C_S} = 6.2 + 80N_R,$$

$$\overline{d_c/d_t} = 0.24: \qquad \overline{C_S} = 8 + 80N_R,$$

$$\overline{d_c/d_t} = 0.28: \qquad \overline{C_S} = 8.8 + 80N_R.$$

When the hematocrit is not zero, the shear force on the white cell fluctuates with time (because the shear force is influenced by the red blood cells whose concentration is never really uniform). The mean shear force, as well as the maximum deviations, increased with increasing velocity of flow. Figure 5.11:5 shows the data for a hematocrit of 30%. The solid circles indicate the mean values averaged over a period of about 25 sec, and the vertical bars indicate maximum deviations from these mean values. For

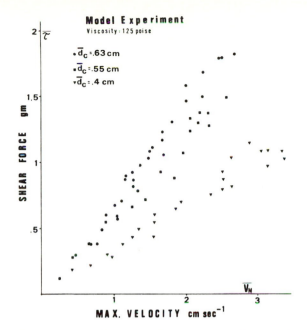

Figure 5.11:4 Shear force as a function of the maximum velocity of the tube flow for model white blood cells of different sizes at zero hematocrit. $\bar{d}_c$ = model white cell diameter. From Schmid–Schöenbein, et al. (1975). Reproduced by permission of the American Heart Association, Inc.

comparison, we also plotted the shear force at zero hematocrit as a straight line, showing the striking effect of the red cells.

On the other hand, the animal experiments yielded micrographs such as those shown in Fig. 5.11:1. These micrographs can be analyzed to obtain data on the velocity of flow in the tube (V_M), the diameter of the white blood cell (d_c), and the diameter of the venule (d_t). From these data and the viscosity of the plasma we can calculate the Reynolds number (N_R). The values of $\overline{C_S}$ were then determined for the corresponding values of N_R and d_c/d_t by interpolating linearly from the experimental values such as those shown in Figs. 5.11:4 and 5.11:5. The results show that the resultant shear force, S, acting on a white blood cell rolling on the endothelial wall lies in the range of 4–45 × 10⁻⁶ dyn at $H = 0$, and

$$8–90 \times 10^{-6} \text{ dyn at } H = 20\%,$$

$$16–180 \times 10^{-6} \text{ dyn at } H = 30\%, \tag{8a}$$

$$21–234 \times 10^{-6} \text{ dyn at } H = 40\%.$$

H is the hematocrit. This is the average shear force (averaged over time); the instantaneous maximum values are higher.

To determine the *stress* of interaction between the white cell and the

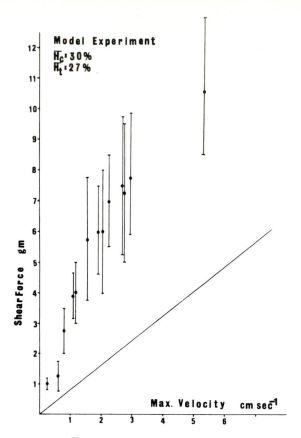

Figure 5.11:5 Shear force $\bar{S}$ acting on a model white cell with diameter $\bar{d}_c = 0.63$ cm plotted as a function of the average center-line velocity $\bar{V}_M$, for a given hematocrit. The hematocrit in the container ($\bar{H}_c$) of 30% corresponds to a hematocrit in the tube ($\bar{H}_1$) of 27%. The solid circles correspond to a mean value integrated over a period of 10–15 sec, and the vertical bars give the maximum deviations during this time period. For comparison, the shear force $\bar{S}$ at zero hematocrit for the same model cell is plotted in the lower part of the figure as a straight line through the origin. From Schmid–Schoenbein et al. (1975). Reproduced by permission of the American Heart Association, Inc.

endothelium of the venule, we must know their area of contact. By estimating the contact length from the photographs and assuming the contact area to be circular, some rough estimation of the shear stress can be obtained. The results are

$$50\text{–}200 \text{ dyn/cm}^2 \text{ at } H = 0,$$

$$100\text{–}400 \text{ dyn/cm}^2 \text{ at } H = 20\%,$$

$$200\text{–}800 \text{ dyn/cm}^2 \text{ at } H = 30\%,$$

$$265\text{–}1060 \text{ dyn/cm}^2 \text{ at } H = 40\%.$$

(8b)

These are again estimated average values (over time). Instantaneous shear stress can be higher.

It would be interesting to estimate the maximum normal stress of interaction that is required to prevent rolling of the white blood cell over the endothelium. For this purpose, let us assume that the normal stress is a linear function of x, as shown in the lower sketch of Fig. 5.11:2. Let the area of contact be a circle of radius a, and let the maximum normal stress at the outer edge be σ_0. Then the total moment is

$$4\int_0^{\pi/2} \sigma_0 a^3 \sin^2\theta \cos^2\theta\, d\theta = \frac{\sigma_0 a^3}{4}\pi, \tag{9}$$

which must be equal to the torque SL as discussed before on p. 273. Hence

$$\sigma_0 = \frac{4SL}{\pi a^3}. \tag{10}$$

For the assumed white blood cell considered previously, with $S = 10^{-5}$ dyn, $a = 2.5\ \mu$m, and $L = 3.5\ \mu$m, we obtain

$$\sigma_0 = 285\ \text{dyn/cm}^2.$$

The corresponding shear stress, assuming a constant stress distribution, is 50 dyn/cm^2. These calculations indicate that the normal stress of interaction is probably of the same order of magnitude as the shear stress, but it may be several times larger.

The calculation of the normal stress is based on the simplifying assumption that the normal stress varies linearly with the distance from the centroid of the contact area. This assumption may very well be incorrect. However, even if we assume a uniform tension for $x < 0$ and a uniform compression for $x > 0$, we will still obtain a stress $\sigma = 3SL/(4a^3)$, which, in the numerical example given previously, amounts to $\sigma_0 = 168$ dyn/cm^2.

Shear rates and shear stresses on the endothelium have been measured previously in large thoracic blood vessels of different species. Ling et al. (1968) calculated the shear stress from measured velocity profiles in the aorta of the dog and the pig, and obtained an average value between 80 and 160 dyn/cm^2 in normal flow. Fry (1968, 1969) created a high-shear flow by means of a plug and showed that acute changes occur in vascular endothelium of dog's aorta when the shear stress exceeds 379 ± 85 (SD) dyn/cm^2 on the basis of certain histological criteria, or 420 dyn/cm^2 on the basis of certain chemical response criteria. It is suspected that these endothelial cell changes due to shear stresses are related to the genesis of atherosclerosis. We now see that Fry's yield stress is of the same order of magnitude as the interacting shear force between white blood cells and vascular endothelium. These facts suggest that the shear stresses in large arteries and small veins are of the same order of magnitude under *in vivo* flow conditions.

It is well known that the number of white blood cells sticking to the endothelium varies with the degree of injury to the tissue and the time after injury, but it is not generally appreciated how small a disturbance will qualify as "injury." The white blood cells examined and reported on in this article were found in the rabbit omentum and mesentery after these tissues had been gently taken out of the animal and laid out under the microscope. This handling was sufficient to cause accumulation, sticking, and rolling of white blood cells on the endothelium of the venule. The reaction subsides in time. Atherton and Born (1972) have reported on the course of events.

5.12 Local Control of Blood Flow

The vascular smooth muscles respond to many substances as well as to mechanical and nervous stimulations. In the microvascular bed, changes in chemical environment of the vascular smooth muscle cells occur due to metabolism of the tissue, release of catacholamines from the nerve fibers, or material transfer across the endothelium. These changes may affect the muscle tone which in turn controls the vessel diameter and flow resistance. Exercise, drugs, metabolic conditions, and nutritional needs can thus affect local blood flow in an organ.

The vascular smooth muscle cells also respond to stress and strain. A step increase in tension may stimulate the muscle to contract and shorten. A step decrease in tension may cause the muscle to relax and lengthen. A step shortening of the muscle stimulates it to relax. A step stretch of the muscle causes it to contract. These active myogenic properties are called *Bayliss phenomena* (Bayliss, 1902). They are opposite to what one would expect from a passive material. We see them in some other muscles, e.g. in the earthworm. If you press your finger on an earthworm, it will swell up when you take your finger off. If you stretch the earthworm it will contract when you release it.

In most organs the factors mentioned above act to control the arteriolar segment of the vascular tree in such a way that the capillary pressure remains relatively constant when blood pressure in the aorta changes. The following phenomena are evidences of local control of blood flow.

Autoregulation of Blood Flow

Autoregulation is the tendency for blood flow to remain constant in face of changes in local arterial pressure to the organ. It is seen in virtually all organs of the body. It is most pronounced in brain and kidney. It is also evident in myocardium, intestine, skeletal muscle, and liver. Figure 5.12:1 shows the pattern of steady-state flow in the kidney along with the transient values obtained immediately after pressure was altered. After a sudden change of arterial pressure in the range 90–160 mmHg the flow changed instantaneously but subsequently returned to its initial level. If the arterial

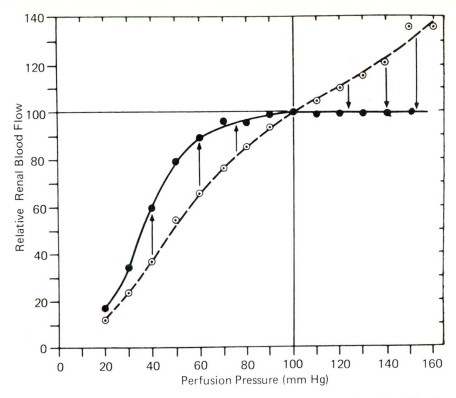

Figure 5.12:1 Autoregulation of renal blood flow. The two curves show blood flow in steady-state conditions (continuous line) and transient values following a sudden shift of perfusion pressure from the control level of 100 mmHg (dashed line). From Rothe et al. (1971). Reproduced by permission.

pressure is reduced, there is often an initial decrease in diameter of the arterioles followed by a dilation which causes the diameter to be increased above control levels, although the intravascular pressure is reduced. Periodic vasomotion of the arteriolar vessels often stops when arterial pressure is reduced.

Autoregulation is due to diameter control of precapillary vessels. Since the resistance and pressure in the post capillary vessels do not change much it follows that the pressure in the capillaries is maintained in spite of large changes in arterial pressure. This is a feature shown in Fig. 5.3:3.

Reactive Hyperemia

Reactive hyperemia is the period of elevated flow that follows a period of circulatory arrest. It exists in every vascular bed in peripheral circulation. It is rapid in onset, with a notable flow elevation following even a few seconds of flow arrest in some vascular beds. The magnitude of the hyperemia is related to the duration of ischemia.

Venous-Arteriolar Response

The arteriolar beds of some organs (intestine, liver, and certain skeletal muscles) constrict when venous pressure is elevated. It is most likely due to an inherent sensitivity of precapillary vessels to blood pressure (myogenic response).

Functional Hyperemia

Functional hyperemia is the increase in blood flow that accompanies increase in tissue activity. It occurs in skeletal and cardiac muscle, brain, intestine, stomach, salivary glands, kidney, and adipose tissue. There is evidence that end-products of tissue metabolism play a role in functional hyperemia. PCO_2, H^+, lactate and pyruvate, adenosine, and sympathetic vasodilator (cholinergic and β-adrenergic) have vasodilator influences. Furthermore, potassium released from depolarized skeletal muscle cells at the initiation of exercise may diffuse to the vicinity of the vascular smooth muscle cells to cause vascular relaxation and a rapid increase in blood flow. Release of potassium may also contribute to the vasodilation in brain during increased cerebral activity.

Hormonal factors may also be important (see Johnson, 1978). Physical factors may play a role too. For example, extravascular compression during muscular contraction may cause a relaxation of myogenic vascular tone in the arterioles of skeletal muscle. Emptying of the veins during muscle contraction increases flow in limbs during exercise.

Myogenic Control

Figure 5.12:2 shows a quantitative evidence of Bayliss mechanism: elevation of static intravascular pressure in the arteriole during no-flow condition leads to a sustained contraction of the arteriole in mesentery (Johnson and Intaglietta, 1976). The reactive hyperemia described earlier showing vasodilation after brief periods of arterial occlusion is another evidence of Bayliss phenomenon. So is the venous–arteriolar response. A fourth evidence is that the reduction of ambient pressure around an organ leads to sustained vasoconstriction (Greenfield, 1964). In all these cases the flow is not increased so that the metabolites changes cannot be a significant factor. It has been reported also that rapid pressure transients lead to powerful contraction, and that pulsatile perfusion leads to increased vascular tone.

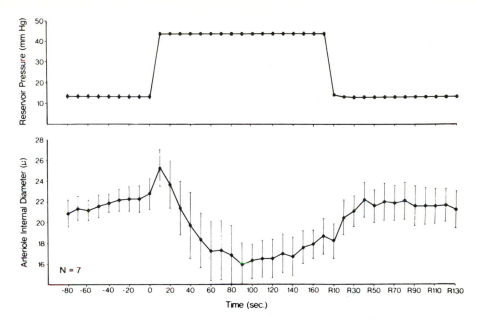

Figure 5.12:2 Effect of static pressure elevation in the vasculature of cat mesentery on arteriolar diameter. Data obtained during total flow arrest and equalization of arterial and venous pressure. From Johnson and Intaglietta (1976). Reproduced by permission.

Two mechanisms have been proposed to underlie the myogenic response. Folkow (1964) has suggested that passive stretch leads to an increase in the spontaneous firing rate of the smooth muscle, inducing contraction. When the cells shortens, it is no longer stretched beyond its normal length, and the stimulus for contraction disappears, and the muscle relaxes. However, as the muscle relaxes, the elevated pressure causes the cell to be stretched beyond its normal resting length, which brings on a second contraction earlier than it would occur normally. As a consequence the smooth muscle fires more frequently and it spends more time in the contracted state. The time-averaged vessel diameter decreases.

Johnson (1978) proposed that the smooth muscle is a tension receptor (as opposed to Folkow's hypothesis of being a length receptor), and that the tension leads to an increase in the spontaneous firing rate of the smooth muscle, inducing contraction. The rest of the argument is similar to Folkow's. Support has been drawn from Bülbring's observation that in guinea pig taenia coli the electric changes correlate closely to tension but poorly to length. Under Johnson's hypothesis, whether the vessel radius increases, decreases, or does not change when intravascular pressure is elevated depends on the "gain" of the feedback loop. The tension and vessel radius are related by the Laplace relationship $T = p \cdot r$, in which p is the transmural pressure, r is the radius, and T is the tension.

Johnson (1980) introduced an important concept that the resistance vessels should be considered as a series-coupled arrangement of independent effectors, each unit responding to change in its own wall tension. According to this concept, a rise in arterial pressure leads to contraction and narrowing of the proximal myogenic vessels, increased resistance and pressure fall through this segment, and thereby largely prevents the stimulus for contraction from reaching the more distal arterioles.

Determination of Vessel Diameter

From the discussions above it is seen that the current concept about the vascular smooth muscle is that there exists a basal vascular tone in all peripheral blood vessels in resting condition, and that in dynamic conditions the tension in the muscle is influenced by a number of metabolic and myogenic factors. According to this concept, we may write the stress in the blood vessel wall as

$$\sigma_{ij} = \sigma_{ij}^{(P)} + \sigma_{ij}^{(S)} \tag{1}$$

in which $\sigma_{ij}^{(S)}$ is the stress tensor due to active contraction of the vascular smooth muscle, $\sigma_{ij}^{(P)}$ is the stress tensor in the blood vessel at resting state, σ_{ij} is the resultant stress tensor. The indexes i and j range over 1, 2 and 3. The muscle stress due to basal tone at the resting state is lumped with $\sigma_{ij}^{(P)}$ because in experimental determination of σ_{ij} at the resting state one cannot distinguish the contributions from smooth muscle from that of the connective tissues. Equation (1) is the same as that presented in the author's book *Biomechanics* (Fung, 1981, p. 319, Eq. 8), and is based on Hill's three-element model. $\sigma_{ij}^{(P)}$ is a function of the strains in the vessel wall. $\sigma_{ij}^{(S)}$ is a function of time, strain, and the history of strain. $\sigma_{ij}^{(P)}$ is said to be the "parallel" element, or "passive" element. $\sigma_{ij}^{(S)}$ is called the "active" stress, or "series" element.

   If we wish to determine the diameter of a long circular cylindrical tube subjected to internal and external pressures in dynamic condition, we need to be concerned only with the circumferential stress alone, if the length of the tube may be considered fixed. In this case the axial strain is fixed; the radial strain can be determined from the axial and circumferential strains by the condition of incompressibility; hence the circumferential strain is the only independent variable. The condition of equilibrium is shown in Fig. 3.8:2, on p. 107. Let the circumferential strain be expressed in terms of the strech ratio λ, which is the ratio of the radius of a point in the deformed configuration divided by that at the resting state. Let the corresponding circumferential stress be denoted by σ_θ. Then according to Eq. (1), we may write

$$\sigma_\theta(\lambda, t) = \sigma_\theta^{(P)}(\lambda) + \sigma_\theta^{(S)}(\lambda, \lambda(\tau), t). \tag{2}$$

Here the idea that σ_θ is a function of the stretch ratio λ and time t is exhibited. $\sigma_\theta^{(P)}$ is a function of the stretch ratio λ. The active stress $\sigma_\theta^{(S)}$ at the instant of time t is a function of the current stretch ratio λ, the stretch history $\lambda(\tau)$ for $\tau < t$ before the current time and the time t. σ_θ should have been written as $\sigma_\theta(\lambda, \lambda(\tau), t)$ also, but we shall omit $\lambda(\tau)$ in the equations below for simplicity.

In Sec. 3.8, we have shown that the condition of equilibrium of the vessel wall (Fig. 3.8:2) leads to the so-called Laplace relation

$$h\langle\sigma_\theta\rangle = p_i a_i - p_e a_e, \tag{3}$$

where h is the wall thickness, a_i is the inner radius, a_e is the outer radius, p_i is the intravascular pressure, p_e is the external pressure, and $h = a_e - a_i$. The symbol $\langle\sigma_\theta\rangle$ means the average value of σ_θ averaged over the thickness of the wall. σ_θ is in general variable over the cross section; see Fig. 2.9:1, p. 56, for the results of a theoretical analysis, and pp. 57, 59 for a discussion on the effect of residual stresses.

The blood vessel wall material may be considered incompressible. Hence Eq. (3.8:22) applies and all λ's can be expressed in terms of the inner radius a_i. With this understanding, we can combine Eqs. (2) and (3) to obtain the basic equation

$$h\langle\sigma_\theta^{(P)}(a_i)\rangle + h\langle\sigma_\theta^{(S)}(a_i, t)\rangle = p_i a_i - p_e a_e. \tag{4}$$

From this equation the radius of the vessel, a_i, can be determined as a function of time, pressures, and muscle action.

The passive stress, $\sigma_\theta^{(P)}$, has been discussed thoroughly in the author's *Biomechanics* (Fung, 1981, Chap. 8). It is best expressed as a derivative of a strain energy function.

The solution of Eq. (4) may be illustrated graphically by an example. In Fig. 5.12:3, the dashed line represents $h\langle\sigma_\theta^{(P)}\rangle$ as a function of the inner

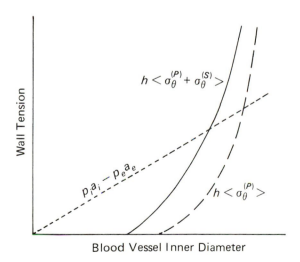

Figure 5.12:3 Graphical solution of Eq. (4). See text.

radius a_i; the solid line represents the left hand side of Eq. (4); the dotted line represents the right hand side of Eq. (4). The point of intersection, A, is the solution of Eq. (4), giving the arteriolar radius and the blood vessel wall tension. Since the solid line will change with time as the muscle is influenced by myogenic and metatolic factors, the vessel radius will change with time.

Burton (1951) assumed that the smooth muscle tone is independent of the vessel radius a_i so that the solid curve is obtained by shifting the dashed curve of Fig. 5.12:3 vertically upward. In that case it is easy to see that for each state of vascular tone there exists a minimal p_i below which the line $p_i a_i - p_e a_e$ will not intersect the wall tension curve $h\langle\sigma_\theta^{(p)} + \sigma_\theta^{(s)}\rangle$. Then Eq. (4) has no solution. This is interpreted as "critical closing", at which the vessel is closed. Burton's hypothesis is questionable since active tension in smooth muscle does in fact vary with muscle length.

Example of an Autoregulation Model

The metabolic and myogenic factors influence the active tension in the vascular smooth muscle. It remains to be shown that their action indeed leads to the control of *flow* as exhibited by the experimental results (e.g. those shown in Fig. 5.12:1). Øien and Aukland (1983) has presented a mathematical analysis of a model of the renal blood flow based on the myogenic hypothesis and showed that autoregulation can be explained under the following hypotheses: (1) Each preglomerular vessel segment reacts to a step-change in pressure p_i by altering the radius a_i until the initial change in wall tension $p_i a_i$ is *reduced* by a factor of G (gain factor). (2) Postglomerular structural resistance remains unchanged. (3) Extravascular tissue pressure equals intrarenal venous pressure. (4) The renal vascular system can be represented by one unbranched tube. The authors show that a gain factor of around 1 is required in order to obtain autoregulation.

Problems

5.3 Give a complete mathematical formulation of the following problem. Write down all the required differential equations and boundary conditions. State all the assumptions clearly and explicitly.

A series of equally spaced rigid spheres suspended in an incompressible Newtonian viscous fluid flowing down a rigid circular cylindrical cylinder in a single file, symmetric fashion. (Ref. Wang and Skalak, 1969.)

5.4 Replace the rigid spheres in the preceding problem by a series of droplets of oil which is immiscible with the carrying fluid. Surface tension should be considered.

5.5 Now consider flexible pellets resembling red blood cells. Revise the theory. (Ref. Zarda et al., 1977.)

5.6 Relax further. First, let the tube be elastic but impermeable to the fluid. Then let the wall of the tube be permeable so that fluid exchange between the fluid, the tube wall, and the medium outside the tube takes place. Make suitable assumptions with regard to the transport characteristics of the membrane and the movement of fluid outside the tube.

5.7 Further generalize the problems named above, let the particles be red blood cells and the tube be capillary blood vessels. Formulate a mathematical theory.

5.8 Discuss conditions in capillary blood flow that are nonstationary in nature. Formulate these transient problems. One example is the famous Landis experiment in which the flow is suddenly stopped by compressing the capillary blood vessel with a microneedle. The movement of the red cell is then recorded and the result is used to study the permeability of the blood vessel wall. (Ref. Lew and Fung, 1969c).

5.9 Again, think of the real capillary bed. Formulate a theory in which the blood vessels are not represented by cylindrical tubes. Discuss the practical significance of such an investigation.

Capillary blood vessels are usually not circular in cross section. Nor are they cylindrical. The asymmetry and unevenness of the wall have significant effect on the force of interaction between vessel walls and blood cells, especially the leucocytes. This is an important problem for future investigation.

5.10 Formulate a mathematical problem to analyze the tank-treading of a red cell flowing in a capillary blood vessel. Cf. Sec. 5.10, and Secomb and Skalak (1982).

5.11 Formulate a mathematical theory for the leucocyte problem discussed in Sec. 5.11.

References

Aroesty, J. and Gross, J. F. (1970). Convection and diffusion in the microcirculation. *Microvascular Res.* **2**: 247–267.

Atherton, A. and Born, G. V. R. (1972). Quantitative investigations of the adhesiveness of circulating polymorphonuclear leucocytes to blood vessel walls. *J. Physiol.* **222**: 447–474.

Baker, M. and Wayland, H. (1974). On-line volumetric flow rate and velocity profile measurement for blood microvessels. *Microvascular Res.* **7**: 131–143.

Bayliss, W. M. (1902). On the local reactions of the arterial wall to changes in internal pressure. *J. Physiol. (London)* **28**: 220–231.

Bülbring, E. (1955). Correlation between membrane potential, spike discharge and tension in smooth muscle. *J. Physiol. (London)* **128**: 200–221.

Bungay, P. M. and Brenner, H. (1973). The motion of a closely-fitting sphere in a fluid-filled tube. *Int. J. Multiphase Flow* **1**: 25–56.

Burton, A. C. (1951). On the physical equilibrium of small blood vessels. *Am. J. Physiol.* **164**: 319–329.

Caro, C. G., Pedley, T. J., Schroter, R. C. and Seed, W. A. (1978). *The Mechanics of the Circulation*, Oxford University Press, Oxford, New York.

Chen, T. C. and Skalak, R. (1970). Spheroidal particle flow in a cylindrical tube. *Appl. Sci. Res.* **22**: 403–441.

Fischer, T. M., Stohr-Liesen, M., and Schmid–Schoenbein, H. (1978). The red cell as a fluid droplet: tank tread-like motion of the human erythrocyte membrane in shear flow. *Science* **202**: 894–896.

Folkow, B. (1964). Description of the myogenic hypothesis. *Supplements to Circ. Res.* **15**: pp. I.279–I.285.

Folkow, B. and Neil, E. (1971). *Circulation*. Oxford University Press, London.

Fronek, K. and Zweifach, B. W. (1974). The effect of vasodilatator agents on microvascular pressures in skeletal muscle. *Angiologia*, **3**: 35–39, Unione Intern. di Angiologia.

Fronek, K. and Zweifach, B. W. (1975). Microvascular pressure distribution in skeletal muscle and the effect of vasodilation. *Amer. J. Physiol.* **228**: 791–796.

Fry, D. L. (1968). Acute vascular endothelial changes associated with increased blood velocity gradients. *Circulation Res.* **22**: 165–197.

Fry, D. L. (1969). Certain histological and chemical responses of the vascular interface of acutely induced mechanical stress in an aorta of the dog. *Circulation Res.* **24**: 93–108.

Fung, Y. C. (1973). Stochastic flow in capillary blood vessels. *Microvascular Res.* **5**: 34–48.

Fung, Y. C. (1981). *Biomechanics: Mechanical Properties of Living Tissues*. Springer-Verlag, New York, Heidelberg, Berlin.

Gaehtgens, P. (1980). Flow of blood through narrow capillaries: Rheological mechanisms determining capillary hematocrit and apparent viscosity. *Biorheology J.* **17**: 183–189.

Greenfield, A. D. M. (1964). Blood flow through the human forearm and digits as influenced by subatmospheric pressure and venous pressure. *Supplements to Circ. Res.* **14**: pp. I.70–I.75.

Hochmuth, R. M. and Sutera, S. P. (1970). Spherical caps in low Reynolds-number tube flow. *Chemical Eng. Sci.* **25**: 593–604.

Hyman, W. A. and Skalak, R. (1972). Non-Newtonian behavior of a suspension of liquid drops in fluid flow. *Amer. Inst. Chem. Eng. J.* **18**: 149–154.

Jendrucko, R. J. and Lee, J. S. (1973). The measurement of hematocrit of blood flowing in glass capillaries by microphotometry. *Microvascular Res.* **6**: 316–331.

Johnson, P. C. (1978). *Peripheral Circulation*. Wiley, New York.

Johnson, P. C. (1980). The myogenic response. In *Handbook of Physiology*, Sec. 2. *The Cardiovascular System*, Vol. 2. *Vascular Smooth Muscle* (D. F. Bohr, A. P. Somlyo, and H. V. Sparks, Jr., eds.) Amer. Physiological Society, Bethesda, Md., pp. 409–442.

Johnson, P. C. and Intaglietta, M. (1976). Contributions of pressure and flow sensitivity to autoregulation in mesenteric arterioles. *Am. J. Physiol.* **231**: 1686–1698.

Kaley, G. and Altura, B. M. (1977). *Microcirculation*, Vols. 1 & 2. University Park, Baltimore, MD.

Lamb, H. (1932). *Hydrodynamics*. 6th ed. Cambridge Univ. Press. Reprinted by Dover, New York.

Lee, T. Q., Schmid-Schoenbein, G. W., and Zweifach, B. W. (1983). An application of an improved dual-slit photometric analyzer for volumetric flow rate measurements in microvessels. *Microvascular Res.* **26**: 351–361.

Lew, H. S. and Fung, Y. C. (1969a). On the low-Reynolds-number entry flow into a circular cylindrical tube. *J. Biomechanics* **2**: 105–119.

Lew, H. S. and Fung, Y. C. (1969b). The motion of the plasma between the red blood cells in the bolus flow. *J. Biorheology* **6**: 109–119.

Lew, H. S. and Fung, Y. C. (1969c). Flow in an occluded circular cylindrical tube with permeable wall. *Zeit angew. Math. Physik* **20**(5): 750–766.

Lew, H. S. and Fung, Y. C. (1970a). Plug effect of erythrocytes in capillary blood vessels. *Biophysical J.* **10**: 80–99.

Lew, H. S. and Fung, Y. C. (1970b). Entry flow into blood vessels at arbitrary Reynolds number. *J. Biomechanics* **3**: 23–38.

Lighthill, M. J. (1968). Pressure-forcing of tightly fitting pellets along fluid-filled elastic tubes. *J. Fluid Mech.* **34**: 113–143.

Ling, S. C., Atabek, H. B., Fry, D. L., Patel, D. J. and Janicki, J. S. (1968). Application of heated-film velocity and shear probes to hemodynamics studies. *Circulation Res.* **23**: 789–801.

Lipowsky, H. H. and Zweifach, B. W. (1977). Methods for the simultaneous measurement of pressure differentials and flow in single unbranched vessels of the microcirculation for rheological studies. *Microvascular Res.* **14**: 345–361.

Lipowsky, H. H. and Zweifach, B. W. (1978). Application of the "two-slit" photometric technique to the measurement of microvascular volumetric flow rates. *Microvascular Res.* **15**: 93–101.

Lipowsky, H. H., Usami, S. and Chien, S. (1980). In vivo measurements of "apparent viscosity" and microvessel hematocrit in the mesentery of the cat. *Microvascular Res.* **19**: 297–319.

Majno, G. (1965). Ultrastructure of the vascular membrane. In W. F. Hamilton and P. Dow (eds.). *Handbook of Physiology*, Sec. 2 *Circulation*, Vol. 3. American Physiological Soc., Washington, D.C. pp. 2293–2375.

Nellis, S. N. and Zweifach, B. W. (1977). A method for determining segmental resistances in the microcirculation from pressure-flow measurements. *Circulation Res.* **40**(6): 546–556.

Norberg, K. A. and Hamberger, B. (1964). The sympathetic adrenergic neuron. *Acta Physiol. Scandinav.* **63** (Suppl. 238).

Ogawa, Y. (1976). A morphological study of microvascular beds in the cutaneous area. *J. of Yokohama City Univ. Ser. Sport Sci. and Med.* **5**: 1–37.

Oseen, C. W. (1910). Über die Stokessche Formel und über die verwandte Aufgabe in der Hydrodynamik. *Arkiv. Mat. Astron. Fysik.* **6**(29).

Øien, A. H. and Aukland, K. (1983). A mathematical analysis of the myogenic hypothesis with special reference to autoregulation of renal blood flow. *Circ. Res.* **52**: 241–252.

Prothero, J. and Burton, A. C. (1961, 1962). The physics of blood flow in capillaries. I. The nature of the motion. *Biophysical J.*, **1**: 567–579. II. The capillary resistance to flow. *ibid*, **2**: 199–212.

Proudman, I. and Pearson, J. R. A. (1957). Expansions at small Reynolds number for the flow past a sphere and a circular cylinder. *J. Fluid Mechanics* **2**: 237–262.

Rothe, C. F., Nash, F. D. and Thompson, D. E. (1971). Patterns in autoregulation of renal blood flow in the dog. *Am. J. Physiol.* **220**: 1621–1626.

Rouse, H. (1959). *Advanced Fluid Mechanics*. Wiley, New York.

Sagawa, K., Kumoda, M. and Schramm, L. P. (1974). Nervous control of the circulation. In *Cardiovascular Physiology* (A. C. Guyton and C. E. Jones, eds.). Butterworths, London, University Park Press, Baltimore, Vol. 1, p. 197–232.

Schlichting, H. (1962). *Boundary Layer Theory*. McGraw–Hill, New York.

Schmid–Schoenbein, G. W., Fung, Y. C. and Zweifach, B. (1975). Vascular endothelium-leucocyte interaction: Sticking shear force in venules. *Circulation Res.* **36**: 173–184.

Schmid–Schoenbein, G. W., Skalak, R., Usami, S. and Chien, S. (1980a). Cell distribution in capillary networks. *Microvascular Res.* **19**: 18–44.

Schmid–Schoenbein, G. W., Usami, S., Skalak, R. and Chien, S. (1980b). The interaction of leukocytes and erythrocytes in capillary and postacpillary vessels. *Microvascular Res.* **19**: 45–70.

Schmid–Schoenbein, H. and Wells, R. E. (1969). Fluid drop-like transition of erythrocytes under shear. *Science* **165**: 288–291.

Secomb, T. W. and Skalak, R. (1982). A two-dimensional model for capillary flow of an asymmetric cell. *Microvas. Res.* **24**: 194–203.

Skalak, R., Chen, P. H. and Chien, S. (1972). Effect of hematocrit and rouleaux on apparent viscosity in capillaries. *Biorheology* **9**: 67–82.

Skalak, R., Tozeren, A., Zarda, P. R. and Chien, S. (1973). Strain energy function of red cell membranes. *Biophysical J.* **13**: 245–264.

Smaje, L., Zweifach, B. W. and Intaglietta, M. (1970). Micropressures and capillary filtration coefficients in single vessels of the cremaster muscle of the rat. *Microvascular Res.* **2**: 96–110.

Stokes, G. G. (1851). On the effect of the internal friction of fluids on the motion of pendulums. *Trans. Cambridge Philosophical Soc.* **9**: p. 8. *Mathematical and Physical Papers*, Vol 3, pp. 1–141.

Svanes, K. and Zweifach, B. W. (1968). Variations in small blood vessel hematocrits produced in hypothermic rats by microocclusion. *Microvascular Res.* **1**: 210–220.

Targ, S. M. (1951). *Basic Problems of the Theory of Laminar Flows* (in Russian). Moskva.

Tong, P. and Fung, Y. C. (1971). Slow viscous flow and its application to biomechanics. *J. Appl. Mechanics* **38**: 721–728.

Tözeren, H. and Skalak, R. (1978). The steady flow of closely fitting incompressible elastic spheres in a tube. *J. Fluid Mechanics* **87**: 1–16.

Tözeren, H. and Skalak, R. (1979). Flow of elastic compressible spheres in tubes. *J. Fluid Mechanics* **95**(4): 743–760.

Wang, H. and Skalak, R. (1969). Viscous flow in a cylindrical tube containing a line of spherical particles. *J. Fluid Mechanics* **38**: 75–96.

Wayland, H. (1982). A physicist looks at the microcriculation. *Microvascular Res.* **23**: 139–170.

Wiedeman, M. P., Tuma, R. F. and Mayrovitz, H. N. (1981). *An Introduction to Microcirculation*. Academic Press, New York.

Wiederhielm, C. A., Woodbury, J. W., Kirk, S. and Rushmer, R. F. (1964). Pulsatile pressure in microcirculation of the frog's mesentery. *Amer. J. Physiol.* **207**: 173–176.

Yen, R. T. and Fung, Y. C. (1978). Effect of velocity distribution on red cell distribution in capillary blood vessels. *Amer. J. Physiol.* **235**(2): H251–H257.

Yih, C. S. (1969). *Fluid Mechanics*. McGraw–Hill. New edn., West River Press, Ann Arbor, MI.

Zarda, P. R., Chien, S. and Skalak, R. (1977). Interaction of a viscous incompressible fluid with an elastic body. In *Computational Methods for Fluid-Structure Interaction Problems* (Belytschko, T. and Geers, T. L. (eds.)). American Society of Mechanical Engineers, New York, pp. 65–82.

Zweifach, B. W. (1974). Quantitative studies of microcirculatory structure and function. I. Analysis of pressure distribution in the terminal vascular bed. *Circulation Res.* **34**: 843–857. II. Direct measurement of capillary pressure in splanchmic mesenteries. *Circulation Res.* **34**: 858–868.

Zweifach, B. W. and Lipowsky, H. H. (1977). Quantitative studies of microcirculatory structure and function. III. Microvascular hemodynamics of cat mesentery and rabbit omentum. *Circulation Res.* **41**(3): 380–390.

CHAPTER 6

Blood Flow in the Lung

6.1 Introduction

We shall now apply the general principles discussed in the preceding chapters to one organ, the lung. The purpose is to illustrate, in one concrete example, the use of physical principles, with the help of anatomy and histology, to explain and predict the function of an organ in quantitative terms.

A mathematical analysis of any system requires a set of hypotheses. A good theory uses as few hypotheses as possible. The solution of any system of equations requires the specification of boundary conditions. The solution will be more valuable if the boundary conditions are realistic. The basic equations must contain descriptions of the geometry, structure, and materials properties of the system. The more closely these descriptions are based on experiments and less idealized, the more truthful will be the solutions. This is the creed of theoreticians. This is our aim.

Let us consider first the general nature of the pulmonary circulation. The function of the lung is to oxygenate the blood and to remove CO_2. Nature chooses to do this by the principle of diffusion; and for this purpose blood is spread out into very thin layers or sheets so that the blood–gas interfacial area becomes very large. In an adult human lung with a pulmonary capillary blood volume on the order of 150 ml, the pulmonary capillary blood-gas exchange area is of the order of 70 m^2, so that the average computed thickness of the sheets of blood in the pulmonary capillaries is only about 4 μm. The thin membrane that separates the blood from the air is less than 1 μm thick; it consists of a layer of endothelial cells, an interstitium, and a layer of epithelial cells. Each sheet of blood, bounded by two membranes, forms an *interalveolar septum*. Several billion septa form a space structure which may be compared to the honeycomb (Malpighi, 1661), or a bowl of soap

290

bubbles. The smallest unit of space bounded by *interalveolar septa* is called the *alveolus*. In an adult man there are 300 million alveoli. Each alveolus, like a cell of a honeycomb, is polyhedral. It is bounded by interalveolar walls which, however, do not form a closed polyhedron because one or more sides must be missing in order to ventilate. Though the open side, every alveolus is ventilated to the atmosphere through a branching airway system.

The blood vessels of the lung must be so arranged as to provide an adequate transit time for the erythrocytes to go through the capillary sheets so that the gas exchange process can be completed. Oxygenation of hemoglobin requires the oxygen to move across the alveolar-capillary membrane, through the plasma and across the erythrocyte membrane. About half of the total time for the diffusion of oxygen from the alveolus to the red cell is spent in traversing the alveolar-capillary membrane. Of the total of approximately 3 sec required to move blood from the pulmonary valve to the left atrium in man, about 1 sec is spent in the alveolar capillary bed. To accomplish complete oxygenation in such a short period of time requires not only a fast oxygenation and CO_2 exchange process in the blood, but also a low resistance system of pulmonary blood vessels to handle the output of the heart. (The resting cardiac output is very close to one total blood volume per minute in nearly all mammals, or about 4.4 l/min in man.) Furthermore, this low resistance system must be flexible, because cardiac output in strenuous exercise can increase fivefold! Nature provides a remarkable factor of safety for physiological stress loading.

Pulmonary vasculature is a low pressure system. This can be seen by comparing the pressures in the pulmonary artery and the aorta in Fig. 2.4:2. The pressure in the windkessel vessels (pulmonary artery) oscillates between 10–25 mmHg; that in the capacitance vessels (pulmonary veins) is only 4 or 5 mmHg. A low-pressure system does not need a very strong container. Thus, the wall of the pulmonary artery is found to be thinner than that of the aorta. The structures of the smaller pulmonary arteries are similarly flimsier. The arteriole, which in systemic circulation is thick-walled (compared with its diameter) and muscular, is thin walled in the lung. The capillary blood vessels, which in systemic circulation are embedded in gel-like tissues, are exposed to gas in the lung. The capillary blood vessels in the systemic circulation are quite rigid, and show negligible change in diameter in normal variation of blood pressure. In contrast, the capillary blood vessels in the lung are quite flexible: the thickness of the capillary sheet varies almost linearly with the blood pressure. Pulmonary venules and veins are similarly thin walled. Thus, the container of the pulmonary blood is quite flexible, and the flow is significantly influenced by the elastic deformation. The resistance of the pulmonary capillaries does not remain constant, it is strongly influenced by blood and air pressures. Pulmonary blood flow is not a linear function of the blood pressure gradient, because an increase in blood pressure distends the blood vessels, reduces the resistance, and increases the flow out of proportion.

The flexibility of the lung structure reveals itself also in other ways. One of the most dramatic effects is the influence of gravity on the distribution of blood flow in the lung. The flow per unit volume increases greatly in the direction of gravity. The reason is rather simple: Gravity affects the hydrostatic pressure in the blood. For man in upright position, the hydrostatic head may equal or exceed the pulmonary arterial pressure. The blood pressure (sum of the hydrostatic head and the pressure in the pulmonary artery minus the resistance loss to the point in question) at the apex of the lung may become smaller than the air pressure, whereas that at the base may become more than twice that of the arterial pressure. As a result, the capillary blood vessel sheet thickness is reduced at the apex and increased at the base; and the flow at the apex may become choked off whereas that at the base is much increased.

The major determinants of pulmonary blood flow are therefore (a) the topology of the blood vessels, (b) the pressures of alveolar gas and blood, (c) the viscosity of blood as affected by hematocrit and other factors, (d) the elasticity of blood vessels, and (e) the intrapleural pressure that affects the size of the lung. These factors interact to produce a peculiarly nonlinear pressure–flow relationship.

The lung, however, is a very complex organ. It has two systems of circulation: (a) the low-pressure pulmonary circulation discussed above, and (b) the high pressure bronchial circulation. It has an extensive lymphatic system. Although the pulmonary blood vessels are richly supplied with nerve fibers and have one or more chemoreceptor areas, the vascular bed of the lung normally is largely free from neural and chemical control. However, it responds promptly to hypoxia, retains the features of potential neural and humoral control in disease, and responds to pharmacological doses of catecholamines, histamine, serotonin, and other agents. The pulmonary arterial system and the bronchial arterial system have some connections, and collateral circulation develops in abnormal states. Connections between the pulmonary arterial ramifications and pulmonary venous tributaries larger than the capillary beds are not seen in the normal individual; but in some disease states arterio-venus shunts can be quite prominent. Thus the study of pulmonary blood flow has many ramifications.

The objective of the present chapter is limited to the analysis of the main features of the mechanics of pulmonary circulation. It will be shown that after certain anatomical, histological, and rheological data are obtained, the problem can be formulated and solved analytically, and the results of theoretical analysis are in reasonable agreement with those of physiological experiments.

6.2 Pulmonary Blood Vessels

Figure 6.2:1 shows the relationship between the heart and lung. Blood flows from the right ventricle to the pulmonary artery, then to capillary blood vessels, then to veins, and finally to left atrium. Figure 6.2:2 shows an en-

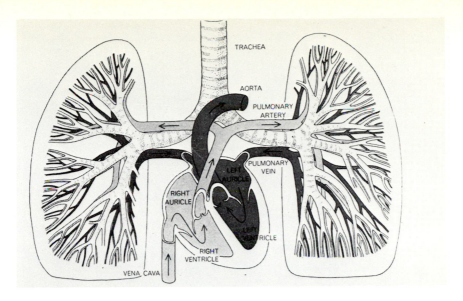

Figure 6.2:1 Relationship between the heart and the lung. Note that the pulmonary arteries lie close to the bronchi, whereas the pulmonary veins stand alone. Only the first few generations of the large pulmonary blood vessels and bronchi are shown in the figure. For smaller vessels, see Figs. 6.2:2 and 6.2:3.

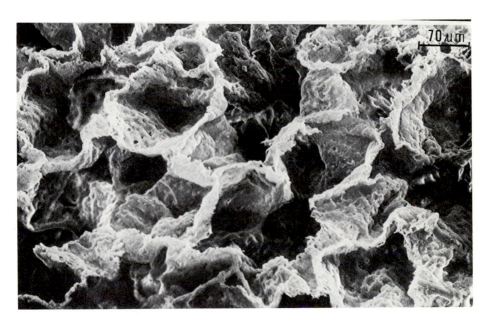

Figure 6.2:2 Scanning electron micrograph of cat lung illustrating how each interalveolar septum is shared by two alveoli. These septa are sheets of pulmonary capillary blood vessels. The wrinkly appearance of the septa is an artifact due to the cutting of the specimen and relieving of the stresses, thereby causing the elastin fibers which cannot be fixed by commonly known fixing agents (see *Biomechanics*, Fung, 1981, p. 198) to contract.

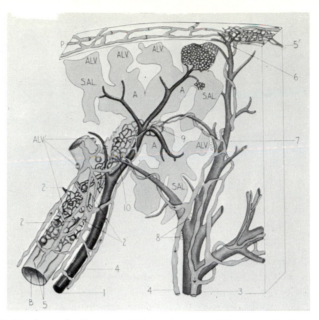

Figure 6.2:3 A schematic diagram of the pulmonary blood vessels, bronchial blood vessels, and lymphatic vessels in the lung and in the pleural surface. Drawing by William S. Miller (1947, p. 75). Reproduced by permission. B is *bronchiole*, leading to two *alveolar ducts* one of which is shown here. A = atrium, ALV, ALV′ = *alveoli*, S. AL. = *alveolar sac*. P = *pulmonary pleura*. 1 = *pulmonary artery*, dividing into capillaries. 2 = branches of pulmonary arteries distributed to bronchioles and ducts and then broken up into capillaries which unite with capillaries derived from the bronchial arteries. 3 = *pulmonary vein*. 4 = *lymphatics*. 5 = *bronchial artery* and capillaries. 5′ = bronchial arterial supply in the pleura (in animals with a *thick* pleura). 6 = *pulmonary venule*. 7, 8, 9, 10 are situations in which lymphoid tissue is found.

larged view of capillary blood vessels in the interalveolar septa. Figure 6.2:3 shows a schematic diagram of a lobule of the lung drawn by Miller (1947, p. 75) to illustrate the relation of the blood vessels to the air spaces. Note that arteries are adjacent to bronchi, whereas the veins stand alone. Bronchial vessels and lymphatics are also shown in the figure. It is seen that the vessels *in* the pleura are bronchial vessels. A photograph of a silicone cast of the venous tree of a cat's lung is shown in Fig. 4.9:1 in Chap. 4.

The geometry of the pulmonary arterial and venous trees can be described by the Strahler system (see Sec. 4.9). In this system the capillaries are counted as vessels of order 0. The smallest arterioles are called vessels of order 1. Two order 1 vessels meet to form a larger vessel of order 2, and so on. But if an order 2 vessel meets a vessel of order 1, the order number of the combined vessel remains as 2. A similar counting is done for the venous tree. The ratio of the number of vessels of order n to that of order $n + 1$ is called the branching ratio. The ratio of the diameter of the vessels of order n to

TABLE 6.2:1 Integrated Data for the Total Pulmonary Arterial System of Man. From Singhal et al. (1973)

Order	Number of branches	Diameter (mm)	Length (mm)	End branches	Capillary bed[a] (%)
17	1.000	30.000	90.50	3.000×10^8	1.000×10^2
16	3.000	14.830	32.00	1.000×10^8	3.333×10
15	8.000	8.060	10.90	3.021×10^7	1.007×10
14	2.000×10	5.820	20.70	1.376×10^7	4.588
13	6.600×10	3.650	17.90	3.983×10^6	1.328
12	2.030×10^2	2.090	10.50	1.159×10^6	3.863×10^{-1}
11	6.750×10^2	1.330	6.60	3.470×10^5	1.157×10^{-1}
10	2.290×10^3	0.850	4.69	8.916×10^4	2.972×10^{-2}
9	5.861×10^3	0.525	3.16	4.805×10^4	1.602×10^{-2}
8	1.756×10^4	0.351	2.10	1.604×10^4	5.437×10^{-3}
7	5.255×10^4	0.224	1.38	5.358×10^3	1.786×10^{-3}
6	1.574×10^5	0.138	0.91	1.787×10^3	5.957×10^{-4}
5	4.713×10^5	0.086	0.65	5.975×10^2	1.992×10^{-4}
4	1.411×10^6	0.054	0.44	1.995×10^2	6.650×10^{-5}
3	4.226×10^6	0.034	0.29	6.664×10	2.221×10^{-5}
2	1.266×10^7	0.021	0.20	2.370×10	7.900×10^{-6}
1	3.000×10^8	0.013	0.13	1.000	3.333×10^{-7}

[a] Capillary bed (%) is the calculated percent of the total capillary bed supplied by one branch of a given order.

that of order $n + 1$ is called the diameter ratio. Similarly, a length ratio is defined. Yen et al. (1983) have measured the branching pattern of the pulmonary arteries and veins of the cat, and their results are presented in Tables 6.11:1 and 6.11:2, pp. 337, 338. Singhal et al. (1973) have measured the branching pattern of human pulmonary arteries; their results are given in Table 6.2:1. For the smallest arterioles (of order 1), Singhal et al. assumes that each alveolus is supplied by one arteriole. For the cat we know this assumption is untrue. Each terminal arteriole of the cat supplies an average of 24 alveoli, and about 18 alveoli drain into one venule (Zhuang et al., 1983).

6.3 Pulmonary Capillaries

In the lung, the smallest unit of the air space is the alveolus. The alveolus is bounded by networks of capillary blood vessels. The walls of each alveolus are shared by neighboring alveoli, and are called *interalveolar septa*. The overriding fact that determines the topology of the capillary blood vessels is that all pulmonary alveolar septa in adult mammalian lungs are similar. Each septum contains one single sheet of capillary blood vessels, and is exposed to air on both sides.

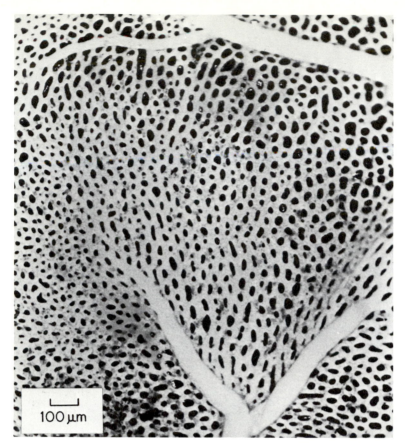

Figure 6.3:1 Photograph of a network of capillary blood vessels in the frog by Maloney and Castle (1969). Reprinted by permission.

The dense network of the capillary blood vessels in an alveolar wall of the frog is shown in Fig. 6.3:1 (Maloney and Castle, 1969). A similar picture of the cat's lung is shown in Fig. 6.3:2, whereas cross-sectional views of the cat's lung can be found in *Biomechanics* (Fung, 1981, Fig. 5.2:1 on p. 141, Fig. 5.2:2 on p. 142, and Figs. 8.8:1, 8.8:2 on p. 288). To characterize the geometry of such a network, we idealize the vascular space as a sheet of fluid flowing between two membranes held apart by a number of more or less equally spaced "posts;" see Fig. 6.3:3. In the plane view (A) this is a sheet with regularly arranged obstructions. The plane may be divided into a network of hexagons, with a circular post at the center of each hexagon. The "sheet-flow" model is therefore characterized by three parameters: L, the length of each side of the hexagon; h, the average height or thickness of the sheet; ε, the diameter of the posts.

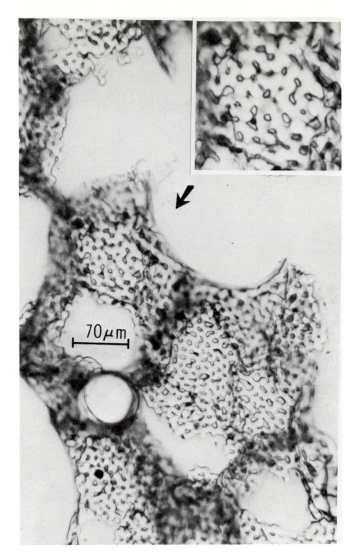

Figure 6.3:2 Cat lung. Flat view of interalveolar wall with the microvasculature filled with a silicone elastomer. This photomicrograph illustrates the tight mesh or network of the extensively filled capillary bed. The circular or elliptical enclosures are basement membrane stained with cresyl violet and are the nonvascular posts. Frozen section from gelatin-embedded tissue; glycerol-gelatin mount. The insert shows a detail from the region indicated by the arrow. From Fung and Sobin (1969), by permission.

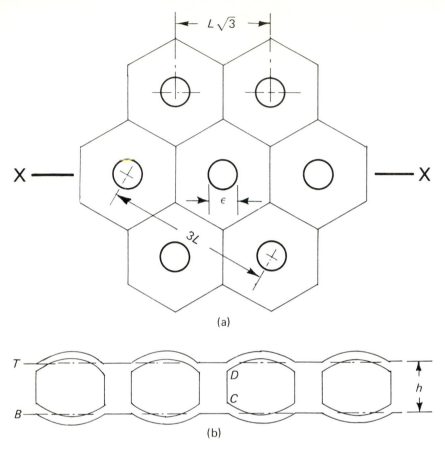

(a)

(b)

Figure 6.3:3 Sheet-flow model. (a) Plane view. (b) Cross section through X—X of (a). The cylindrical elements (circular in (a) and rectangular in (b)) are the "post." The space between the top and bottom walls is the flow channel. For bounding surfaces only, T, top, and B, bottom. Sheet thickness, h. C and D, contact of posts with endothelial surface at T and B. From Sobin et al. (1970). Reprinted by permission of the American Heart Association, Inc.

We shall define a "*vascular-space–tissue ratio*" (VSTR) as the ratio of the vascular lumen volume to a certain circumscribing volume defined below. As illustrated in Fig. 6.3:3(b), the circumscribing volume is that enclosed between surfaces T and B. The tissues (epithelial, interstitial, and endothelial) external to the surfaces T and B are excluded. Thus VSTR does not represent the volumetric fraction of the total interalveolar septum occupied by blood; it represents only the fraction of the blood volume over a sum of the volumes of the vascular space and the posts. For the sheet model, the VSTR is independent of the height h and is equal to the percentage of the area occupied by blood in the plane cross section. From Fig. 6.3:3(a), we have

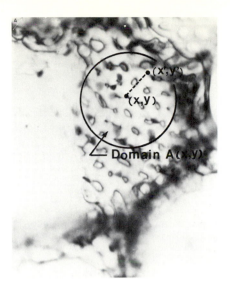

Figure 6.3:4 Domain of averaging around a point (x, y) in an alveolar sheet. From Fung and Sobin (1969). Reprinted by permission.

$$\text{The area of a hexagon} = \frac{3\sqrt{3}}{2}L^2.$$

$$\text{The area of a circle} = \pi\frac{\varepsilon^2}{4}.$$

(1)

Hence for the sheet flow,

$$\text{VSTR} = 1 - \frac{\pi}{6\sqrt{3}}\frac{\varepsilon^2}{L^2}.$$

(2)

In actual practice, it is difficult to measure and evaluate L, ε, and h from microscopic preparations because of the random irregularities in the geometric appearance of the specimens. The VSTR, however, can be determined with greater confidence by planimetry and random sampling. The dimension of the obstructing posts (ε) can be calculated from Eq. (2) by determining the VSTR and measuring $3L$ as indicated in Figure 6.3:3(a). Then

$$\frac{\varepsilon}{L} = \sqrt{\frac{6\sqrt{3}}{\pi}(1 - \text{VSTR})}.$$

(3)

The idea is illustrated in Fig. 6.3:4. We choose an area that is large compared with the individual posts, and measure the area ratio of the vascular space and the circumscribing area, thus obtaining VSTR directly. ε/L is then calculated from Eq. (3). Let the measured average area of the posts be A_p, and that of the basic hexagon be A_s; then

TABLE 6.3:1 Summary of Data for Elastomer-Filled Lungs of Vertically
Positioned Cats at a Transpulmonary Pressure (= Alveolar − Pleural
Pressures) of 10 cm H_2O*. From Sobin et al. (1970)

Δp	VSTR (%)	Hexagon area (μ^2)	Post diameter (μ)	Interpost distance (μ)	No. fields analyzed
6.3	90.94 ± 1.94	239.51 ± 27.06	5.25 ± 0.83	10.21 ± 0.30	6
6.8	88.81 ± 2.10	275.34 ± 37.80	6.22 ± 0.66	10.34 ± 0.99	6
7.3	91.16 ± 1.50	256.53 ± 45.58	5.35 ± 0.80	10.60 ± 0.89	6
10.3	90.16 ± 1.84	202.08 ± 43.34	5.01 ± 0.82	9.15 ± 0.91	18
14.3	90.59 ± 2.12	193.25 ± 63.07	4.74 ± 1.02	8.99 ± 1.38	18
18.3	90.43 ± 2.64	203.54 ± 38.75	4.96 ± 1.11	9.24 ± 0.51	18

* Values are means ± SD. Δp is the transmural pressure difference, i.e., vascular pressure
minus alveolar air pressure; VSTR is vascular space–tissue ratio expressed in percent;
hexogon area is planimetered sheet area divided by the number of posts in area; and interpost
distance is the distance between posts' edges.

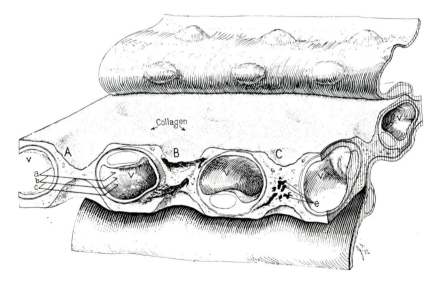

Figure 6.3:5 A composite drawing of the pulmonary interalveolar wall of the dog
showing the interalveolar microvascular sheet composed of a vascular compartment (V)
(the capillary bed) and the avascular (intercapillary) posts (A, B, C). The alveolar
epithelium has been pulled back to show the connective tissue matrix of the wall.
Collagen converges on the post from the surrounding capillary wall. In post B collagen
fiber bundles pass around within the post in a curving arrangement. From Rosenquist
et al. (1973), by permission.

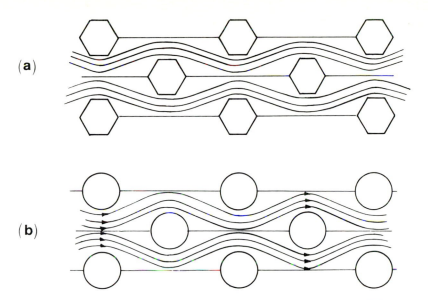

Figure 6.3:6 Streamlines of flow in an alveolar capillary network. (a) Flow in the middle plane of a tube model. Note that although the capillaries are considered as tubes the flow is entirely different from Poiseuillean pattern. (b) Flow in sheet model. Note the similarty in the flow patterns between (a) and (b). From Fung and Sobin (1969), by permission.

$$L = \sqrt{\frac{2}{3\sqrt{3}} A_s} \tag{4a}$$

$$\varepsilon = 2\sqrt{\frac{A_p}{\pi}}. \tag{4b}$$

The interpost distance (the distance between post edges) is $L\sqrt{3} - \varepsilon$, which is the width of the channel for the passage of red cells in the plane of the alveolar wall.

The data for the cat lung are presented in Table 6.3:1. The VSTR for each individual lobe is not influenced by the blood pressure; the average value is 0.91. These data indicate that in the plane of the interalveolar wall, the capillary bed can occupy 91% of the area of the wall.

This high value of VSTR applies to the interalveolar septa. It does not apply to those alveoli which were noted by Miller (1947) to have capillary beds with a "coarse" mesh, such as pleura, peribronchial, and perivascular septa, and those abutting connective tissues.

To help visualize the vascular space in the pulmonary alveolar sheet, we present a composite drawing Fig. 6.3:5. The epithelium is lifted from the interstitium and pulled back. The elastin and collagen fibers in the interstitium are indicated but not drawn in detail. The cross section of an individual capillary blood vessel appears like a tube, but overall the vascular space is represented as a sheet. From the point of view of fluid mechanics the sheet representation is particularly appropriate, because the streamlines will occupy the vascular space as sketched in Fig. 6.3:6, as if in a sheet. Each segment is so short that the Poiseuillean velocity profile discussed in Sec. 3.2 does not have a chance to develop. The Poiseuillean formula, Eq. (17) of Sec. 3.2, certainly does not apply.

6.4 Elasticity of Pulmonary Arteries and Veins

A complete set of data on the elasticity of pulmonary arteries and veins of all orders exists for the cat, although scattered data for larger vessels do exist for several other animals. Two methods were used to obtain these data in the author's laboratory. For pulmonary blood vessels larger than 100 μm in diameter, the method of x-ray photography was used (Yen et al. 1980, 1981). The lung was hung in a lucite box, and inflated by negative pleural pressure while the airway was exposed to atmosphere. The pulmonary vessels were first perfused with saline, then with a suspension of radio-opaque $BaSO_4$, either from the artery, or from the vein. The $BaSO_4$ particles will not pass through the capillaries; hence, either the arterial tree or the venous tree can be photographed in x-ray. Photographs were taken while the perfusion pressure were varied step by step. Then the vessel diameters were measured and the pressure and diameter relationship was determined. For blood vessels smaller than 100 μm in diameter, including the capillaries, the silicone elastomer method was used (Sobin et al. 1966, 1972, 1980). The lung was inflated and perfused with a liquid silicone rubber of low viscosity, freshly catalyzed with 3% stannous ethylhexoate and 1.5% ethyl silicate. Then the flow was stopped and the perfusion pressure equilibrated at a selected value. The elastomer was allowed to solidify. After solidification, histological specimens were prepared and the vessel diameters were measured. The pressure–diameter relationship was then determined for vessels of identified hierarchy (order number).

Figure 6.4:1 shows the results of Yen et al. (1980) for the pulmonary arteries of the cat. The diameter of each vessel, D, plotted on the ordinate, is normalized with respect to the diameter of that vessel when $p_a - p_{PL}$ is equal to zero, p_a being the blood pressure, p_{PL} being the pleural pressure. Each vessel is identified by its diameter at $p - p_{PL}$ equal to zero and classified into groups as shown in the figure. The abscissa is the pressure difference $p_a - p_{PL}$. The lung inflation pressure $p_A - p_{PL}$ was 10 cm H_2O.

Note that the pressure–diameter relationship for the pulmonary arteries is very different from that of the systemic arteries discussed in Chapter 8 of *Biomechanics* (Fung, 1981). Curves for the systemic arteries are very nonlinear, with pressure an exponential function of diameter. Curves for pulmonary arteries are straight lines. The reason for this difference is that

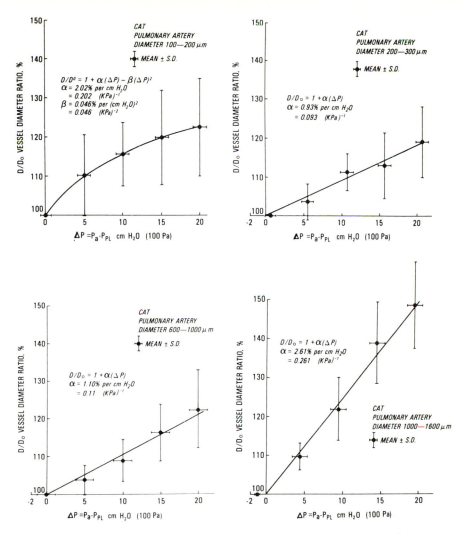

Figure 6.4:1 (a) Percentage change in diameter of the pulmonary arteries of the cat as functions of the pressure difference of the arterial blood pressure and the pleural pressure, $\Delta p = p_a - p_{PL}$, for vessels in the size range 100–200 μm. (b) Vessels in 200–300 μm range. (c) Vessels in 600–1000 μm range. (d) Those in 1000–1600 μm range. The alveolar gas pressure, p_A, was zero (atmospheric). The pleural pressure, p_{PL}, was -10 cm H_2O. The vertical bars indicate the scatter (S.D.) of D/D_0 in different lungs studied. The horizontal bars indicate the S.D. of the pressures in different vessels. From Yen et al. (1980). Reproduced by permission.

the systemic arteries are tested as isolated tubes, whereas the pulmonary arteries are embedded in lung parenchyma. Hence, the pressure–diameter curves shown in Fig. 6.4:1 are not that of the arteries alone, but the artery–parenchyma combination. The lung parenchyma, consisting of the alveolar walls, are attached to the outside of the blood vessel. They are an integral part of the vessel. The vessels are tethered, embedded in an elastic medium.

From the regression lines of Fig. 6.4:1, the slope, i.e., the *compliance constants*, are determined and listed in Table 6.11:1, on p. 337.

The corresponding results for the pulmonary veins of the cat are shown in Fig. 4.9:2, on p. 214, in which the ordinate is the vessel diameter (projected width) normalized with respect to D_{10}, the diameter of the vessel when $p - p_A = 10$ cm H_2O. This value of 10 cm H_2O was chosen because it was worried that the cross sectional shape of the pulmonary veins may not be circular when $p - p_A$ is zero; but when $p - p_A$ is 10 cm H_2O the cross section will not deviate far from being a circle; hence D_{10} serves better as a normalizing factor. A source of scatter of data is thus minimized.

A remarkable feature revealed by Fig. 4.9:2 on p. 214 is the gentle change of the slope of the curves when $p - p_A$ is negative. The implication of this has been discussed at length in Sec. 4.9. It is an indication that the pulmonary veins do not collapse when the transmural pressure is negative. This stability is, again, due to tethering of the lung parenchyma, in which the veins are embedded.

If a linear relationship between blood pressure and vessel diameter is assumed for the data shown in Fig. 4.9:2, then the slope of the regression line is called the compliance constant. This constant has been determined for all orders of pulmonary veins, and is listed in Table 6.11:3 on p. 339, for several specified sets of values of p_A and p_{PL}. When the pleural pressure changes, the degree of lung inflation changes, and the compliance constant will change. Figure 6.4:2 shows the variation of the compliance constant with changing pleural pressure when p_A is zero (atmospheric).

For vessels smaller than 100 μm in diameter, reading diameter from x-ray film becomes increasingly difficult. Hence we used the silicone elastomer method mentioned earlier. In this method it is not possible to follow a single vessel and observe its change of diameter with changing blood pressure. The best one can do is to identify the hierarchy of the vascular tree, measure the mean diameter of the vessels of each order, and examine the change of the mean diameter with changing pressure difference $p - p_A$. Our results are presented in Table 4.9:1 on p. 212. The estimated compliance constants of these small vessels are also listed in Table 6.11:3.

One special vessel in each histological photograph is easily identified: namely, the smallest noncapillary blood vessel; either the smallest arteriole or the smallest venule. To these smallest vessels, the *extreme-value* statistics (see Fung (1981), p. 108) can be applied. An accurate statement of the expected diameter of the smallest noncapillary vessel in a given size of the sample can be made. Figure 6.4:3 shows an example of the data plotted on

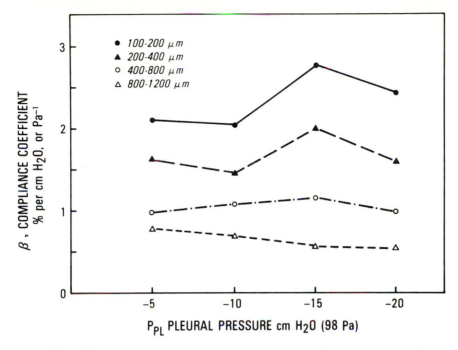

Figure 6.4:2 Variation of the compliance constant of the pulmonary veins of the cat with the transpulmonary pressure, $p_A - p_{PL}$. In the experiment, the alveolar gas pressure p_A was zero. Hence the compliance coefficient β is plotted against the pleural pressure for four groups of vessels in the diameter ranges 100–200, 200–400, 400–800, 800–1200 μm. From Yen and Foppiano (1981). Reproduced by permission.

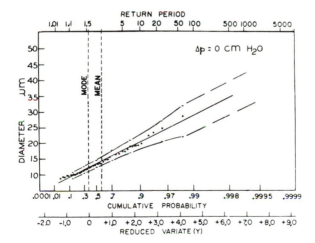

Figure 6.4:3 Extreme-value distribution of the smallest noncapillary pulmonary blood vessels. Solid circles are the experimentally observed blood vessel diameters. The regression line is a visual best fit. From Sobin et al. (1978). Reproduced by permission.

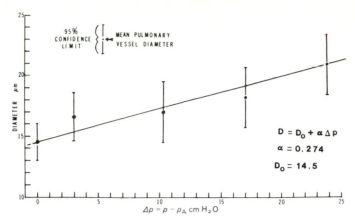

Figure 6.4:4 Plot of the mean diameter and 95% confidence level of the smallest vessels obtained by extreme-value statistics for the five transmural pressures $p - p_A = 0, 3,$ 10.25, 17, and 23.75. p, p_A are blood and airway pressures, respectively. From Sobin et al. (1978). Reproduced by permission.

the Gumbel extreme-value probability distribution paper. Figure 6.4:4 shows the variation of the mean diameter of the smallest noncapillary blood vessel in each of 50 histological slides with the transmural pressure $p - p_A$. From this curve we obtain a compliance constant of these vessels of the cat to be 0.274 μm per cm H_2O, or 1.61% per cm H_2O, quite consistent with the values listed in Table 6.11:3 obtained by an entirely different method.

For other animals only scattered data are available. See the list of references in Yen et al. (1980).

6.5 Elasticity of the Pulmonary Alveolar Sheet

As is common to most topics in science, the question of elasticity can be formulated in many different forms, varying in degree of generality and difficulty. For the blood flow problem, the question of elasticity we are concerned with is this: When the pressure in the blood vessel is changed, how much does the blood volume change? In the sheet-flow model of the pulmonary alveoli, the problem is translated to the following: when the pressures of the blood and of the alveolar air change, (1) how does the thickness of the sheet change, and (2) how does the plane area of the sheet change? Note that the blood volume in an alveolar sheet is equal to

$$\text{thickness} \times \text{area} \times \text{VSTR},$$

where the VSTR is the vascular-space–tissue ratio discussed before. The morphometric data presented in Sec. 6.3 show that the VSTR remains constant when blood pressure changes. Hence the elasticity problem can be limited to the consideration of thickness and area.

It turns out that these questions have both a simple answer and a com-

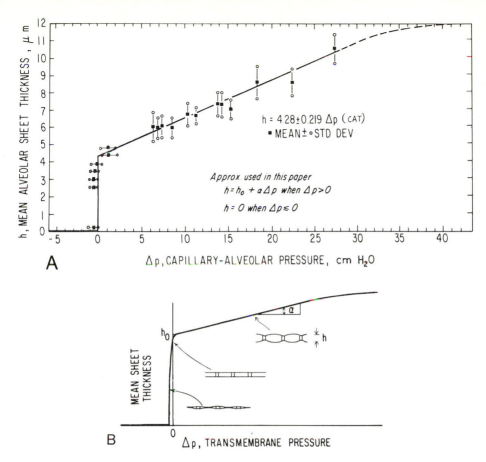

Figure 6.5:1 A. Sheet thickness-pressure relationship of the cat. Equations (1a)–(1d) approximate this curve by a discontinuous cu.. ve that is composed of four line segments: a horizontal line $h = 0$ for Δp negative, which jumps to $h = h_0$ at Δp slightly greater than 0, then continues as a straight line for positive Δp until some upper limit is reached, beyond which it bends down and tends to a constant thickness. B, The elastic deformation of the alveolar sheet is sketched for three conditions: $\Delta p < 0$, $\Delta p = 0$, and $\Delta p > 0$. The relaxed thickness h_0 of the sheet is equal to the relaxed length of the posts. Under a positive internal (transmural) pressure, the thickness of the sheet increases; the posts are lengthened; the membranes deflect from the planes connecting the ends of the posts; and the mean thickness becomes h. From Fung and Sobin (1972a, b). Reproduced by permission of the American Heart Association, Inc.

plicated answer. In simple terms, the thickness h varies with the pressure difference Δp (equal to the static pressure of blood minus the pressure of the alveolar air) as follows, (Fig. 6.5:1):

$h = 0$ if Δp is negative, and smaller than $-\varepsilon$, where ε is a small number about 1 cm H_2O. (1a)

TABLE 6.5:1 The Compliance Constant, α, and the Thickness at Zero Transmural Pressure, h_0, of the Pulmonary Alveolar Vascular Sheet at Specified Values of Transpulmonary Pressure, $p_A - p_{PL}$ (p_A = alveolar gas pressure, p_{PL} = pleural pressure)

Animal	h_0 (μm)	α (μm/cm H_2O)	Reference	$p_A - p_{PL}$ (cm H_2O)
Cat	4.28	0.219	Fig. 6.5:1	10
Dog	2.5	0.122	Fung, Sobin (1972)*	10
	2.5	0.079	Fung, Sobin (1972)*	25
Man	3.5	0.127	Sobin et al. (1979)	10

* Based on the data of Glazier et al. (1969) and Permutt et al. (1969).

$h = h_0 + \alpha \Delta p$, if Δp is positive and smaller than certain limiting value.

$$(1b)$$

h tends to a limiting value h_∞ if Δp increases beyond the limiting value.

$$(1c)$$

In the small range $-\varepsilon < \Delta p < 0$, h increases from 0 to h_0. A rough approximation is $h = h_0 + (h_0/\varepsilon)\Delta p$.

$$(1d)$$

Here α, h_0, h_∞, and ε are constants independent of Δp. The parameter h_0 is the sheet thickness at zero pressure difference when the pressure decreases from positive values. The parameter α is called the *compliance coefficient* of the pulmonary capillary bed. The thickness h is understood to be the mean value averaged over an area that is large compared with the posts, but small relative to the alveoli. The known values of h_0 and α are given in Table 6.5:1.

Also, in simple terms, the answer to the second question is that if A_0 represents the area of certain region of an alveolar septa when the static pressure of the blood is some physiologic value p_0, then the area of the same region A when blood pressure is changed to p is

$$A \doteq A_0. \qquad (2)$$

In other words, the area is unaffected by the blood pressure.

The answers to our questions become more complex when we try to relate the constants h_0, α, h_∞, and A_0 to the airway pressure, the intrapleural pressure, the surfactants on the alveolar septa, the geometric parameters of the septa, the structure of the entire lung and the shape of the thoracic cage and the diaphragm, and whether a pathologic condition such as edema or emphysema exists. In order to unravel these relationships, we may take a two-pronged approach: we may study the problem theoretically and derive these relationships from the principles of mechanics, or we may lay out an extensive program of experiments in order to deduce empirical correlations among various parameters. It is easy to see that the required experimental program would be very large. For pragmatism, one should take a combined approach: to deduce as much as possible from theoretical considerations, and to test as often as possible by experiments.

A theoretical analysis of the sheet elastic compliance α as a function of geometric parameters is presented by Fung and Sobin (1972a). Of major concern is the dependence of the compliance coefficient α on the tension T, (dyn/cm^{-1}), in the alveolar septa. T increases when lung volume increases. It can be shown that the larger the tension, the smaller is the compliance coefficient. Since T is the sum of the surface tension and elastic tension, an increase of surface tension would cause an increase in T and a decrease in the compliance of the alveolar sheet, thus causing a decrease in blood flow. An expansion of the lung also increases T, and, if other things remain equal, would also decrease blood flow in the alveolar sheet.

6.6 Apparent Viscosity of Blood in Pulmonary Capillaries

We need to know the flow behavior of blood before we can formulate the pulmonary blood flow problem mathematically. The general problem of blood viscosity has been discussed in *Biomechanics* (Fung, 1981). To understand the flow of blood in pulmonary capillary sheet we must study the interaction of red blood cells with the capillary sheet. As Ernest Sechler used to say: "When you design an airplane, you must think like an airplane", we may wish to think of blood flow by picturing ourselves as a red blood cell. As a red cell moving through the lung, what do we see? At first we see a big tunnel. Then the tunnel divides and divides again and again, and becomes smaller. At the arteriolar level the tunnel diameter is only two or three times our own diameter. Then you enter the capillary sheet and the scenery suddenly changes. You seem to have entered an underground parking garage. You are a car. The celling is low and there is bumper-to-bumper traffic. You have to swing right and left in order to avoid the posts.

Figure 6.6:1 shows my interpretation of a scene in a pulmonary alveolar sheet as seen by a red cell. Many red cells float in this space. One on the right is caught on a post. The picture would have been more faithful if the cells had been drawn bigger. To clarify the view, I have drawn them too small and too sparsely. In reality the cells should fill the height almost entirely.

To analyse the motion of the red cells in such an environment, we may begin with a dimensional analysis (see *Biomechanics*, (Fung, 1981), p. 143). For our problem the variables of interest are: the pressure p, the pressure gradient ∇p, the coefficient of viscosity of the plasma μ_0, the mean velocity of flow U, the angular frequency of oscillation ω, the sheet thickness, h, the width of the sheet w, the diameter of the posts ε, the distance between the posts a, the angle between the mean flow and a reference line defining the postal pattern shown in Fig. 6.3:3, θ, the hematocrit H, the diameter of the red cell D_c, and the characteristic elastic modulus of the red cell membrane E_c. By simple trial we see that the following parameters are dimensionless:

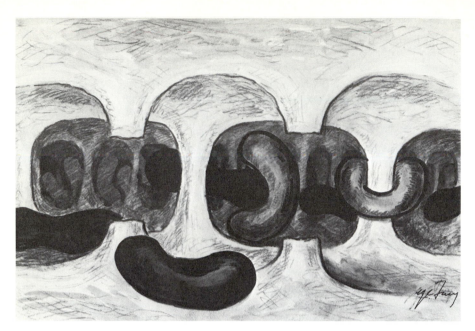

Figure 6.6:1 Conceptual drawing of pulmonary alveolar blood flow. The red cells move in the pulmonary alveolar vascular space that has some resemblance to an underground parking garage.

$$\frac{h^2}{\mu_0 U}\nabla p, \qquad \frac{Uh\rho}{\mu_0} = N_R \text{ (Reynolds number)},$$

$$\frac{D_c}{h}, \qquad \frac{\mu_0 U}{E_c h} \equiv \text{cell membrane strain parameter,}$$

$$\frac{h}{2}\sqrt{\frac{\omega\rho}{\mu_0}} \equiv \text{Womersley number,}$$

$$H, \frac{w}{h}, \frac{h}{\varepsilon}, \frac{\varepsilon}{a}, \theta, \text{VSTR (see Eq. (2) of Sec. 6.3).}$$

Hence, according to the principle of dimensional analysis, any relationship between the variables p, U, ... must be a relationship between these dimensionless parameters. In particular, the parameter we are most interested in, that connecting the pressure gradient and the flow velocity, may be written as

$$\frac{h^2}{\mu_0 U}\nabla p = F\left(\frac{D_c}{h}, \frac{\mu_0 U}{E_c h}, N_R, \frac{h}{2}\sqrt{\frac{\omega\rho}{\mu_0}}, H, \frac{w}{h}, \frac{h}{\varepsilon}, \frac{\varepsilon}{a}, \theta, \text{VSTR}\right), \qquad (1)$$

where F is a certain function that must be determined either theoretically or experimentally.

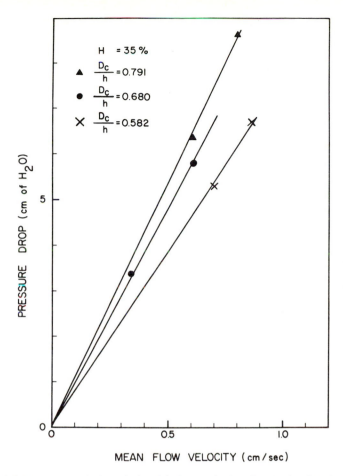

Figure 6.6:2 Pressure–velocity relationship for particulate flow in simulated pulmonary alveolar capillary blood vessels at a hematocrit (H) of 35%. D_c is the diameter of the red blood cell. h is the thickness of the vascular space of the interalveolar sheet. From Yen and Fung (1973). Reprinted by permission.

In capillary blood flow, the Reynolds number and Womersley number are much smaller than 1, and their effects may be neglected. The cell membrane strain parameter is the ratio of the typical shear stress in the fluid, $\mu_0 U/h$, to the elasticity modulus of the cell membrane, E_c. Its effect and the effect of D_c/h have been discussed in *Biomechanics* (Fung, 1981, pp. 153, 157, 158). In general, in narrow circular cylindrical tubes the effects of these parameters make the pressure–flow relationship nonlinear. In the pulmonary alveolar sheet, however, the red cells are far less constrained than they are in the tube, and a model experiment by Yen and Fung (1973) shows that the pressure–flow relationship is linear when D_c/h is smaller than 0.80. See Fig. 6.6:2. This is fortunate. We can then write Eq. (1) as

$$\nabla p = -\frac{\mu_0 U}{h^2} F\left(\frac{D_c}{h}, \frac{\mu_0 U}{E_c h}, H, \frac{w}{h}, \frac{h}{\varepsilon}, \frac{\varepsilon}{a}, \theta, \text{VSTR}\right). \tag{2}$$

To investigate the function, F, Lee and Fung (1968), Lee (1969), Fung (1969), and Yen and Fung (1973) made theoretical and experimental studies on particulate flow in alveolar sheet. They isolate the effects of D_c/h, $\mu_0 U/E_c h$, H, w/h, and the rest of the parameters separately, and write

$$\nabla p = -\frac{\mu_0 U}{h^2} F'\left(\frac{D_c}{h}, \frac{\mu_0 U}{E_c h}, H\right) k\left(\frac{w}{h}\right) f\left(\frac{h}{\varepsilon}, \frac{\varepsilon}{a}, \theta, \text{VSTR}\right). \tag{3}$$

This is further abbreviated to

$$\nabla p = -\frac{U}{h^2} \mu k f, \tag{4}$$

where μ stands for the apparent viscosity:

$$\mu = \mu_0 F'\left(\frac{D_c}{h}, \frac{\mu_0 U}{E_c h}, H\right), \tag{5}$$

and k and f are functions of the parameters indicated in Eq. (3). The ratio μ/μ_0 is called the "relative" viscosity. Yen and Fung (1973) write

$$\mu = \mu_0(1 + aH + bH^2), \tag{6}$$

where H is the hermatocrit, a, b are functions of the ratio of the cell diameter D_c and sheet thickness h. μ_0 is the viscosity of plasma. Their experimental results are presented in Fig. 5.2:3, p. 145 of *Biomechanics* (Fung, 1981), the effect of the parameter $\mu_0 U/E_c h$ has not been investigated in detail so far.

The function k is well known, (see, for example, Purday, 1949). When $h/w < 0.2$, it is given by the equation

$$k = 12 \Big/ \left(1 - 0.63\frac{h}{w}\right). \tag{7}$$

Hence for all practical purposes k can be replaced by 12. The function f is called the *geometric friction factor*. Lee (1969) made a theoretical calculation of the function f. Yen and Fung (1973) confirmed Lee's results. f as a function of h/ε is given in Fig. 6.6:3, which is obtained with the parameters ε/a, θ, and VSTR pertinent to the cat's lung, (Table 6.3:1). In the case of cat's lung, θ has little effect, and f is independent of the orientation of the flow.

These experimental results were obtained in steady state flow. Their applicability to pulmonary microcirculation is based on the smallness of the Womersley number and Reynolds number (in the order of 10^{-2}) in alveolar sheet. Experimental verification that at low Reynolds number no flutter will occur when the local blood pressure is smaller than the alveolar gas pressure has been presented by Fung and Sobin (1972b).

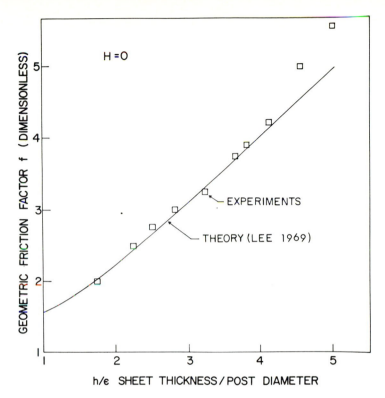

Figure 6.6:3 The geometric friction factor f as a function of the alveolar sheet structure. Theoretically and experimentally determined values of f are compared for an alveolar sheet for which the values of ε/a, θ, and VSTR are those of the cat's and human lung, whereas the sheet thickness/post diameter ratio is varied. From Yen and Fung (1973). Reprinted by permission.

6.7 Formulation of the Analytical Problems

"Local Mean Flow" and "Local Mean Disturbances"

To analyze the blood flow in an alveolar sheet, we introduce first the concept of local mean velocity of flow. The detailed flow field is, of course, very complicated when the disturbances of individual posts, red cells, membrane deflections, and other phenomena are considered. Therefore mathematically it is expedient to separate the flow field into two parts: a local mean flow and local disturbances. It is expected that the local mean flow field will be relatively smooth and can be determined from the boundary conditions. The present chapter is concerned with the local mean flow. When the mean flow field is known, the local disturbances can be computed separately in a much simplified manner.

To be precise, we now define the local mean flow and the perturbations. Let us first define a Cartesian frame of reference x, y, z. We take the origin at a point on the midplane of the sheet, x, y axes in the sheet, and z axis perpendicular to the sheet. See Fig. 6.3:4, p. 299. At a point x, y, z, the velocity vector has three components $u(x, y, z)$, $v(x, y, z)$, $w(x, y, z)$ in the directions of the coordinate axes. We break u, v, w into two parts, and write

$$u(x,y,z) = U(x,y) + u'(x,y,z),$$

$$v(x,y,z) = V(x,y) + v'(x,y,z), \qquad (1)$$

$$w(x,y,z) = W(x,y) + w'(x,y,z),$$

where $U(x,y)$, $V(x,y)$, $W(x,y)$ are functions of x, y alone. We call $U(x,y)$, $V(x,y)$ the local mean velocity if they represent the average value of $u(x,y,z)$, $v(x,y,z)$ over a small volume around $(x,y,0)$; i.e., if

$$U(x,y) = \frac{1}{Ah} \iint_{A(x,y)} dx'\, dy' \int_{-h/2}^{h/2} u(x',y',z)dz$$

$$V(x,y) = \frac{1}{Ah} \iint_{A(x,y)} dx'\, dy \int_{-h/2}^{h/2} v(x',y',z)dz. \qquad (2)$$

The mean velocity $W(x,y)$, defined by a similar equation, vanishes when the area A is chosen large enough. In these equations, h is the thickness of the sheet, $A(x, y)$ is a domain of integration containing the point (x, y), and A is the area of $A(x, y)$ as illustrated in Fig. 6.3:4. The points (x', y') lie in the area A. The domain A is chosen to be large enough that it contains a number of posts and red cells so that the velocities U and V represent the smoothed out velocity field, and yet small enough that the variation of U, V over the entire alveolar sheet still reflects the significant features of the flow field. In practical calculations an area containing, say, 10 posts would be satisfactory for such a local averaging.

The velocity components $u'(x, y, z)$, $v'(x, y, z)$, $w'(x, y, z)$ in Eq. (1) are called the local perturbations. According to Eqs. (2) the mean values of the local perturbations $u'(x, y, z)$, $v'(x, y, z)$, and $w'(x, y, z)$ are zero.

The local mean pressure and the mean sheet thickness are defined in a similar manner.

Basic Equations

In the development of our theory, the first basic relation we seek is that relating the local mean pressure $p(x, y)$ to the velocities $U(x, y)$, $V(x, y)$. This can be derived from the basic equations of hydrodynamics, or alternatively

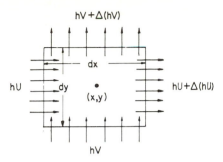

Figure 6.7:1 A rectangular element of the sheet showing the balance of the flow. From Fung and Sobin (1969). Reprinted by permission.

by model testing with the help of dimensional analysis. As it is shown in Sec. 6.6, a dimension analysis leads to Eq. (4) of Sec. 6.6, or

$$\frac{\partial p}{\partial x} = -\frac{\mu U}{h^2} k f_x \left(\frac{h}{\varepsilon}, \frac{\varepsilon}{a}, \theta, \text{VSTR} \right),$$

$$\frac{\partial p}{\partial y} = -\frac{\mu V}{h^2} k f_y \left(\frac{h}{\varepsilon}, \frac{\varepsilon}{a}, \theta, \text{VSTR} \right). \tag{3}$$

In this equation, μ is the apparent viscosity of blood, h is the sheet thickness and the numerical factors k, f_x, f_y are functions of the sheet geometry as discussed in Sec. 6.6. k is equal to 12 in practical cases, and f lies in the range 2–3.

The second basic relation we need is one that describes the conservation of mass. Consider a small rectangular element of the alveolar sheet (see Fig. 6.7:1). Blood enters the left-hand side and leaves the right-hand side. In a time interval dt, the mass entering the left-hand side is equal to the product of the density, velocity, area, and dt. The velocity is U and the area is hdy; h being the thickness of the sheet and dy the length of the edge. The density is ρ. Hence

$$\text{mass inflow at left} = \rho h U \, dy \, dt. \tag{4}$$

On the right-hand side, the mass outflow in the same time interval is

$$\left[\rho h U + \frac{\partial(\rho h U)}{\partial x} dx \right] dy \, dt. \tag{5}$$

Similarly, the mass inflow at the bottom edge is $\rho h V \, dx \, dt$, and the outflow at the top is

$$\left[\rho h V + \frac{\partial(\rho h V)}{\partial y} dy \right] dx \, dt.$$

Summing up all the inflow and outflow, we have

$$\text{net mass outflow} = \left[\frac{\partial(\rho h U)}{\partial x} + \frac{\partial(\rho h V)}{\partial y}\right] dx\, dy\, dt. \tag{6}$$

By the law of conservation of mass, this net mass outflow must be equal to the net decrease of the mass of the element. For a *steady flow* in a sheet with impermeable walls there can be no change in the mass of the element; hence we must have

$$\frac{\partial(\rho h U)}{\partial x} + \frac{\partial(\rho h V)}{\partial y} = 0. \tag{7}$$

If the sheet thickness h is variable, then the equation of continuity, Eq. (7), combined with the equation of motion of the fluid, Eq. (3), yields the following equation:

$$\frac{\partial}{\partial x}\left(\frac{h^3}{kf_x}\frac{\partial p}{\partial x}\right) + \frac{\partial}{\partial y}\left(\frac{h^3}{kf_y}\frac{\partial p}{\partial y}\right) = 0. \tag{8}$$

Now p is related to h by the constitutive Eq. (6.5:1a–d). Using Eq. (6.5:1b or d), we obtain

$$\frac{\partial}{\partial x}\left(\frac{h^3}{kf_x}\frac{\partial h}{\partial x}\right) + \frac{\partial}{\partial y}\left(\frac{h^3}{kf_y}\frac{\partial h}{\partial y}\right) = 0. \tag{9}$$

If we ignore the spatial variation of k and f, and assume $f_x = f_y$ for practical purposes we obtain

$$\frac{\partial}{\partial x}\left(h^3\frac{\partial h}{\partial x}\right) + \frac{\partial}{\partial y}\left(h^3\frac{\partial h}{\partial y}\right) = 0, \tag{10}$$

or

$$\left(\frac{\partial^2}{\partial x^2} + \frac{\partial^2}{\partial y^2}\right)h^4 = 0. \tag{11}$$

Thus the fourth power of h is governed by a Laplace equation. Expressed in terms of pressure, we have, on defining

$$\Phi = h^4 = [h_0 + \alpha(p - p_A)]^4, \tag{12}$$

the result

$$\left(\frac{\partial^2}{\partial x^2} + \frac{\partial^2}{\partial y^2}\right)\Phi = 0. \tag{13}$$

This completes the mathematical formulation for the steady-state case of sheets with impermeable wall.

If p is smaller than the alveolar gas pressure p_A, then $h = 0$ and there will be no flow. If p is greater than the upper limiting value, then the linear relation Eq. (6.5:1b) ceases to hold, and Eqs. (11) and (13) are no longer valid. When p becomes sufficiently large, h tends to a constant: Then Eq. (8) can be used again with the factor h^3 eliminated. Thus in this limiting case the differential equation is again linear, and the pressure distribution satisfies the Laplace equation.

Generalization to Nonstationary Case and Permeable Vessel

For a nonstationary flow, and in the case in which fluid movement in or out of the endothelium of the capillary blood vessel takes place, the equation of continuity Eq. (7) must be modified. This modification can be obtained by considering the balance of inflow and outflow in a control volume that consists of the sides $x = \text{const.}, x = \text{const.} + dx, y = \text{const.}, y = \text{const.} + dy$, and the membranes $z = \pm h/2$, and the rate of change of the control volume:

$$\text{Rate of change of volume} = \left[\frac{\partial(\rho h U)}{\partial x} + \frac{\partial(\rho h V)}{\partial y}\right] dx\, dy\, dt. \qquad (14)$$

The control volume is changed by (a) the transient change in thickness h, and (b) the filtration across the blood–tissue barrier. The rate of increase of thickness is $\partial h/\partial t$, which induces, in a time interval dt, an increase of control volume equal to $(\partial h/\partial t)dt\, dx\, dy$. The mass transfer across the blood–tissue barrier may be assumed to obey Starling's hypothesis* $\dot{m} = K_p(\Delta p - \sigma \Delta \pi)$, where $\dot{m}$ is the rate of mass transfer per unit time per unit area, K_p is the filtration coefficient, Δp is the difference in hydrostatic pressure on the sides of the barrier, $\Delta \pi$ is the corresponding difference in osmotic pressure, and σ is the reflection coefficient. Since our attention is focused on the flow of blood, we may write

$$\dot{m} = K_p(p - p^*). \qquad (15)$$

where p refers to the local mean pressure in the blood, and

$$p^* = \sigma \Delta \pi + \text{pressure in tissue space.} \qquad (16)$$

Summing up both contributions we obtain, from Eq. (14),

$$\left[\frac{\partial(\rho h U)}{\partial x}\right] + \left[\frac{\partial(\rho h V)}{\partial y}\right] = -\rho\left(\frac{\partial h}{\partial t}\right) - 2K_p(p - p^*). \qquad (17)$$

The factor 2 in the last term is added because the capillary wall area is about twice the area of the sheet. Eliminating U, V from Eqs. (17) and (3), we obtain

$$\frac{\rho}{\mu}\left[\frac{\partial}{\partial x}\left(\frac{h^3}{kf_x}\frac{\partial p}{\partial x}\right) + \frac{\partial}{\partial y}\left(\frac{h^3}{kf_y}\frac{\partial p}{\partial y}\right)\right] = \rho\left(\frac{\partial h}{\partial t}\right) + 2K_p(p - p^*). \qquad (18)$$

---

* This is a linear phenomenologic law for mass transport across a membrane. See chap. 2, sec. 2.5, of the companion volume *Biodynamics: Flow, Motion, and Stress* (Fung, 1984).

To complete the analysis we again use the equation that describes the elasticity of the alveolar sheet in the physiologic range when $p - p_{alv}$ is positive:

$$h = h_0 + \alpha(p - p_{alv}). \tag{6.5:1b}$$

Then we obtain the following basic equation:

$$\frac{\partial}{\partial x}\left(\frac{h^3}{kf_x}\frac{\partial h}{\partial x}\right) + \frac{\partial}{\partial y}\left(\frac{h^3}{kf_y}\frac{\partial h}{\partial y}\right) = \mu\alpha\left[\frac{\partial h}{\partial t} + \frac{2}{\rho}K_p\left(\frac{h - h_0}{\alpha} - p^* + p_{alv}\right)\right]. \tag{19}$$

This is a nonlinear "diffusion" equation, basically different from the usual "wave" equation that describes pulsatile flow in large arteries. The impedance characteristics of the capillaries are therefore different from those of the arteries.

In general, we may use the approximation $f_x = f_y = f$. If the variation of h is not too large, we may regard k and f as constant and simplify Eq. (19) to

$$\left(\frac{\partial^2}{\partial x^2} + \frac{\partial^2}{\partial y^2}\right)h^4 = 4\mu kf\alpha\left[\frac{\partial h}{\partial t} + \frac{2K_p}{\rho\alpha}(h - h^*)\right], \tag{20}$$

where

$$h^* = h_0 + \alpha(p^* - p_{alv}). \tag{21}$$

Solutions of these equations are considered in the next sections.

6.8 An Elementary Analog of the Theory

The sheet-flow equation contains a great deal of information that can be revealed through solutions with various boundary conditions. This equation is nonlinear. But the nonlinearity is of a special kind, through the fourth power of h which is operated on by the Laplace operator.

The nature of the solution can be brought out easily if we use a one-dimensional analog. Consider two uniform, parallel, horizontal, elastic strings as shown in Fig. 6.8:1. At finite intervals these strings are tied by vertical cross members. If we pull on the horizontal strings with a tension T, the strings are stretched uniformly, and the ratio of the lengths of segments bc and ac remains a constant. This ratio is an analog of VSTR: the segments ab and cd are analogs of the posts, and bc and de are the analog of the alveolar–capillary membrane.

On the other hand, if the post segments were replaced by springs of different compliance than the strings, then the VSTR (bc/ac) would change with the tension T(Fig. 6.8:1B). The constancy of VSTR observed in the pulmonary alveolar sheets of the cat suggests that the elasticity of the postal region (segments ab, cd, etc.) is represented by the analog shown in Fig. 6.8:1A.

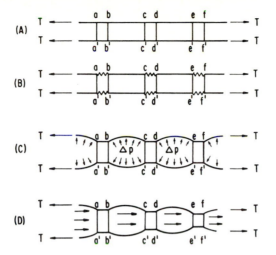

Figure 6.8:1 Simplified one-dimensional analog of the alveolar sheet. A, stretching of the membrane. B, stretching of the post. C, deflection under internal pressure. D, deflection due to variable internal pressure when blood flows in the channel. From Fung and Sobin (1977). Reprinted by permission.

Let the strings be loaded by an internal vertical loading of Δp per unit length, as shown in Fig. 6.8:1C. The equilibrium of the string requires that

$$T \times \text{curvature of string} = \Delta p.$$

If the tension remains constant and the deflection is small, then the vertical deflection of the string is proportional to Δp.

The change of the average distance between the strings (analog of the sheet thickness) is given by the sum of the distention of the posts aa', bb', etc. and the average deflection of the strings.

Now consider flow in a channel of unit width represented by Fig. 6.8:1 D (replace the strings by channel walls). Let the average speed of flow be U, the volume flow rate per unit width be Q, the local thickness be h, and the pressure be p. Then

$$U = -\frac{h^2}{12\mu}\frac{dp}{dx} \tag{1}$$

$$Q = hU. \tag{2}$$

In the range of p in which $h = h_0 + \alpha p$, we have

$$\frac{dh}{dx} = \alpha\frac{dp}{dx}. \tag{3}$$

Hence,

$$Q = -\frac{h^3}{12\mu\alpha}\frac{dh}{dx} = -\frac{1}{48\mu\alpha}\frac{dh^4}{dx}. \tag{4}$$

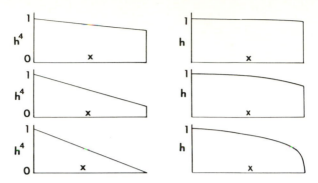

Figure 6.8:2 Plot of Eqs. (8) and (9) showing the variation of h^4 and h with x. With an appropriate choice of units, we assume that the thickness h_a is 1. h_v^4 at $x = L$ is assumed to be 0.75, 0.25, and 0 for the three cases shown in the figure. The corresponding values of h_v are 0.931, 0.707, and 0, respectively.

For a steady flow, Q is a constant. Differentiating Eq. (4) with respect to x, we obtain, because $dQ/dx = 0$, the differential equation

$$\frac{d^2 h^4}{dx^2} = 0, \tag{5}$$

which is a special case of the sheet-flow equation, Eq. 6.7:11. This differential equation is easily integrated. The general solution is

$$h^4 = c_1 x + c_2, \tag{6}$$

where c_1, c_2 are arbitrary constants. To determine c_1, c_2, we notice the boundary conditions

(a) at the "arteriole," $x = 0$, the thickness of the "sheet" is h_a.
(b) at the "venule," $x = L$, the thickness of the "sheet" is h_v.

Hence,

$$h_a^4 = c_2, \qquad h_v^4 = c_1 L + h_a^4. \tag{7}$$

Solving for c_1, c_2 and substituting into Eq. (6), we obtain

$$h^4 = h_a^4 - (h_a^4 - h_v^4)x/L, \tag{8}$$

or

$$h = [h_a^4 - (h_a^4 - h_v^4)x/L]^{1/4}. \tag{9}$$

This is the full solution. For various combinations of h_a and h_v the distribution of the thickness h is shown in Fig. 6.8:2. It is seen that the exponent $\frac{1}{4}$ makes h rather flat near the arteriole, and constricts rather rapidly toward the venule if h_v is small.

We can obtain the flow Q from Eq. (4). If the channel length is L, then the mean flow in the whole channel is

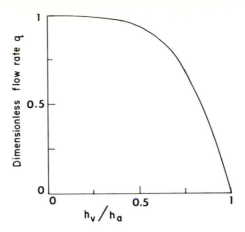

Figure 6.8:3 The variation of the volume flow rate with the thickness ratio h_v/h_a. q is dimensionless, defined by Eq. (12). h_v and h_a are sheet thickness at the venule and arteriole, respectively.

$$\frac{1}{L}\int_0^L Q\,dx = \frac{1}{48\mu\alpha L}[h^4(0) - h^4(L)]. \tag{10}$$

For a one-dimensional channel flow of an incompressible fluid, the conservation of mass requires Q to be constant. Hence the left-hand side of Eq. (10) is exactly Q. In this case, we can also integrate Eq. (4) to obtain

$$h^4 = -48\mu\alpha Qx + \text{constant}.$$

But $h = h_a$ when $x = 0$. Hence the constant equations h_a^4, and we have the channel thickness distribution:

$$h(x) = (h_a^4 - 48\mu\alpha Qx)^{1/4}$$

which is, of course, equivalent to Eq. (9). When $x = L$, the thickness h becomes h_v, and we obtain the exact result

$$Q = \frac{h_a^4 - h_v^4}{48\mu\alpha L}. \tag{11}$$

The last equation is a remarkable result. It shows that the flow depends on the difference of the fourth power of the sheet thickness at the arteriole from the fourth power of the sheet thickness at the venule. Thus if h_v is considerably smaller than h_a, its influence on the volume flow rate would be small. This is exhibited in Fig. 6.8:3, in which we have plotted the dimensionless volume flow rate

$$q = \frac{48\mu\alpha L}{h_a^4}\dot{Q} \tag{12}$$

against the ratio h_v/h_a. From Eqs. (11) and (12) we have, obviously,

$$q = 1 - \left(\frac{h_v}{h_a}\right)^4. \tag{13}$$

It is seen clearly that q is significantly reduced by h_v only if h_v approaches h_a. If h_v is less than one-half of h_a, q differs from 1 by less than 6%; hence the flow is controlled essentially by h_a, the sheet thickness at the arteriole.

6.9 General Features of the Sheet Flow

Rapid Variation of Sheet Thickness at the Venule, and Nearly Uniform Hydrostatic Pressure near the Arteriole

In the more general case, the nature of the solution may be illustrated by an idealized example as shown in Fig. 6.9:1. In the upper figure, we have sketched a hypothetical rigid alveolar sheet ($h_0 \neq 0$, $\alpha = 0$), which is opened to an arteriole and a venule at regularly spaced intervals. The pattern is periodic and three segments are shown in the figure. At the left are shown a

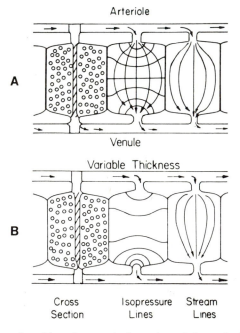

Figure 6.9:1 A type of problem that can be investigated theoretically. With given sheet dimensions and boundary conditions, the variation of the average sheet thickness, velocity distribution, and pressure distribution can be computed. Figure shows streamlines and pressure contours. From Fung and Sobin (1969). Reprinted by permission.

plan view and a vertical cross section. The thickness of the sheet is assumed to be constant. At the right are shown the streamlines, i.e., the lines tangential to the velocity vectors. In the center are shown the lines of constant blood pressure. These contours of equipressure lines are drawn at intervals of constant pressure drop. The pressure at the horizontal line in the middle is halfway between the arteriole pressure and venule pressure. Other equipressure lines are orthogonal to the streamlines. The pressure gradient is inversely proportional to the distance between the equipressure lines. The velocity of flow is inversely proportional to the spacing between streamlines. These contours thus show the velocity and pressure distribution in the alveolar walls.

In the lower panel of Fig. 6.9:1 we consider a different situation. We relax the assumption that the alveolar wall is rigid, and assume instead that the sheet thickness varies linearly with the difference between the blood pressure and the air pressure in the alveolar space. In this case the pressure and velocity distributions are significantly modified. Fig. 6.9:1(b) is drawn for the case in which the arteriole pressure is greater than the airway pressure, but the venule pressure is equal to the airway pressure. In the left panel, the sheet thickness is seen to contract rapidly in the neighborhood of the venule. In the middle panel, the equipressure contours are seen to crowd toward the venule. The pressure in the sheet is much more uniform than that in Fig. 6.9:1(a) except in the neighborhood of the venule, where rapid pressure drop occurs. The streamlines sketched in the figure on the right show a similar increase in the velocity near the drain into the venule.

The detailed information on velocity and pressure distribution has important bearings on pulmonary physiology. The velocity distribution is relevant to the blood transit time in alveoli and oxygenation of the red cells. The pressure distribution is important to the question of fluid transport across the alveolar wall and hence is relevant to the question of edema and homeostasis. The thickness distribution is directly related to the flow resistance.

The mathematical details of the solution are given below.

Computation of Flow Field

Let us consider first the problem shown in Fig. 6.9:1(a), *the flow in a sheet of constant thickness.* This is an artificial problem, but its solution provides a stepping stone to the real problem of flow in an elastic sheet governed by Eq. (6.7:11).

By the periodicity of spatial geometry, it is sufficient to consider a single rectangular sheet. Let us assume that the sheet is of uniform thickness. The boundary conditions are that the borders of the sheet are streamlines except at the openings to the arteriole and venule, where pressures are specified. To satisfy these boundary conditions, it is convenient to introduce a *stream function* $\psi(x, y)$ so that

$$hU = \frac{\partial \psi}{\partial y}, \qquad hV = -\frac{\partial \psi}{\partial x}, \tag{1}$$

which satisfy the equation of continuity, Eq. (6.7:7), identically. The equation of motion is satisfied if pressure is computed from velocity through Eq. (6.7:3). On the other hand, according to Eq. (6.7:3) the pressure p may be regarded as a *velocity potential*. Furthermore, for $h = $ constant and $f_x = f_y$, Eq. (8) of Sec. 6.7 becomes a harmonic equation

$$\frac{\partial^2 p}{\partial x^2} + \frac{\partial^2 p}{\partial y^2} = 0. \tag{2}$$

The potential lines $p = $ constant and the streamlines $\psi = $ constant are mutually orthogonal. Since p and ψ are conjugate to each other, ψ is governed by a harmonic equation too. The boundary condition on a boundary where a constant pressure is specified is, therefore,

$$p = \text{constant}, \quad \text{or} \quad \frac{\partial p}{\partial s} = 0, \quad \text{or} \quad \frac{\partial \psi}{\partial n} = 0, \tag{3}$$

where s and n denote tangential and normal directions, respectively. On a boundary which coincides with a streamline, the normal velocity vanishes; then the boundary condition is

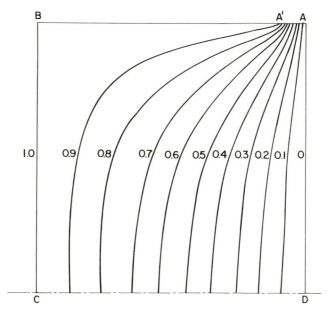

Figure 6.9:2 Streamlines of flow corresponding to the case (a) in Fig. 6.9:1. The fluid enters the sheet at AA′. No fluid penetrates the borders of A′B, BC, and the center line AD. The boundary CD is a line of symmetry on which the pressure is constant. Numerals are the values of the stream function ψ on the streamlines $\psi = $ const. Reproduced by permission from Fung and Sobin (1969).

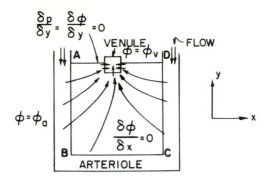

Figure 6.9:3 Geometry of an elastic alveolar sheet.

$$\psi = \text{constant}, \quad \text{or} \quad \frac{\partial \psi}{\partial s} = 0, \quad \text{or} \quad \frac{\partial p}{\partial n} = 0. \tag{4}$$

Consider a square alveolar sheet of uniform thickness as shown in Fig. 6.9:2, which is one-quarter of a panel of Fig. 6.9:1(a). The flow enters the sheet at the arteriole opening A-A′, and leaves the sheet at the venule, which is shown in Fig. 6.9:1(a) but not in Fig. 6.9:2. The streamlines of the draining flow are mirror images of those shown in Fig. 6.9:2 reflected in the plane at the base. Let the width of the arteriole and venule opening be 1/10 of the width of the sheet. By symmetry of the boundary conditions, it is easy to see that the center line and the solid boundaries are streamlines. Without loss of generality, let us choose the units of measurement in such a way that the boundary value of ψ on the center line is 0, and that on the solid boundary is $\psi = 1$. If the flow entering and leaving the sheet is uniform, then ψ increases linearly from 0 to 1 at the arteriole opening AA′ and venule opening BB′. With these known boundary values, the values of ψ can be found easily by several standard methods. The results in Fig. 6.9:2 were obtained by the relaxation method. The streamlines can then be plotted by interpolation. Since the pattern is symmetric, only one-quarter of the sheet is shown in Fig. 6.9:2.

From the stream functions, the velocities can be deduced according to Eq. (1). Contours of constant blood pressure lines ($p = \text{constant}$) are lines orthogonal to the streamlines, and thus can be deduced very easily from Fig. 6.9:2.

Next, let us consider the case of real interest: *flow in an elastic sheet*. Examples in this case will demonstrate the rapid thickness variation and pressure drop in the neighborhood of the venule, especially when the so-called zone 2 condition prevails (see Sec. 6.12). Let us consider an example as shown in Fig. 6.9:3. Here we assume that the precapillary forms the outer border ABCD, in which the pressure is a constant. The postcapillary drains the blood at the upper center in a rectangular opening. The upper horizontal border is assumed to be a streamline.

Let us examine a case in which the exit pressure at the venule is so much decreased that the sheet thickness at the venule becomes very small. With an appropriate choice of units, let the thickness of the sheet at the opening into the precapillary be $h_a = 1$, and that at the opening to the postcapillary be $h_v = \varepsilon$, which is a small number approaching zero. We consider the function $\Phi' = h^4$ and set the boundary conditions

$$\Phi' = h_a^4 = 1 \text{ at border adjacent to precapillary,}$$

$$\Phi' = h_v^4 = 0 \text{ at border adjacent to postcapillary,} \tag{5}$$

$$\frac{\partial \Phi'}{\partial n} = 0 \text{ along the top horizontal streamline.}$$

The last boundary condition, that the normal derivative vanishes on a streamline, can be derived from the following equations:

$$\Phi = h^4 = [h_0 + \alpha(p - p_A)]^4$$

$$p - p_A = \frac{h}{\alpha} - \frac{h_0}{\alpha}, \tag{6}$$

and

$$\operatorname{grad} p = \frac{kf}{h^2} V, \tag{7}$$

whence the vanishing of normal velocity implies

$$(\operatorname{grad} p)_n = (\operatorname{grad} h)_n = (\operatorname{grad} \Phi)_n = 0. \tag{8}$$

By symmetry, the vertical center line is another streamline. Setting $\partial \Phi'/\partial n = 0$ on the center line, we need to consider only half of the alveolar sheet. We then solve the harmonic equation $\nabla^2 \Phi' = 0$ subjected to the boundary conditions listed above. By the relaxation method, this can be done quickly. When the solution is obtained, we compute $h = (\Phi')^{1/4}$, and plot the contour lines $h(x, y) = \text{constant}$ in Fig. 6.9:4 (left panel). Note that the thickness drops very sharply near the drain into the venule, but over most of the sheet the thickness is quite uniform. The line representing a thickness of 90% of h_a lies about the border of the upper right quadrant of the sheet. The thickness drops another 10% to the 0.8 h_a line in about 20% of the length of the edge. Then the drop becomes faster. The 50% thickness line is seen to be very close to the opening. The final drop of 50% of thickness takes place within the last 2% of the distance.

Next let us consider a sequence of boundary thickness h_v at the venule drain:

$$h_v = 0.2, 0.4, 0.6, 0.8,$$

and a corresponding sequence of thickness h_a at the precapillary:

$$h_a = \sqrt[4]{1 + h_v^4}$$

$$h_a \cong 1.0004, 1.0063, 1.0309, 1.0896. \tag{9}$$

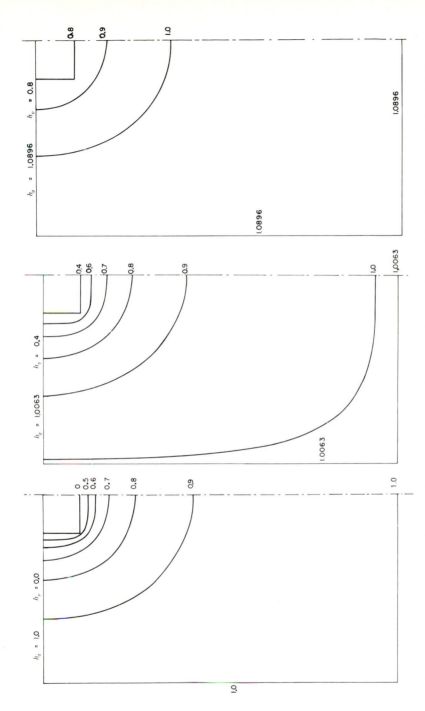

Figure 6.9:4 Mean sheet thickness distribution for boundary conditions specified in Fig. 6.9:3. Left panel: $h_a = 1.0$, $h_v = 0$. Middle panel: $h_a = 1.0063$, $h_v = 0.4$. Right hand panel: $h_a = 1.0896$, $h_v = 0.8$. Numerals associated with each contour are values of the sheet thickness as a fraction of the thickness at the arteriole, h_a, of the first case. Reproduced by permission from Fung and Sobin (1969).

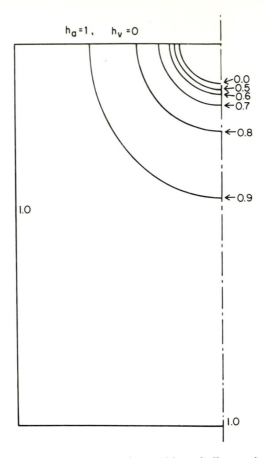

Figure 6.9:5 Solution to a boundary value problem similar to that shown in Figs. 6.9:3 and 6.9:4 except that the draining site is changed from a square to a circle. The mean thickness contours are shown for the case $h_a = 1$, $h_v = 0$. Note the similarity of the contours to those of Fig. 6.9:4. Reproduced by permission from Fung and Sobin (1969). Numerals are values of the sheet thickness as fractions of h_a.

We define $\Phi = h^4$, and set the boundary conditions

$$\Phi = h_a^4 = 1 + h_v^4 \text{ on precapillary borders,}$$

$$\Phi = h_v^4 \text{ on postcapillary borders,} \qquad (10)$$

$$\frac{\partial \Phi}{\partial n} = 0 \text{ on streamlines.}$$

To solve the equation $\nabla^2 \Phi = 0$ subjected to these boundary conditions let us define

$$\Phi = \Phi' + h_v^4. \qquad (11)$$

Then it is seen that Φ' is exactly what was solved above and $\Phi'^{1/4}$ has been presented in the left hand panel of Fig. 6.9:4. Hence Φ can be computed without further analysis, and contours $h(x, y) = \Phi^{1/4} = $ constant can be plotted. Two examples are presented in the middle and right-hand panels of Fig. 6.9:4.

An inspection of these figures shows that the thicker the sheet at the venule opening, the gentler is the thickness reduction. For example, the 50% reduction in thickness takes place at a distance from the drain opening at the following percentage of edge length:

h_v/h_a	0	0.199	0.397	0.582	0.734
50% line	2.1	4.1	7.9	11.1	16.8

This table shows the distance on the center line between the contour $h = h_v + \frac{1}{2}(h_a - h_v)$ and the venule drain opening, expressed as percentage of the length of the edge AB in Fig. 6.9:3. Incidentally, we see from these figures that the shape of the draining hole is not too important: the effect of the corner of the square is quickly rounded off. A circular drain will yield essentially the same result. Figure 6.9:5 illustrates the point. Compare it with Fig. 6.9:4. Note the similarity of the contours in these two figures. This is a basic property of the partial differential equations of the elliptic type. The square boundary is used in Figs. 6.9:3 and 6.9:4 to save a little computational labor.

6.10 Pressure–Flow Relationship of the Pulmonary Alveolar Blood Flow

We have derived a nonlinear pressure–flow relationship in the very simple case of one-dimensional flow in Sec. 6.8. We have shown by the examples given in Sec. 6.9 that the features of two-dimensional sheets are quite similar to the one-dimensional case. By integrating the equation of motion along the streamlines over the entire field, we shall derive an expression for the average flow over a sheet in the general, two-dimensional case.

We have shown in Eq. (4) of Sec. 6.6 that the mean flow velocity in a pulmonary alveolar sheet is

$$U = -\frac{1}{\mu k f} h^2 \text{ grad } \Delta p. \tag{1}$$

Here Δp stands for the transmural pressure, $p - p_{\text{alv}}$, μ is the apparent coefficient of viscosity of blood, k and f are numeric factors which depend on the details of the sheet structure, h is the local mean sheet thickness, and the symbol "grad" stands for the gradient operator. The flow per unit width is therefore

$$\dot{Q} = hU = -\frac{1}{\mu k f} h^3 \text{ grad } \Delta p \tag{2}$$

Apply this to a streamtube. Let s denote the arc length along the tube, and w be the width of the streamtube. Then the rate of flow in the tube is $\dot{Q}w$, which does not vary along the length of the streamtube, although both $\dot{Q}$ and w individually are functions of s. Now, on multiplying Eq. (2) with w, using Eq. (1b) of Sec. 6.5, which holds in the linear range of elasticity, and integrating from the arteriole to the venule, we obtain, with ds representing length along the streamline,

$$\int \dot{Q}w\,ds = -\int \frac{1}{\mu kf}[h_0 + \alpha \Delta p]^3 \frac{d\Delta p}{ds} w\,ds. \tag{3}$$

The integral on the left hand side is equal to the flow in the streamtube multiplied by $\int ds = L$, the length of the streamtube. The integral on the right hand side can be simplified according to the mean value theorem of the integral calculus. Because $w(s)$ and μkf are finite and are functions of bounded variation, we can write the right hand side of Eq. (3) as

$$-\frac{\overline{w}}{\overline{\mu kf}} \int [h_0 + \alpha \Delta p]^3 \frac{d\Delta p}{ds} ds \tag{3a}$$

where $\overline{w}$ and $\overline{\mu kf}$ are the values of $w(s)$ and $\mu kf(s)$ evaluated at some value of s on the streamtube. $\overline{w}$ is a characteristic width of the streamtube, and can be approximated by the area of the streamtube divided by the length, L. In accordance with these remarks, and carrying out the integration in Eq. (3a), we can write Eq. (3) as

$$\text{Flow in tube} = \frac{\text{tube area}}{4\overline{\mu kf} L^2 \alpha}[(h_0 + \alpha \Delta p_{\text{art}})^4 - (h_0 + \alpha \Delta p_{\text{ven}})^4]. \tag{4}$$

Here the subscripts "art" and "ven" refer to arteriole and venule, at the entry and exit to the capillary sheet, respectively.

A comparison of Eq. (4) with the familiar Poiseuille formula given in Eq. (17) of Sec. 3.2 shows a great difference between the flow in an elastic sheet and the flow in a rigid rube. In a rigid tube the flow is linearly proportional to the pressure drop $(p_{\text{art}} - p_{\text{ven}})/L$. In an elastic sheet this is not: Eq. (4) shows that

$$\text{Flow} = \frac{\text{area}}{4\mu kf L^2}(p_{\text{art}} - p_{\text{ven}})[(h_0 + \alpha \Delta p_{\text{art}})^3 + (h_0 + \alpha \Delta p_{\text{art}})^2(h_0 + \alpha \Delta p_{\text{ven}})$$

$$+ (h_0 + \alpha \Delta p_{\text{art}})(h_0 + \alpha p_{\text{ven}})^2 + (h_0 + \alpha \Delta p_{\text{ven}})^3]. \tag{5}$$

The factor in the brackets is the *conductance* of the flow and depends on the blood pressure.

Because a field of flow can be wholly covered by streamtubes, we can sum up the flow in all the streamtubes between an arteriole and a venule to obtain the flow between these two vessels. Let A be the area of alveolar sheet in question and S be the vascular–space–tissue ratio; then the total area of the vascular space is SA, and the total flow may be written as

$$\text{Flow} = \frac{SA}{4\mu k f \bar{L}^2 \alpha}[(h_0 + \alpha \Delta p_{\text{art}})^4 - (h_0 + \alpha \Delta p_{\text{ven}})^4]. \tag{6a}$$

where $\bar{L}$ is an average length of the streamtubes defined by the relation

$$\frac{SA}{\bar{L}^2} = \sum \frac{\text{area of streamtube}}{(\text{length of streamtube})^2} \tag{6b}$$

in which the summation covers all individual streamtubes of the sheet whose area is SA. Expressed in terms of sheet thickness, Eq. (6) is

$$\text{Flow} = \frac{1}{C}[h_a^4 - h_v^4], \tag{7}$$

where

$$C = \frac{4\mu k f \bar{L}^2 \alpha}{SA}, \tag{8}$$

$$h_a = h_0 + \alpha \Delta p_{\text{art}}, \quad h_v = h_0 + \alpha \Delta p_{\text{ven}}, \tag{9a}$$

$$\Delta p_{\text{art}} = p_{\text{art}} - p_{\text{alv}}, \quad \Delta p_{\text{ven}} = p_{\text{ven}} - p_{\text{alv}}. \tag{9b}$$

We may compute $\bar{L}$ by associating each streamline with a specific value of the stream function, ψ, and obtain

$$\frac{1}{\bar{L}^2} = \frac{1}{\psi_2 - \psi_1} \int_{\psi_2}^{\psi_1} \frac{1}{L^2(\psi)} d\psi, \tag{10}$$

where ψ_1 and ψ_2 are the dividing streamlines that enclose the whole field of flow between the arteriole and venule in question.

Equation (6) provides an explicit formula of blood flow in the pulmonary alveoli as related to the blood rheology (through μ), alveolar area (A), alveolar structural geometry (through k, f, which depend on a, c, etc.), the vascular–space–tissue ratio (S), the arteriole and venule transmural pressures ($p_{\text{art}}, p_{\text{ven}}$), the average length of streamlines between an arteriole and a venule ($\bar{L}$), the compliance of the alveolar sheet with respect to blood pressure (α), and indirectly, through α, to the tension of the alveolar septa (T, which is the sum of tissue stress and surface tension).

If we write Eq. (6) in the form

$$p_{\text{art}} - p_{\text{ven}} = R \cdot (\text{Flow}), \tag{11}$$

then R can be called the *resistance* of the capillary blood vessels. If both Δp_{art} and Δp_{ven} are positive, then the resistance is given by

$$R = \frac{C}{h_a^3 + h_a^2 h_v + h_a h_v^2 + h_v^3}, \tag{12}$$

which is a nonlinear function of the blood pressure.

Equation (7) is derived under the assumption of a linear thickness–pressure relationship, Eq. (1b) of Sec. 6.5, and is valid as long as $\Delta p_{\text{ven}} \geq 0$

or $p_{ven} \geq p_{alv}$. If the pressure in the venule is less than the alveolar gas pressure (see Sec. 6.12), then "sluicing" or "waterfall" occurs. The condition of sluicing is discussed in Sec. 6.13, where we conclude that the sluicing gate must be located either in the capillary sheet or at the junction of the capillary sheet and the draining venule. The flow in this case depends on how negative is $p_{ven} - p_{alv}$ and on the transpulmonary pressure $p_{alv} - p_{PL}$. It is in fact theoretically non-unique. However, a good approximation of the maximum flow in waterfall condition is given by Eq. (7) with the h_v term omitted. Thus

$$\text{Flow} = \frac{1}{C}h_a^4. \tag{13}$$

Equation (7) exhibits the essence of pulmonary alveolar blood flow. Because of the fourth power, the flow depends much more on the pressure at the entry (p_{art}) than that at the exit (p_{ven}). If the pressures are such that h_v is one-half of h_a, then h_v^4 is only 1/16 of h_a^4, and Eq. (7) shows that the flow varies almost as the fourth power of the pressure at the entry, p_{art}. Figure 6.10:1 shows the theoretical pressure–flow relationship given by Eq. (7) and

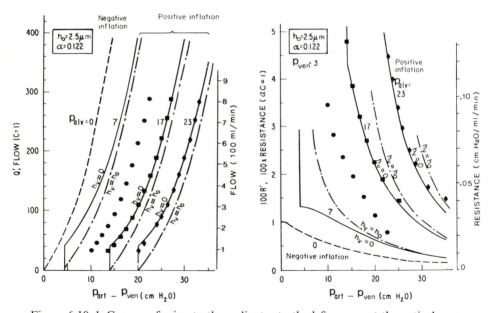

Figure 6.10:1 Curves referring to the ordinates to the left represent theoretical pressure–flow relationship given by Eqs. (7) and (13), and resistance given by Eq. (12). See text for explanation. Q' is the flow when $C = 1$, and $R' = \alpha R$ is resistance when $\alpha C = 1$. Points associated with the ordinate to the right correspond to experimental data of Roos et al. (1961) on isolated lung of the dog with left atrium pressure equal to 3 cm H_2O, pleural pressure equal to 0, and alveolar pressure equal to 23 ($\blacklozenge$), 17 ($\blacksquare$), and 7 ($\bullet$) cm H_2O. From Fung and Sobin (1972a). Reproduced by permission of American Heart Assoc. Inc.

the resistance given by Eq. (12). The constants used are pertinent to the dog, $h_0 = 2.5 \, \mu m$, $\alpha = 0.122 \, \mu m/cm \, H_2O$. The pressure p_{ven} is fixed at 3 cm H_2O; the alveolar gas pressure p_A is 0, 7, 17, or 23 cm H_2O. The entry pressure p_{art} is varied. The pleural pressure is assumed to be zero in the case of positive inflation and negative in the case of negative inflation represented by the curve for $p_{alv} = 0$. In the case of positive inflation, sluicing occurs (Sec. 6.12), and we have exhibited the results with either $h_v = h_0$ or $h_v = 0$. The constant C is set to be 1 for the scale on the ordinate to the left.

There is no direct experimental result on pulmonary alveolar blood flow available for comparison. Data on blood flow in a whole lung do exist. The flow in a whole lung will be analyzed in the following Section (6.11). In Fig. 6.10:1 we plotted the experimental results by Roos et al. (1961) on an isolated lung of the dog on the same graph, except with a scale (ordinate on the right-hand side) so adjusted that one of the experimental point falls exactly on the theoretical curve for the alveolar blood flow. The figure shows that the trends of the variations of flow and resistance with blood pressure are roughly the same for the whole lung as for the alveolar bed alone.

6.11 Blood Flow in Whole Lung

The results of the preceding section, together with the results of Sec. 3.4, will enable us to analyze the blood flow in a whole lung. For the pulmonary alveolar sheets, experimental results on their elasticity can be summarized by Eq. (1b) of Sec. 6:5:

$$h = h_0 + \alpha(p - p_A), \tag{1}$$

where h denotes the thickness of capillary sheet, p is the blood pressure, p_A is the airway pressure, h_0 is the thickness of capillary sheet when $p = p_A$, and α is the compliance constant of the capillary sheet. Eq. (1) is valid when $p - p_A > 0$ and smaller than an upper limit of about 25 cm H_2O (for cat) or 15 cm H_2O (for man), beyond which h tends to a constant asymptotically. When $p - p_A < 0$, the capillaries are collapsed and h tends to zero. Using Eq. (1), together with the equations of continuity and motion, and an experimentally verified linear relationship between local velocity of flow and pressure gradient, we obtain the volume flow (Eq. (6.10:7)):

$$\dot{Q} = \text{const.} \, [h_{art}^4 - h_{ven}^4] = \text{const.} \, \{[h_0 + \alpha(p_{art} - p_A)]^4$$
$$- [h_0 + \alpha(p_{ven} - p_A)]^4\}, \tag{2}$$

where $\dot{Q}$ is the volume flow rate, h_{art} is the sheet thickness at the arteriole where blood enters into the sheet, h_{ven} is the sheet thickness at the venule where blood exits from the sheet, p_{art} and p_{ven} are the pressures at the corresponding arterioles and venules. The constant in Eq. (2) is equal to $1/C$, with C given by Eq. (6.10:8).

For pulmonary arteries and veins, the results presented in Sec. 6.4 show that the vessel diameter D changes linearly with blood pressure p:

$$D = D_0 + \alpha p. \tag{3}$$

Here D_0 is the tube diameter when p is zero; α is the compliance constant. Then for steady flow of a viscous incompressible fluid in such a tube the analysis of Sec. 3.4 yields the result Eq. (3.4:13):

$$\frac{640\mu\alpha L}{\pi} \dot{Q} = [D(o)]^5 - [D(L)]^5 = [D_0 + \alpha p_{\text{entry}}]^5 - [D_0 + \alpha p_{\text{exit}}]^5. \tag{4}$$

Equations (2) and (4) are called the *fourth* and *fifth power laws* respectively. Equation (4) may be corrected for losses due to turbulence and bifurcation by replacing μ with the "apparent" viscosity which depends on the Reynolds number. To account for the effect of change of kinetic energy along the stream, we may add a pressure drop at the end of a vessel of order n by an amount equal to $\frac{1}{2}\rho v_{n+1}^2 - \frac{1}{2}\rho v_n^2$; see Eq. (18) on p. 18. Then a repeated application of Eqs. (4) and (2) will synthesize the flow in different segments into that of the whole lung. In the following, we shall apply these equations to the cat's lung, because morphological and elasticity data for the cat are available.

Application of Experimental Data on Vessel Elasticity

Experimental data on the elasticity of pulmonary arteries and veins of the cat are presented in Sec. 6.4. These data were obtained by measuring the vessel dimensions at different values of blood pressure while the pressures in the airway (p_A) and pleura (p_{PL}) were fixed. Hence the constants h_0, D_0, and α in Eqs. (1) and (3) must depend on p_A and p_{PL} because these parameters were not varied in the experiments. This dependence has not been determined fully at this time. The only data available are given in Fig. 6.4:3. However, some theoretical studies of this dependence are available. Fung and Sobin (1972a) analyzed h_0 and α as functions of membrane tension in the sheet (interalveolar septa), which depends on the transpulmonary pressure $p_A - p_{\text{PL}}$. Yen et al. (1980) argued that for pulmonary vessels whose diameter is much larger than the alveolar diameter, the vessel diameter may be written as

$$D = D_0[1 + \beta(p - p_{\text{PL}})], \tag{5}$$

whereas for vessels whose diameter is smaller than the alveolar diameter, we should have

$$D = D_0[1 + \beta(p - p_A)], \tag{6}$$

where D_0 and β are functions of $p_A - p_{\text{PL}}$. (We changed the notation α of Yen et al. (1980, 1981) to β to avoid a conflict with Eq. (3).) The reasoning is that the pulmonary vessel diameter varies with the internal pressure p, the external pressure p_A, and the tension in the attached alveolar walls which is approximately equal to $p_A - p_{PL}$ if averaged over a unit area. For large vessels, use of the average stress $p_A - p_{PL}$ for tethered alveolar wall is applicable, hence the "transmural" pressure becomes $p - [p_A - (p_A - p_{PL})]$ $= p - p_{PL}$ which is exhibited in Eq. (5). For small vessels, use of the average stress in alveolar wall as tethering force outside the vessel is inappropriate. Such a small vessel is shown in Fig. 4.9:3, p. 217, to be tethered by three interalveolar septa, spaced at approximately 120°. Across the vessel wall between the septa the "transmural" pressure is $p - p_A$; hence Eq. (6). Lai-Fook (1979) has shown that the parenchyma stress is affected in the neighborhood of a large blood vessel by the elasticity of the vessel to a value which may be written as $k(p_A - p_{PL})$. Usually, $k > 1$. If this is assumed, then the "transmural" pressure across a large pulmonary vessel is $p - [p_A - k(p_A - p_{PL})]$ and Eq. (5) may be replaced by

$$D = D_0[1 - \beta(1 - k)p_A + \beta(p - p_{PL})]. \tag{7}$$

Since the available data are expressed in terms of Eqs. (5) and (6), these equations will be used in the following analysis: Eq. (5) for vessels $> 100\ \mu m$, Eq. (6) for vessels $< 100\ \mu m$. On using Eq. (4), note that $\alpha = D_0\beta$.

Application of Morphometric Data of Vascular Tree

Morphological data on pulmonary venous and arterial tree of the cat are given in Sec. 6.2. Strahler system is used to describe the branching pattern statistically. To analyze blood flow, however, one must have a definite vascular circuit every time. The creation of a circuit from statistical data on branching, is, unfortunately, a non-unique process. An infinite number of circuits can be created that are consistent with the statistical data, but not uniquely specified by them.

As an example, consider the two patterns shown in Fig. 6.11:1. They have the same branching ratio of 3 for the three orders depicted. In pattern 1, the flow in a larger vessel is distributed equally into three daughter vessels every time. If we apply Eq. (4) to this pattern, Q being equal to the total flow divided by the number of branches of each order, we can calculate the pressure drop one order at a time. In contrast, consider a vascular tree shown in pattern 2. Assume that, at the entrance into the vessels at the top, one-third of the flow is diverted into a group of vessels of lower orders. When the remaining 2/3 of the flow in the main trunk arrives at the next node, it is divided equally into the two daughter groups. In each daughter group, one-third again enters the smaller vessels of the next order. With such an assumption, it is possible to calculate the pressure distribution throughout the lung; but all vessels of the same order do not have the same pressure.

The same reasoning is used to devise two circuits consistent with the statistical morphometric data. We consider two models similar to those

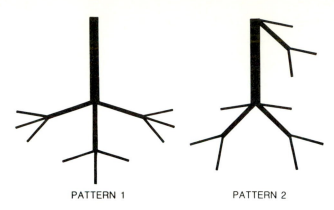

PATTERN 1   PATTERN 2

Figure 6.11:1 Two patterns of branching considered in the present article. Three orders are depicted. Vessels of the same diameter belong to the same order. From Zhuang et al. (1983a), by permission.

shown in Fig. 6.11:1. In model 1, flow in a branch of order $n + 1$ is divided equally into B_n daughter vessels of order n, B_n being the branching ratio of order n. In model 2, we assume that each vessel of order $n + 1$ bifurcates into two vessels of order n at the exit end as shown in Pattern 2, whereas B_n-2 remaining vessels of order n are attached to the entry end of the parent vessel (of order $n + 1$). We shall use the following approximation to obtain the flow distribution in model 2. Let the total flow be Q_t. Let the total number of vessels of an order n be N_n. The flow in each vessel of order n is Q_t/N_n. For the largest artery, of order 11, some flow is diverted into vessels of order 10 or smaller at the entry section, the remaining flow in the main trunk is equal to $2Q_t/N_{10}$. For the daughter branch of order 10, a similar division is made, and the flow is $2Q_t/N_9$. And so on, until the vessels of the smallest order are reached, in which the flow is of course, Q_t/N_1. From this assumed flow pattern, we compute the pressure distribution.

It is obvious that if the total flow, and the pressures at the left atrium and the airway are the same, the resistance of model 2 is smaller than that of model 1. The resistance of the real system is expected to be closer to that of the model 2.

Data Base

Tables 6.11:1–6.11:3 show the morphometric and elastic data of the cat's right lung, collected from Tables 4.9:2, 6.2:1, 6.4:1, and 6.4:2. D_0 is computed for vessels <100 μm according to Eq. (6), and for vessels >100 μm according to Eq. (5).

For pulmonary capillaries of the cat, Sobin et al. (1972) give $h_0 = 4.28$ μm, $\alpha = 0.219$ μm per cm H_2O, S (vascular space-tissue ratio) = 0.916. Sobin

TABLE 6.11:1 Morphometric Data of Pulmonary Arteries of the Cat Measured at Transpulmonary Pressure $p_A - p_{PL} = 10$ cm H_2O

Order	Number of branches in right lung N_n	Diameter[1] D_{on} (cm)	Length L_n (cm)	Apparent viscosity coefficient μ_n (cp)	Compliance[2] α (10^{-4} cm p_a^{-1})	Compliance[2] β ($10^{-4} p_a^{-1}$)
1	300,358	0.0024	0.0116	2.5	0.00463	1.928
2	97,519	0.0044	0.0262	3.0	0.00848	1.928
3	31,662	0.0073	0.0433	3.5	0.01407	1.928
4	9,736	0.0122	0.0810	4.0	0.02352	1.928
5	2,925	0.0192	0.151	4.0	0.02154	1.122
6	774	0.0352	0.272	4.0	0.02802	0.796
7	202	0.0533	0.460	4.0	0.03807	0.714
8	49	0.0875	0.819	4.0	0.09818	1.122
9	12	0.1519	1.426	4.0	0.4045	2.663
10	4	0.2486	1.187	4.0	0.6620	2.663
11	1	0.5080	2.500	4.0	1.353	2.663

[1] Yen et al. (1983) gives the diameter data of vessels of orders 1–4 measured at $p - p_A = -7$ cm H_2O, whereas those of orders 5–11 were measured at $p - p_{PL} = 3$ cm H_2O. In this Table, D_{on} are the diameters at zero "transmural" pressure, defined as $p - p_A = 0$ for orders 1–4, and $p - p_{PL} = 0$ for orders 5–11, and are computed from the data of Yen et al. (1980) according to the equations $D = D_o[(1 + \beta(p - p_A)]$ for orders 1–4 and $D = D_o[1 + \beta(p - p_{PL})]$ for orders 5–11.

[2] For the method of computing compliance, see notes in Table 6.11.3. $\alpha = \beta D_{on}$.

TABLE 6.11:2 Morphometric Data of Pulmonary Veins of the Cat at
$p_A - p_{PL} = 10$ cm H_2O

Order	Number of branches N_n	Diameter[1] D_{on} (cm)	Length L_n (cm)	Apparent viscosity coefficient μ_n (cp)
1	282,733	0.0025	0.0086	2.5
2	86,241	0.0046	0.0247	3.0
3	26,306	0.0077	0.0496	3.5
4	8,024	0.0127	0.1545	4.0
5	2,348	0.0251	0.2380	4.0
6	656	0.0432	0.3810	4.0
7	171	0.0642	0.4950	4.0
8	46	0.1040	0.7610	4.0
9	13	0.1727	1.5120	4.0
10	4	0.3010	1.9240	4.0
11	1	0.4491	2.5000	4.0

[1] The diameter values are computed from those of Yen and Foppiano (1981) according to the formulas described in footnote (1) of Table 6.11:1.

et al. (1980) give the average path length $\bar{L} = 556 \pm 285$ (SD) μm. Based on the same topological map used by Sobin et al. (1980), we obtained the total capillary area of the right lung of the cat to be 0.42 m^2 by stereological methods.

The apparent viscosity values given in Tables 6.11:1 and 6.11:2 are estimated under the hypothesis that the hematocrit varies from about 45% in larger vessels with diameter > 100 μm (orders 4–11) to about 30% in the capillaries. The variation of the apparent viscosity of blood in pulmonary capillary sheet with hematocrit has been determined by Yen et al. (1973) in model experiments, from whose data we calculate that when the hematocrit is 30%, the apparent viscosity is 1.92 cp. On the other hand, at a hematocrit of 45% in large vessels, an apparent viscosity of 4.0 cp is assumed. The apparent viscosity of blood in small vessels of the orders of 1–3 is obtained by linear interpolation and listed in Tables 6.11:1 and 6.11:2.

Results

Steady flow is considered. With the data presented above, we compute the flow in vessels of successive orders, and then use Eqs. (2) and (4) to calculate the blood pressures, and formulas (5)–(7) to obtain vessel diameters at different pressures. Two circuits are analyzed, called models 1 and 2, analogous to patterns 1 and 2 shown in Fig. 6.11:1. Analysis of steady flow in model 1 is rigorous. Pressure loss due to entry flow and changes due to kinetic energy ($\frac{1}{2}\rho v^2$) are negligible for the cat. The analysis of model 2 is

TABLE 6.11:3 Compliance of Pulmonary Veins of the Cat Obtained in Experiments with $p_A = 0$, p_{PL} Specified, and variable Local Blood Pressure[(1), (2)]

Order	Compliance $p_{PL} = -10$ cm H_2O		Compliance[3] $p_{PL} = -15$ cm H_2O		Compliance[3] $p_{PL} = -20$ cm H_2O	
	α (10^{-4} cm p_a^{-1})	β ($10^{-4} p_a^{-1}$)	α (10^{-4} cm p_a^{-1})	β ($10^{-4} p_a^{-1}$)	α (10^{-4} cm p_a^{-1})	β ($10^{-4} p_a^{-1}$)
1	0.00482	1.928	0.00482	1.928	0.00482	1.928
2	0.00887	1.928	0.00887	1.928	0.00887	1.928
3	0.0148	1.928	0.0148	1.928	0.0148	1.928
4	0.0331	2.080	0.0446	2.806	0.0396	2.490
5	0.0430	1.469	0.0598	2.041	0.0478	1.633
6	0.0528	1.092	0.0484	1.000	0.0469	0.969
7	0.0785	1.092	0.0719	1.000	0.0697	0.969
8	0.0810	0.724	0.0628	0.561	0.0833	0.745
9	0.1346	0.724	0.1043	0.561	0.1385	0.745
10	0.2346	0.724	0.1817	0.561	0.2414	0.745
11	0.3504	0.724	0.2715	0.561	0.3606	0.745

[1] For orders 1 to 3 the data are from Sobin et al. (1978). $\alpha = \beta \cdot D_{on}$.

[2] For orders 4 to 11, Yen and Foppiano (1981) gives the elastic properties by the formular $D = D_{10}[1 + \beta(p - p_{PL} - 10 \text{ cm } H_2O)]$. Hence $\alpha = D_{10}\beta$. Note that, however, β was written as α in Yen and Foppiano (1981).

[3] The compliance at $p_{PL} = -15$ and -20 cm H_2O was measured in Yen and Foppiano (1981) and expressed in terms of β. But the values of D_{on} are unknown at these transpulmonary pressures; hence α is computed by multiplying β with D_{10n} at $p_{PL} = -10$ cm H_2O computed according to the equation in (2) above. There is a dearth of information on the dependence of D_{on} with the transpulmonary pressure.

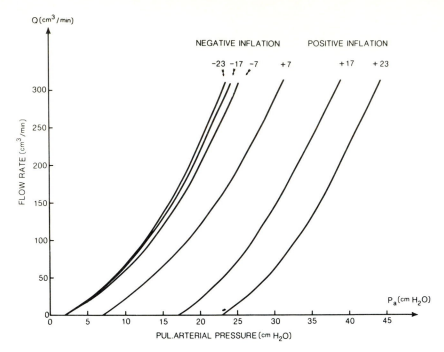

Figure 6.11:2 The relationship between flow and pulmonary arterial pressure under six different transpulmonary pressures. In "negative inflations," the left atrial pressure P_v is fixed at 2 cm H_2O; in "positive inflations," P_v is fixed at 3 cm H_2O. From Zhuang et al. (1983a), by permission. Data refer to the cat.

approximate due to the ad hoc assumption about the flow distribution. In the following, the results refer to model 1 of the right lung of the cat, unless stated otherwise.

Figure 6.11:2 shows the relationship between flow and pulmonary arterial pressure under six different transpulmonary pressures and two left atrial pressures. In the cases labeled as "positive inflations", the pleural pressure p_{PL} is 0 (atmospheric), the airway pressure p_A is indicated in the figure, and the left atrial pressure p_v is fixed at 3 cm H_2O. In "negative inflations", $p_A = 0$, p_{PL} is shown in the figure, and p_v is fixed at 2 cm H_2O. These values of p_A, p_{PL}, and p_v are so chosen that the results may be compared with an experiment to be discussed later.

The curves of Fig. 6.11:2 show that the relationship between flow ($\dot{Q}$) and arterial pressure (p_a) is nonlinear. $\dot{Q}$ increases more rapidly then increasing p_a. At fixed values of p_a, flow decreases with increasing transpulmonary pressure in positive inflation; but it increases with increasing transpulmonary pressure in negative inflation.

Figure 6.11:3 shows the difference between the pressure–flow relationship for the two branching models, 1 and 2, illustrated in Fig. 6.11:1. The calculation is referred to a negative inflation, $p_A = 0$, $p_{PL} = -7$ cm H_2O,

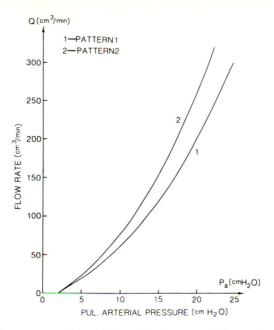

Figure 6.11:3 The pressure–flow relationships for two different branching models 1 and 2 explained in the text. Both curves refer to a negative inflation at $p_A = 0$, $p_{PL} = -7$ cm H_2O, $p_v = 2$ cm H_2O. From Zhuang et al. (1983a), by permission.

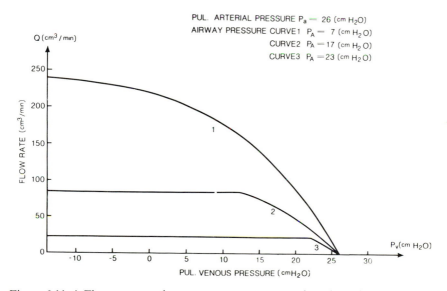

Figure 6.11:4 Flow versus pulmonary venous pressure when the pulmonary arterial pressure is fixed at 26 cm H_2O, the pleural pressure p_{PL} is zero, and the alveolar gas pressure p_A is 7, 17, and 23 cm H_2O. From Zhuang et al. (1983a), by permission.

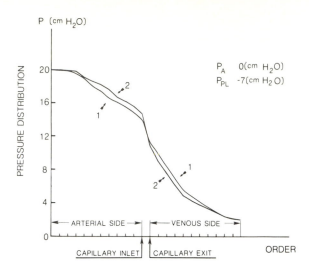

Figure 6.11:5 The longitudinal pressure distributions in pulmonary blood vessels for the case in which $p_a = 20$, $p_v = 2$, $p_A = 0$, $p_{PL} = -7$ cm H_2O. Each tick mark on the horizontal axis represents the location of the exit end of each vessel in a given order. The numerals 1 and 2 refer to branching models 1 and 2, respectively. From Zhuang et al. (1983a), by permission. Data refer to the cat.

$p_v = 2$ cm H_2O. It is seen that at any arterial pressure, p_a, flow is higher in a circuit of model 2 than that in model 1; in other words, the resistance to flow is lower in model 2.

Figure 6.11:4 shows flow versus a variable pulmonary venous pressure, with a fixed arterial pressure of 26 cm H_2O, $p_{PL} = 0$, and three values of p_A: 7, 17, and 23 cm H_2O. By definition, the flow is said to be in zone 2 condition when $p_v \leq p_A$. In the calculation of Fig. 6.11:4, the sluicing gates are assumed to lie at the exit ports of the capillary sheets. This assumption was proposed by Fung and Sobin (1972a) under the hypothesis that the pulmonary venules and veins will not collapse when $p_v < p_A$, because of the support the vessels receive from the tension in the interalveolar septa that attach to the vessel walls. This last hypothesis has received a full experimental verification which is presented in Sec. 4.9.

Figure 6.11:5 shows the pressure distribution in the lung, plotted against the order number of the vessels, for the case in which $p_a = 20$, $p_v = 2$, $p_A = 0$, $p_{PL} = -7$ cm H_2O. Vascular circuits of both patterns 1 and 2 are considered as indicated in the figure.

If the pressure drop from the pulmonary artery of order 11 to the arteriole of order 1 is compared with the drop in the capillaries and veins, we obtain the results shown in Table 6.11:4.

Finally, we show in Fig. 6.11:6 the transit time of blood in the pulmonary capillaries, calculated by the method to be presented in the following Sec.

TABLE 6.11:4 Distribution of Pressure Drop in Pulmonary Blood Vessels of the Cat and Comparison with Data on Dog in the Literature

	Arteries	Capillaries	Veins
Pattern 1	35.9%	15.4%	48.7%
Pattern 2	29.3%	21.9%	48.8%
Brody et al. (1968)	46%	34%	20%
Hakim et al. (1981)*	40.2%	15.6%	44.2%
Gaar et al. (1967)†	56%		44%

* By method of abrupt occlusion of inflow and outflow of blood in selected vessels in dog's lung. Hakim et al. (1981) considered three compartments in the lung: the upstream or arterial compartment, (Δp_a), the downstream or venous compartment, (Δp_v), and the vascular compartment in between (Δp_m).

† Gaar et al. (1967) divided the distribution of pressure into the arterial side and the venous side from the midpoint of the capillaries.

6.13, in which $p_A = 0$, $p_{PL} = -7$, $p_v = 2$ cm H_2O, whereas the pulmonary arterial pressure or flow rate is varied. The figure shows that the transit time decreases when the flow rate increases, but does not follow an inverse proportionality relationship, owing to the distensibility of the capillary blood vessels.

Discussion

The results shown in Fig. 6.11:2 may be compared with the trend shown by Ross et al. (1961) in their experiments on dog's lung, see Fig. 6.10:1. We find that the theoretical trend compares very well with the experimental result except for the case of negative inflation with $p_A = 0$, $p_v = 2$, $p_{PL} = -23$ cm H_2O. Theoretically, the trend is continuous; at a given p_a the flow increases (i.e. the resistance decreases) as p_{PL} changes from -7 to -17 and -23. Ross et al's experimental results, however, show a discontinuous trend: at a given p_a, the flow increases as p_{PL} changes from -7 to -17, then decreases as p_{PL} changes from -17 to -23. The reason for this discrepancy is not clear. It could be due to an inadequate accounting of the changes in vessel diameters and elasticity as functions of p_A and p_{PL}, as discussed earlier. This suggests that the study of D_0 and α as functions of p_A and p_{PL} is an important topic for the future.

From the curves of Fig. 6.11:2, we can estimate the cardiac output. Take the case in which $p_A = 0$, $p_{PL} = -17$, $p_v = 2$, and $p_a = 20$ cm H_2O. Figure 6.11:2 yields a flow of 210 ml/min for the right lung of a cat of 3.6 kg body weight. Thus, the cardiac output is 420 ml/min, or 117 ml/min/kg, a value agreeing quite well with that given by Weiner et al. (1967).

The results shown in Fig. 6.11:4 may be compared with those given by

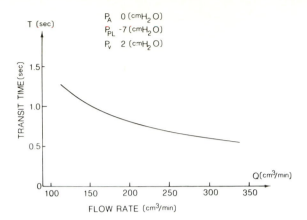

Figure 6.11:6 The transit time of blood in pulmonary capillaries for the case in which $p_A = 0$, $p_{PL} = -7$, $p_v = 2$ cm H_2O. The flow rate in half lung and the pulmonary arterial pressure are varied. From Zhuang et al. (1983), by permission.

Permutt et al. (1962) for the dog. The existence of flow limitation is well exhibited by the theoretical curves of Fig. 6.11:4. The reduction of the maximum flow with increasing p_A is also demonstrated theoretically. But two features shown by Permutt et al. (1962) are not found in the simple theory presented herein: (a) The existence of a hysteresis loop in the pressure–flow relationship when p_v first decreases and then increases. (b) A minor but definite decrease of flow below the maximum as p_v continues to decrease below p_A. Our own experiments on a cat's lung yielded a similar result, see Fig. 6.13:8, p. 355. To explain these discrepancies a refined theory is required. My own theory is presented in Sec. 6.13 under the (verified) hypotheses that the venules remain patent when $p_{ven} < p_A$ and that the interalveolar septa are under tension when the lung is inflated. It is shown that part of the alveolar sheet (capillary blood vessels) can be collapsed ($h = 0$) while other parts remain open, see Fig. 6.13:4. Hysteresis in the pressure–flow relationship when the venous pressure is changed cyclically below airway pressure is explained by the additional energy needed to reopen collapsed capillary blood vessels.

The pressure distribution shown in Fig. 6.11:5 and Table 6.11:4 may be compared with the experimental results by Brody et al. (1968), Hakim et al. (1981), and Gaar et al. (1967). In addition to the comparison shown in Table 6.11:4, we give in Table 6.11:5 a comparison of our theoretical results with the experimental results obtained recently on dog's lung by Bhattacharya et al. (1982) who obtained the data by two methods: micro-puncture and occlusion. The theoretical data in Table 6.11:5 refer to the case in which $p_a = 16.9$, $p_A = 7.0$, $p_v = 10.0$ cm H_2O for zone 3 condition, $p_v = 1.7$ cm H_2O for zone 2 condition, in agreement with Bhattacharya's experimental condition. Our theoretical pressure is calculated at the exit end of a venular vessel of order 2, with a diameter of 46 μm.

TABLE 6.11:5 Comparison of Our Theoretical Results with Experimental Results of Bahattacharya et al. (1982)

Method	Vessels	Pressure in zone 3 cdn. cm H_2O	Pressure in zone 2 cdn. cm H_2O	Reference
Micro-puncture	Venules (20–50 μm)	11.3 ± 0.8	7.4 ± 1.2	Bhattacharya et al. [1982].
Occlusion	Venules (20–50 μm)	11.4 ± 0.5	5.2 ± 1.6	Bhattacharya et al. [1982].
Our theory	Venules of order 2 (46 μm)	11.9	6.48	This report

Arterial pressure = 16.9 cm H_2O, Alveolar pressure = 7.0 cm H_2O, Left atrium pressure for zone 3 condition = 10.0 cm H_2O, Left atrium pressure for zone 2 condition = 1.7 cm H_2O.

From Tables 6.11:4 and 6.11:5, we see that our theoretical results compare quite well with the experimental results of Hakim et al. (1981) and Bhattacharya et al. (1982). But we do not agree with Brody et al. (1968).

Finally, the blood transit time in pulmonary capillaries plotted in Fig. 6.11:6 may be compared with experimental data by Johnson et al. (1960) and Wagner et al. (1982). Figure 6.11:6 shows that at a physiological flow of 200 ml/min for the right lung of the cat, the transit time is about 0.80 sec., which is quite close to the value 0.79 sec. obtained by Johnson et al. (1960), but is considerably shorter than the value given by Wagner et al. (1982).

The example above illustrates the calculation of pulmonary circulation of a whole lung of the cat on the basis of experimental data on the morphology of the vascular tree and elasticity of blood vessels of all orders. Comparison of the theoretical results with experimental results in the literature has yielded good agreement in many cases, but there are a few significant discrepancies which suggest that further work is needed. Among these are: (a) collection of data on vessel dimensions and compliance constants when airway and pleural pressures are varied, especially for small vessels, and for large negative inflation, (b) the hysteresis in pressure–flow relationship and details of flow limitation in zone 2 condition. Furthermore, it is obvious that morphometric and elasticity data for man, dog, and other animals are needed.

6.12 Regional Difference of Pulmonary Blood Flow

In large animals the hydrostatic pressure due to gravitation plays an important role in pulmonary blood flow. Let p_{PA} be the pressure in the pulmonary artery of the highest order immediately next to the pulmonic valve,

p_{LA} be the pressure in the left atrium, z be the height of a point above the level of pulmonic valve, measured along the direction of gravitational acceleration; then the pressure in the flowing blood at the point of height z is

$$p(z) = p_{PA} - \rho g z - \sum_{\text{from } PA} (\Delta p)_i \tag{1}$$

or

$$p(z) = p_{LA} - \rho g(z - z_{LA}) + \sum_{\text{from } LA} (\Delta p)_i \tag{2}$$

where ρ is the density of the blood, g is the gravitational acceleration, $(\Delta p)_i$ is the pressure drop in a blood vessel of order i, and the summation includes all orders of vessels starting from the pulmonary artery of the highest order in Eq. (1), or all orders of vessels starting from the left atrium in Eq. (2). In the preceding section we have shown how to compute $(\Delta p)_i$ using the 5th-power law for arteries and veins and the 4th-power law for the capillaries. We ignored the z-terms in Sec. 6.11. For large animals the z-terms cannot be ignored, and the analysis is more complex, although the principle remains the same.

West (1974, p. 43) divides the lung into three zones:

$$\text{zone 1:} \qquad p_A > p_a > p_v \tag{3}$$

$$\text{zone 2:} \qquad p_a > p_A > p_v \tag{4}$$

$$\text{zone 3:} \qquad p_a > p_v > p_A \tag{5}$$

where the subscripts A, a, and v stands for alveolar gas, arterial blood, and venous blood, respectively. He computes p_a, p_v as static pressures

$$p_a = p_{PA} - \rho g z, \qquad p_v = p_{LA} - \rho g z. \tag{6}$$

The idea is that the "waterfall" phenomenon may occur in zone 2. However, since pulmonary arteries and veins remain patent when p_A exceeds p_v or p_a (Sec. 4.9), whereas the capillaries would collapse in this condition (Sec. 6.5), the waterfall phenomenon will occur only in the capillary sheet. Hence it is the entry and exit condition of the capillary sheet that is significant. Using the notations p_{art} and p_{ven} for the pressures at the capillary entry from an arteriole and exit into a venule, respectively, as in Sec. 6.10, we may define

$$\text{zone 1:} \qquad p_A > p_{\text{art}} > p_{\text{ven}} \tag{7}$$

$$\text{zone 2:} \qquad p_{\text{art}} > p_A > p_{\text{ven}} \tag{8}$$

$$\text{zone 3:} \qquad p_{\text{art}} > p_{\text{ven}} > p_A. \tag{9}$$

In zone 1, we expect little flow in the capillaries. In zone 3, all vessels are patent. In zone 2, waterfall phenomenon occurs. p_{art}, p_{ven} are to be calculated according to Eqs. (1) or (2), and they are functions of z.

Experimental evidences of regional differences in the lung and their physiological and pathological significances are discussed fully in West (1977).

6.13 The "Sluicing" Condition when $p_{ven} < p_A$

Our concept of the sluicing condition at the junctions of capillaries and venules of order 1 is based on anatomical, rheological, mechanical, and mathematical considerations. Anatomically, two features stand out. One is related to the topological structure of the pulmonary arterioles, venules, and capillaries. The other is related to the structure of the capillary–venule junctions. Figure 6.13:1, from Sobin et al. (1979), shows a histological section of the cat's lung. In this montage of micrographs every arterial blood vessel with a diameter less than 100 μm is marked with a bull's eye, and every venous vessel of similar dimension is marked with a black circle. It is seen that the arterial vessels are grouped together. The venous vessels are also grouped together. When overlays are made to cover the areas containing arterial vessels only, we obtain a picture which resembles a map of islands in an ocean. The arterial territories are islands. By stereological methods it is determined that the average distance between an arteriole and the nearest venule is 556 ± 285 μm in the cat (Sobin et al. 1979). The average diameter of cat's alveoli being 163 μm (Zhuang et al., 1983b), blood leaving an arteriole will travel on the average 3.4 alveoli before it enters a venule. Each venule of order 1 drains an average of 18 alveoli in the cat, (Zhuang et al. (1983b)). The path of blood is determined, of course, by the pressure field, and is not predictable from anatomy alone.

Figure 6.13:2 shows the relationship between a terminal venule and capillary sheets. The many junctions are clearly seen. Figure 6.13:3 shows a photograph of a venule draining a capillary sheet, showing the details of the membranes at the junction. A schematic drawing combining the features shown in these figures is given in Fig. 6.13:4. In this idealized drawing, the many alveolar walls from many alveoli draining into a venous tree are combined into a single large sheet. One area of the sheet is shown as collapsed, ($h = 0$, shaded); the remainder is open. One venule is attached to the collapsed sheet; another is draining the open sheet. The justification of these possibilities will be explained later.

Another schematic drawing is given in Fig. 6.13:5(a). Here one interalvolar septum intersects a venule perpendicularly whereas three others tether it longitudinally. Figures 6.13:2 and 6.13:3 suggest that the blood flow in the perpendicular capillary sheet drains into the venule. Whether the flow in the longitudinally tethered sheets drain into the venule along the line of tethering or not is unknown. If they do, then the flow condition can be approximate by the "one-dimensional" case considered in Section 6.8.

Rheologically, the important fact is that the venules (of all orders) will

a

a

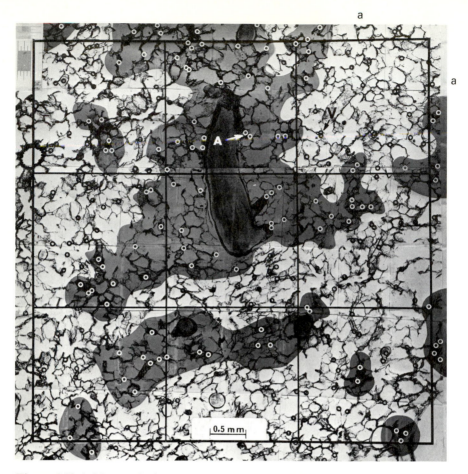

Figure 6.13:1 Map made from montage of individual photomicrographs of a histological section (50 μm thick) of cat lung. Vessels from 15–100 μm diameter are individually identified, arteries by white circles (arrow "A"), veins by black circles (arrow "V"). A large artery lies in the middle of the section. The domains of the arteries are made darker by overlay of the areas with blue transparency film; and they appear as isolated islands. The domain of the veins is continuous. Thus the arterial regions are like islands immersed in an ocenan which contains only pulmonary veins. From Sobin et al. (1980), by permission.

remain patent under the condition $p_{ven} < p_A$, when the pressure in the venules is smaller than the alveolar gas pressure (Sec. 4.9), whereas the capillaries will collapse if the blood pressure is exceeded by p_A (Sec. 6.5). Hence the venule can serve as an anchor for the walls of the alveolar capillary sheet.

Mechanically, we note that all interalveolar septa are subjected to tension when the lung is inflated. Tissue stress exists because inflated lung is larger than that at the unloaded condition. Surface tension exists at the gas-tissue interface.

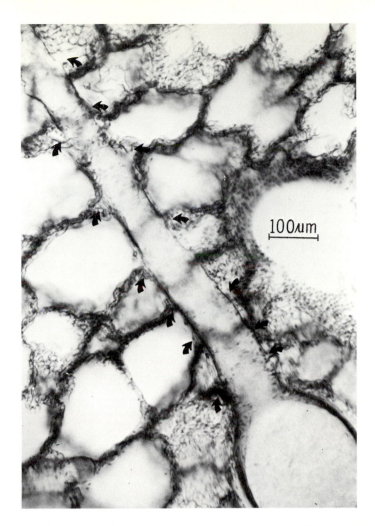

Figure 6.13:2 The connection between a venule and alveolar sheets in cat's lung. Courtesy of Dr. Sidney Sobin.

Mathematically, we note that there exists a simple solution of the basic sheet flow equation (6.7:11) or (6.7:20), namely,

$$h = 0. \tag{1}$$

This simple solution is trivial in the one-dimensional case, because it implies absence of flow. But in the three-dimensional structure of alveoli this is a very significant solution: $h = 0$ can be imposed in any area, provided that the remaining area can handle the flow, because $h = 0$ is an allowable boundary condition for the differential equations (6.7:11) and (6.7:20). In other words, in the three-dimensional structure of the lung, the solution

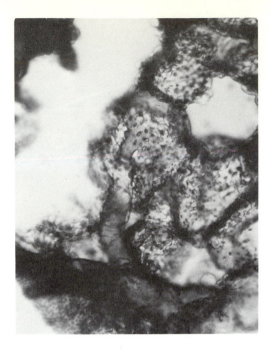

Figure 6.13:3 Another view of the junction of an alveolar sheet and a venule in the cat. From Sobin and Tremer (1966), by permission.

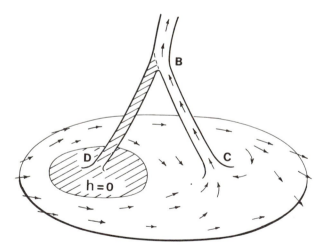

Figure 6.13:4 A schematic drawing showing a possible condition of flow from an alveolar sheet into a venous tree. Two terminal venules (of order 1) intersect the sheet. The blood pressure at the point B is smaller than the alveolar gas pressure, i.e. $p - p_A < 0$. Blood flows from the sheet into the venule BC, the junction C is thus a sluicing gate. A portion of the sheet around the terminal D of the venule BD is, however, closed. The vascular sheet thickness is zero in the shaded region, where there is no flow. The blood pressure at D is equal to that at B, whereas that at C is greater than that at B.

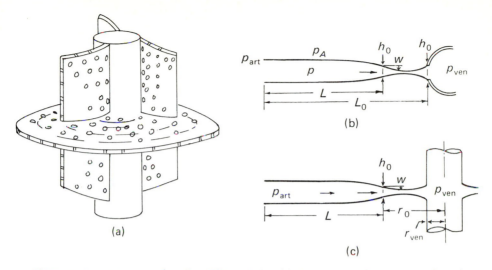

(a)

(b)

(c)

Figure 6.13:5 Schematic drawings of (a) relationship between a pulmonary venule and the neighboring capillary sheets, (b) a sluicing gate in the "one-dimensional" case, in which a sheet drains into a venule along an edge, (c) a sluicing gate in the case of a sheet draining axisymmetrically into a venule perpendicular to its plane.

$h = 0$ can be embedded in limited regions anywhere, as long as the boundary condition permits. Of course, to make the solution $h = 0$ possible the external pressure (p_A) must be greater than the internal pressure in the sheet. This in turn requires that $p_{ven} < p_A$. Figure 6.13:4 illustrates such a case.

Based on these observations, we may examine the sluicing condition mathematically. Figure 6.13:5(b) shows an idealized "one-dimensional" case. The sheet flow coming from the left has a pressure at the entry, p_{art}, greater than the alveolar gas pressure p_A. After flowing in a length L the pressure is so reduced that p becomes equal to p_A so that the sheet thickness becomes h_0. At the exit side the sheet is anchored in the venule which remains patent inspite of $p_{ven} < p_A$. We assume that the sheet thickness is h_0 at the exit section. In the membranous walls of the sheet there is a tensile stress resultant equal to T per unit length. If the membranes are curved, then the product of the tension and curvature is equipolent to a lateral pressure tending to distend the membranes. Let the curvature be denoted by $1/R$, R being the radius of curvature. Normally this term T/R is negligibly small compared with $p - p_A$. In the neighborhood of the sluicing gate, however, it may become significant. If we retain this term, then the sheet thickness—transmural pressure relationship, Eqs. (6.5:1a–d) should be modified by replacing $p - p_A$ by $p - p_A + T/R$. In the one-dimensional case shown in Fig. 6.13:5(b), with w representing the deflection of the wall from the plane $y = h_0/2$, $1/R$ is equal to d^2w/dx^2 if $(dw/dx)^2$ is negligible compared with 1. Hence, since

$$h = h_0 - 2w,$$

$$\frac{1}{R} = \frac{d^2 w}{dx^2} = -\frac{1}{2} \frac{d^2 h}{dx^2}. \tag{2}$$

The thickness–pressure relationship (6.5:1d),

$$h = h_0 + \frac{h_0}{\varepsilon}\left(p - p_A + \frac{T}{R}\right), \tag{3}$$

can be reduced to

$$\frac{T}{2} \frac{d^2 h}{dx^2} = p - p_A + \frac{(h_0 - h)\varepsilon}{h_0}. \tag{4}$$

For the cat, ε is approximately 0.5 cm H_2O. Combining this with the equation of motion (6.6:4),

$$\frac{dp}{dx} = -\frac{\mu k f U}{h^2}, \tag{5}$$

and the equation of continuity

$$hU = \text{const.} = \dot{Q}, \tag{6}$$

we obtain the basic equation,

$$\frac{T}{2} \frac{d^3 h}{dx^3} + \frac{\varepsilon}{h_0} \frac{dh}{dx} + \frac{\mu k f \dot{Q}}{h^3} = 0. \tag{7}$$

The boundary conditions are:

$$h|_{x=L} = h|_{x=L_0} = h_0, \quad \text{and} \quad (p - p_A)|_{x=L} = 0. \tag{8}$$

From these equations we can calculate the distribution of the blood pressure and the thickness distribution of the capillary sheet. The solution has been obtained by Zhuang (unpublished) by iterative numerical integration of the differential equations (4), (5) and (6). The tension T is evaluated by the method of Lee and Flicker (1973) to be 24.5 dyn/cm when $p_A - p_{PL} = 10$ cm H_2O. With the following constants pertaining to the cat,

$$\mu = 1.92 \text{ cp}, \quad k = 12, \quad h_0 = 4.28 \ \mu m, \quad f = 1.6,$$

$$\alpha = 0.219 \ \mu m/cm \ H_2O, \quad \beta = 8.56 \ \mu m/cm \ H_2O, \quad L = 556 \ \mu m,$$

we obtain the typical sluicing gate shape shown in Fig. 6.13:6(a). The flow is a function of p_{art}, p_{ven}, p_A, and p_{PL}.

In the case of axisymmetric draining of a sheet into a circular cylindrical venule as suggested by Fig. 6.13:5(c), we can show that in polar coordinates the equation of equilibrium becomes

$$\frac{T}{2} \frac{1}{r} \frac{d}{dr}\left(r \frac{dh}{dr}\right) = p - p_A + \frac{(h_0 - h)\varepsilon}{h_0}. \tag{9}$$

The term dp/dx in Eq. (5) should be replaced by dp/dr; and Eq. (6) becomes

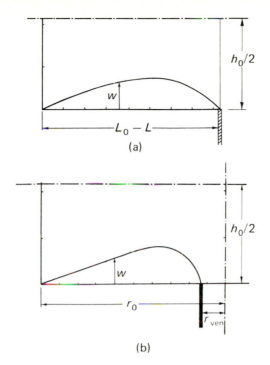

Figure 6.13:6 Theoretical solution of the sluicing gate equation, showing the sheet thickness distribution in the gate. The thickness is assumed to be h_0 at the venule which remains patent. The venule is located at the right hand side in the drawing. Only one-quarter of the cross section is shown. The vertical scale is much enlarged. (a) The "one-dimensional" case of a sheet draining into a venule along an edge, drawn for $h_0 = 4.28$ μm, $L_0 - L$ = the distance from the venular wall to the place where the transmural pressure, $p - p_A$, is zero, is 41.6 μm; $p_{art} = 10$ cm H_2O, $p_A = 0$, $p_{PL} = -20$ cm H_2O, and $hU = 0.836 \times 10^{-4}$ cm^2/sec. (b) The axisymmetric case of a sheet draining into a venule perpendicular to the sheet, drawn for $h_0 = 4.28$ μm, $r_0 = 100$ μm, $r_{ven} = 13$ μm, $p_{PL} = -20$ cm H_2O, $rhU = 0.474 \times 10^{-6}$ cm^3/sec.

$rhU =$ const. $= \dot{Q}$. In this case the solution gives the shape of the sluicing gate as shown in Fig. 6.13:6(b). The pressure–flow relationship is those shown in Fig. 6.13:7.

Patchy Flow in Zone 2 Condition

The solutions just shown and the solution $h = 0$ can co-exist, and together they make the flow condition in zone 2 nonunique. Wherever the solution $h = 0$ applies, there is no flow, and there will be no red blood cell in this region (as discussed in Sec. 5.6). The red cell distribution in the interalveolar septa will be "patchy", containing regions with cells and regions without. Experimental evidence that this does occur has been provided by Warrell et

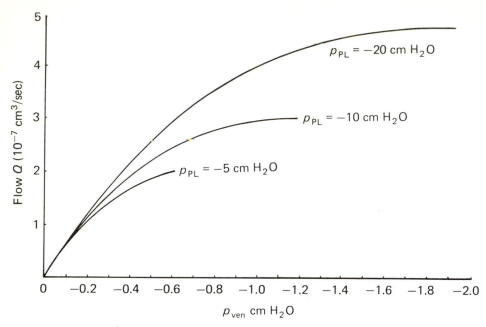

Figure 6.13:7 Theoretical relation between the rate of flow and the venular pressure. The flow depends on the tension in the alveolar wall, which in turn depends on the transpulmonary pressure $p_A - p_{PL}$. This example refers to a venule draining the capillary sheet axisymmetrically, with $p_A = 0$ (atmospheric), p_{PL} indicated in the figure, and the radial distance from the venular axis to the place where the transmural pressure $p - p_A$ is zero, r_0, equal to 100 μm.

al. (1972). Furthermore, for a given left atrium pressure the total flow will be decreased when the capillary sheets attached to some venules of order 1 collapse because the shutting off of flow in these venules causes the remaining venules of order 1 to take on a greater share of the flow, and consequently a higher pressure drop occurs, resulting in a higher p_{ven}, and lower $\dot{Q}$. Evidence of this exists also, see Fig. 6.13:8. In this figure the flow in the lung of a cat is plotted against the pressure in the left atrium while the pressure in the main pulmonary artery was fixed. It is seen that the flow reaches a peak when p_v approaches p_A, then $\dot{Q}$ decreases with further decrease in p_v. A hysteresis loop is clearly seen. An explanation is that the reopening of a collapsed sheet requires additional energy.

6.14 Distribution of Transit Time in the Lung

The length of time it takes for a red cell to go through the lung, i.e., the transit time, depends obviously on the path it takes in the lung. Since different cells take different paths, their transit times are not a constant, but

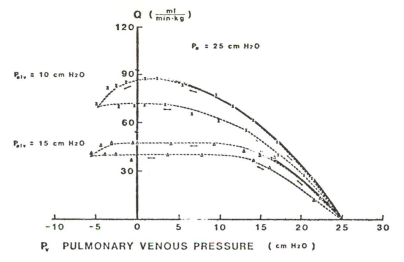

Figure 6.13:8 An experimental result on the relationship between blood flow and a variable pulmonary venous pressure (at the left atrium), p_v, in cat's lung, while the pressures in pulmonary artery (p_a), alveoli (p_{alv}), and pleura (p_{PL}) were fixed. Open chest cat's lung perfused with Macrodex (6% dextran 70 in normal saline) with a high dosage of a smooth muscle relaxing agent papaverine (1 mg/ml of macrodex) added. For this figure, $p_a = 25$ cm H_2O, $p_{alv} = 10$ or 15 cm H_2O, $p_{PL} = 0$. From Yen et al. (1983c), by permission.

vary from streamline to streamline. For a given lung, we speak of the transit time distribution in a manner exactly analogous to the statistical distribution of a random variable. If $f(t)$ is the frequency function of the transit time, then by definition $f(t)dt$ is equal to the fraction of the fluid that enters the lung whose transit time lies between t and $t + dt$.

Since the velocity distribution is given by the sheet-flow theory, we can derive a theoretical transit-time distribution for blood in the pulmonary alveoli. As an example, let us consider the case illustrated in Fig. 6.9:1, whose solution is given in Fig. 6.10:1. In this case, we have $h = $ constant, and the velocity along any streamline, $\psi = $ constant, is $\partial\psi/\partial n$, where n is the distance perpendicular to the streamline. Let s be the distance measured along the streamline, then the transit time, t, for a particle along that stream-line is

$$t = \int \frac{ds}{\text{velocity}} = \int \frac{ds}{\partial\psi/\partial n}. \tag{1}$$

If we consider two neighboring streamlines, $\psi = $ constant $= c$ and $\psi = c + \Delta\psi$, and let the distance between these two streamlines be Δn, then the transit time along these streamlines is

$$t_{\psi=c} \simeq \int_{\psi=c} \frac{\Delta n \, ds}{\Delta \psi} = \frac{1}{\Delta \psi} \int_{\psi=c} \Delta n \, ds \tag{2}$$

$$= \frac{\text{(area between the streamlines)}}{\Delta \psi}.$$

$\Delta \psi$ is by definition equal to the quantity of flow between the streamlines $\psi = c$ and $\psi = c + \Delta \psi$. Hence if we divide up the entire flow field by a succession of streamlines separated by a constant interval $\Delta \psi$ from each other, then Eq. (2) shows that the transit time of each streamtube is proportional to the area between successive streamlines. But if $f(t)$ is the frequency function of the transit time in the alveolar sheet, then $\Delta \psi = f(t) \Delta t$, and we can compute $f(t)$ by dividing through $\Delta \psi$ with $\Delta t = t_{\psi=c+\Delta\psi} - t_{\psi=c}$.

With these relations we can determine the frequency function for the present example as follows. The area between successive streamlines in the sheet shown in Fig. 6.10:1 is determined with a planimeter. Each of the streamtube contains 10% of the flow. The inverse of the difference of areas between successive streamlines is proportional to the frequency function. The result is shown by the histogram of Fig. 6.14:1, which can be represented approximately by the empirical formula

$$f(\tau) = \tfrac{1}{20}\delta(\tau - 1) + 1.678e^{-2(\tau-1)} + \tfrac{1}{45}e^{-0.2(\tau-1)} \tag{3}$$

for $\tau \geq 1$, while $f(\tau) = 0$ for $\tau < 1$. Here $\tau = $ (transit time)/(minimum transit time) and $\delta = $ unit impulse function. If we return to physical units with t in seconds and let $t_{\min}$ denote the minimum transit time, then

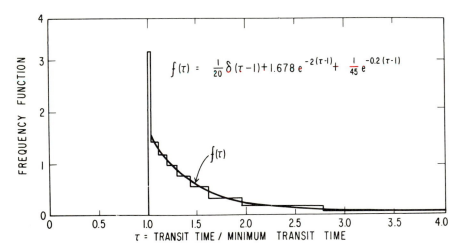

Figure 6.14:1 Theoretical transit time distribution for blood flow in an alveolar sheet illustrated in Fig. 6.9:3. Computation gives the histogram which is fitted by a curve $f(\tau)$. τ is the ratio of transit time to the minimum transit time through the sheet. Reproduced by permission from Fung and Sobin (1972b). © American Heart Association, Inc.

$$f(t) = \frac{1}{t_{min}} f(\tau) = \frac{1}{t_{min}} f\left(\frac{t}{t_{min}}\right). \tag{4}$$

The mean transit time, denoted by $\bar{t}$, is

$$\bar{t} = \int_0^\infty t f(t) dt = t_{min} \int_1^\infty \tau f(\tau) d\tau. \tag{5}$$

For the empirical formula given above, we have

$$\bar{t} = 1.475 t_{min}.$$

These formulas are derived from a sheet of uniform thickness. If the sheet thickness is variable, a stream function can be defined as in Eq. (6.10:1), so that

$$hU = \frac{\partial \psi}{\partial y}, \qquad hV = -\frac{\partial \psi}{\partial x}. \tag{6}$$

Then the transit time along a stream line, $\psi = c$, is given by

$$t = \int \frac{h \Delta n \, ds}{\Delta \psi}. \tag{7}$$

Thus for a field covered by streamlines spaced at constant $\Delta \psi$, the transit time in an individual stream tube is proportional to the volume of the tube. Since we have shown that the alveolar sheet remains quite uniform in thickness over a wide range of pressure, it is expected that the variation in thickness will not affect the frequency distribution function significantly.

We can relate the mean transit time to the physical parameters of the alveolar sheet. By a process entirely analogous to that employed in deriving equation (7) of Sec. 6:10, we obtain the mean velocity of flow in an alveolar sheet:

$$U = \frac{1}{3\mu k f \alpha \bar{L}} [h_a^3 - h_v^3], \tag{8}$$

where $\bar{L}$ is the mean path length of the streamlines between the arteriole and venule:

$$\frac{1}{\bar{L}} = \frac{1}{(\psi_2 - \psi_1)} \int_{\psi_1}^{\psi_2} \frac{1}{L(\psi)} dx. \tag{9}$$

Then

$$\bar{t} = \frac{\bar{L}}{U} = \frac{3\mu k f \alpha \bar{L}^2}{h_a^3 - h_v^3}. \tag{10}$$

It is obvious that $\bar{t}$ should be proportional to the coefficient of viscosity, μ, and the friction factor, f, and increase with increasing length of the path, $\bar{L}$; but the reason for $\bar{t}$ to depend directly on the square of the mean path length between the arteriole and venule, $\bar{L}^2$, and inversely on $h_a^3 - h_v^3 =$

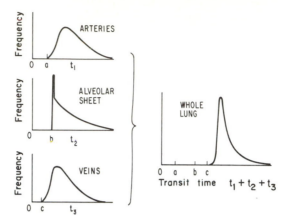

Figure 6.14:2 Convolution of transit times, t_1, t_2, and t_3, of blood in the pulmonary arteries, capillaries, and veins, respectively. Upper left: arterial; from Cumming et al. (1969). Middle left: capillary. Lower left: venous. Right hand side panel: result of convolution. Reproduced by permission from Fung and Sobin, (1972b).

$([h_0 + \alpha \Delta p_{art}]^3 - [h_0 + \alpha \Delta p_{ven}]^3)$, is more subtle, and requires some thinking for its assimilation.

For example, if we take the data of the dog, $\alpha = 0.122$ μm/cm H_2O or 0.122×10^{-3} μm/dyn, $h_0 = 2.5$ μm, $f = 1.8$, $k = 12$, $\bar{L} = 556$ μm (Sobin et al. 1980, for the cat), $p_{ven} = p_A = 0$ so that $h_v = h_0$, then the mean transit time in alveolar sheet is $\bar{t} = 1.89$ sec. when $p_{art} = 10$ cm H_2O, $\bar{t} = 0.811$ sec. when $p_{art} = 20$ cm H_2O. If we use $\bar{L} = 273$ μm according to Miyamoto and Moll (1971), then $\bar{t} = 0.455$ and 0.195 sec in these two cases, respectively.

Transit-Time Distribution in the Whole Lung

Cumming et al. (1969) have computed the transit-time distribution from morphological data of a human lung. Their result for a particle to pass from the pulmonary valve down to terminal branches of the order of 50 μm with a pulmonary blood flow of 80 ml/sec is sketched in the upper left corner of Fig. 6.14:2. Adding to this the transit time in the alveolar sheet and the veins, we can obtain the transit time through the entire lung. Since it is well known that the distribution function of the sum of several random variables is the convolution of the distribution functions of the individual variables, we see that if the transit times, t_1, t_2, and t_3, in the arteries, alveoli, and veins are distributed as shown in Fig. 6.14:2, the transit time in the whole lung from the pulmonary valve to the left atrium will be distributed as shown on the right hand side of the figure.

As an illustration of the mathematical procedure, consider the following case. Let the frequency functions for t_1, t_2, and t_3 be approximated by

$$f_1(t) = \frac{\alpha^3}{2}(t - a)^2 e^{-\alpha(t-a)} H(t - a),$$

$$f_2(t) = \varepsilon\delta(t - b) + (1 - \varepsilon)\beta e^{-\beta(t-b)} H(t - b), \tag{11}$$

$$f_3(t) = \frac{\gamma^3}{2}(t - c)^2 e^{-\gamma(t-a)} H(t - c),$$

where $H(t - a)$ is the unit-step function which equals 0 when $t < a$ and 1 when $t \geq a$. The characteristic function of $f_1(t)$ is*

$$\int_{-\infty}^{\infty} e^{ixt} f_1(t) dt = \frac{\alpha^3 e^{ixa}}{(\alpha - ix)^3}. \tag{12}$$

Similarly the characteristic function of f_2 and f_3 are, respectively,

$$f_2 = \varepsilon e^{ixb} + (1 - \varepsilon)\frac{\beta e^{ixb}}{(\beta - ix)} \quad \text{and} \quad f_3 = \frac{\gamma^3 e^{ixc}}{(\gamma - ix)^3}. \tag{13}$$

Since the frequency function of $t_1 + t_2 + t_3$ is the convolution $f_1 * f_2 * f_3$, the characteristic function of $t_1 + t_2 + t_3$ is the product of the three characteristic functions

$$\frac{\alpha^3\gamma^3 e^{ix(a+b+c)}}{(\alpha - ix)^3(\gamma - ix)^3}\left[\varepsilon + (1 - \varepsilon)\frac{\beta}{(\beta - ix)}\right]. \tag{14}$$

The frequency function of $t_1 + t_2 + t_3$ is the inverse Fourier transformation of the above. The calculation becomes very simple in the case $\alpha = \beta = \gamma$; then the frequency function of $t_1 + t_2 + t_3$ is

$$f(t) = \frac{\varepsilon\alpha^6}{5!}\tau^5 e^{-\alpha\tau} + (1 - \varepsilon)\frac{\alpha^7}{6!}\tau^6 e^{-\alpha\tau} \tag{15}$$

for $t \geq a + b + c$, while it is 0 for $t < a + b + c$, where

$$\tau = t - (a + b + c). \tag{16}$$

The frequency function Eq. (15) is more peaky than $f_1(t)$ and $f_2(t)$. The general case in which $\alpha \neq \beta \neq \gamma$ can be resolved by using partial fractions.

The frequency function of transit times through the lung can be measured by the indicator-dilution method. Tancredi and Zierler (1971) reported that at a given p_{alv} and p_{LA} a family of the density functions of transit times can be transformed to a nearly coincident function, $f(t/\bar{t})$ as described in

---

* See, for example, Cramer (1946) p. 235. The f_1, f_2, and f_3 are the famous χ^2 distributions of degrees of freedom 6, 2, and 6, respectively. The resultant of convolution of the functions given in equation (11) is a sum of two χ^2 distributions of degrees of freedom 12 and 14. These functions are tabulated.

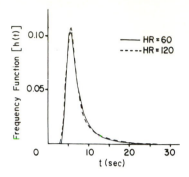

Figure 6.14:3 The frequency function, $h(t)$, of transit times in pulmonary circulation in open-chest dogs at constant cardiac output and left atrial pressure, showing the lack of effect of heart rate. Reproduced by permission from Maseri et al. (1970). © American Heart Association, Inc.

our Eq. (4). Figure 6.14:3 shows a frequency function of transit times through the whole pulmonary circulation from pulmonary artery to left atrium, obtained by Maseri et al. (1970) for the dog. Its general form is in agreement with the theoretic curve. Among other things it shows that the frequency function is not affected by heart rate or by the presence or absence of respiratory movements.

6.15 Other Investigations

Pulmonary Blood Volume

By integrating the sheet thickness over the sheet area, we obtain the vascular volume. The features shown in Fig. 6.9:1 and the discussion in Sec. 6.9 suggest that the alveolar blood volume would be directly related to the pulmonary arterial pressure, whereas the pulmonary venous pressure would have only a minor effect, because any decrease in sheet thickness due to a lowering of p_{ven} is localized to the immediate neighborhood of the venule.

A theoretically predicted pulmonary capillary blood volume as a function of p_{art}, p_{ven}, and p_{alv} is shown in the left-hand panel of Fig. 6.15:1 with the constants and geometry pertinent to dog's lung. It is seen that the blood volume varies almost linearly with $p_{art} - p_{alv}$, whereas very little effect is shown by $p_{ven} - p_{alv}$. This result may be compared with the experimental results of Permutt et al. (1969), which are shown on the right-hand side of the figure. The pulmonary blood volume shown here, however, is the total pulmonary blood volume obtained by the indicator-dilution method, not merely the capillary blood volume. But the related work of Permutt et al. (1969) on the steady-state carbon-monoxide diffusing capacity, which is proportional to the capillary blood volume, shows the same trend.

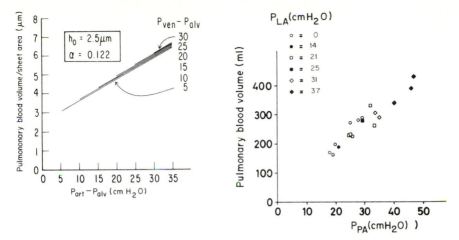

Figure 6.15:1 *Left:* Theoretical relationship between the pulmonary alveolar blood volume and the arterial and venous pressures. Ordinate is the pulmonary blood volume per unit area of the sheet. Abscissa is the transmembrane pressure at the arteriole end of the sheet. The transmembrane pressure at the venule end is seen to have only a minor effect on the blood volume. Data correspond to Fig. 4 of Fung and Sobin (1972*b*). *Right:* Experimental results showing the relationship between pulmonary blood volume and pulmonary artery pressure in one dog at a variety of left atrial pressures. From Permutt et al. (1969). Reprinted by permission.

Pulsatile Blood Flow in the Lung

A typical set of records of pulmonary pressures and flows in a conscious dog is shown in Fig. 6.15:2. In the large pulmonary arteries and veins the Reynolds and Womersley numbers are much larger than 1, and the premises assumed in Chap. 3 apply. Hence the general method of pulse waves analysis presented in Chap. 3 can be used. Extensive theoretical and experimental studies have been reported by Bergel and Milnor (1965), Wiener et al. (1966), Skalak (1969), Pollack et al. (1968), Milnor (1972) and others.

For blood flow in pulmonary capillaries, the Reynolds and Womersley numbers are much smaller than 1, so that the inertial forces are much smaller than the forces from pressure and viscous stresses. Hence the equation of motion of the blood in the capillaries is the same as if the flow were steady. But the balance of mass is described by Eq. (7) of Sec. 6.7, which depends on the rate of change of sheet thickness $\partial h/\partial t$. The basic equation of sheet flow, Eq. (20) of Sec. 6.7, involves the time-derivative $\partial h/\partial t$, and is not quasi-steady. If permeability of water across the endothelium can be neglected, the basic equation is

$$\left(\frac{\partial^2}{\partial x^2} + \frac{\partial^2}{\partial y^2}\right) h^4 = 4\mu k f \alpha \frac{\partial h}{\partial t}. \tag{1}$$

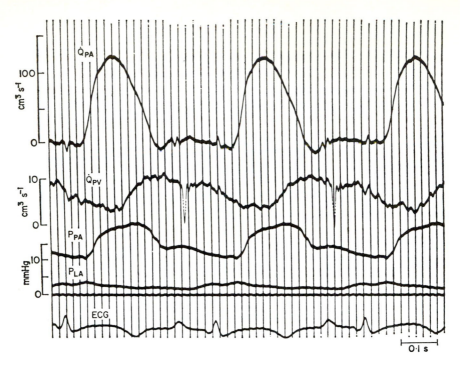

Figure 6.15:2 Experimental records of pulmonary pressures and flows in a conscious dog, at rest. Symbols: Q, blood flow; P, pressure; PA, pulmonary artery; PV, pulmonary vein, within 2 cm of the left atrium; LA, left atrium; ECG, electrocardiogram, lead I. Sharp downward spikes in the pulmonary venous flow tracing and smaller spikes in the pulmonary arterial flow during diastole are electrocardiographic signals. Timing lines appear at intervals of 0-02 s. From Milnor (1972). Reproduced by permission.

This is a nonlinear differential equation and does not have a harmonic solution with respect to time. Hence, strictly speaking, the usual concept of impedance does not apply. Only in small perturbations can the basic equations be linearized and the concept of impedance be useful. Linearization can be justified if and only if the amplitude of the thickness fluctuations is small compared with the mean pulmonary alveolar sheet thickness. This condition is met if the amplitude of the pressure oscillation is small compared with the mean pulmonary arterial pressure. Under this restriction, the solution of Eq. (1) may be set in the following form:

$$h(x, y, t) = h_{SI}(x, y) + e^{i\omega t} H(x, y). \tag{2}$$

We assume $H(x, y)$ to be much smaller than $h_{SI}(x, y)$, which is the solution of the equation for a steady flow between impervious walls:

$$\left(\frac{\partial^2}{\partial x^2} + \frac{\partial^2}{\partial y^2}\right) h_{SI}^4 = 0. \tag{3}$$

Equation (3) has been treated in Sections 6.8–6.10. The subscripts SI stand for steady and impervious. Substituting Eq. (2) into Eq. (1) and retaining only the first powers of H, we obtain the basic equation,

$$\left(\frac{\partial^2}{\partial x^2} + \frac{\partial^2}{\partial y^2}\right) h_{\text{SI}}^3 H = \mu k f \alpha \omega i H. \tag{4}$$

Similar to Eq. (2) the pressure and flow per unit width (with components q_x, q_y) can also be represented as the sum of the steady-impervious terms and the oscillatory terms

$$p(x, y, t) = p_{\text{SI}}(x, y) + e^{i\omega t} P(x, y),$$
$$q_x(x, y, t) = Uh = q_{x\text{SI}}(x, y) + e^{i\omega t} Q_x(x, y), \tag{5}$$
$$q_y(x, y, t) = Vh = q_{y\text{SI}}(x, y) + e^{i\omega t} Q_y(x, y).$$

We introduce the dimensionless frequency parameter:

$$\Omega = \mu k f \alpha \omega L^2 / h_0^3 \tag{6}$$

where L is the length of the sheet, and h_0 is the sheet thickness as the transmural pressure tends to zero from positive values. Blood enters each sheet at the arteriole and exits at the venule. Let the oscillatory pressure and flow at the arteriolar and venular edges of the sheet be denoted by P_a, Q_a, P_v, Q_v, respectively. The relationship between these quantities can be expressed in the following matrix form:

$$\begin{Bmatrix} P_a \\ P_v \end{Bmatrix} = \begin{Bmatrix} Z_{11} Z_{12} \\ Z_{21} Z_{22} \end{Bmatrix} \begin{Bmatrix} Q_a \\ Q_v \end{Bmatrix}, \tag{7}$$

$$\begin{Bmatrix} Q_a \\ Q_v \end{Bmatrix} = \begin{Bmatrix} Y_{11} Y_{12} \\ Y_{21} Y_{22} \end{Bmatrix} \begin{Bmatrix} P_a \\ P_v \end{Bmatrix}, \tag{8}$$

$$\begin{Bmatrix} P_a \\ Q_a \end{Bmatrix} = \begin{Bmatrix} A_{11} A_{12} \\ A_{21} A_{22} \end{Bmatrix} \begin{Bmatrix} P_v \\ Q_v \end{Bmatrix}. \tag{9}$$

With P as the analog of voltage and Q the analog of current, we can use the terminology of the "four-terminal" network theory and call the Z_{ij} impedances, the Y_{ij} conductances, and the A_{ij} the elements of a transfer matrix (i, $j = 1$ and 2). For example, $Z_{11} = P_a/Q_a$ when $Q_v = 0$; hence it is the impedance between the arterial pressure and arterial flow when oscillation in venous flow is eliminated. $Z_{12} = P_a/Q_v$ when $Q_a = 0$; hence it is the transfer impedance between arterial pressure and venous flow when there is no fluctuation in arterial flow. Other coefficients can be similarly interpreted. The A matrix is the most useful, because with it the capillary network can be inserted between arteries and veins and thus completing the circuit.

Further details and extension to three-dimensional cases are presented in Fung (1972).

Fluid Movement in the Interstitial Space of the Pulmonary Alveolar Sheet

The basic equation of sheet flow, Eq. (19) of Sec. 6.7, takes into account the permeability of the endothelium and the exchange of fluid between the vascular and tissue spaces. To deal with the problem of pulmonary edema in the interstitium or alveoli, it is necessary to solve this equation. The solution forms part of the general theory of fluid movement in the tissue space treated in Chapter 2 of the companion volume, *Biodynamics: Flow, Motion, and Stress* (Fung, 1984).

The subject of lung water and solute exchange has an extensive literature, see reviews in Fishman (1972), Fishman and Hecht (1968), Giuntini (1970), Staub et al. (1967), Staub (1978). Compared with tissue space in other organs, the interstitium of the pulmonary alveolar sheets has the unique feature that its volume is considerably smaller than that of the vascular space. The solution of Eq. (6.7:19) is presented by Fung (1974), and the results corroborate well with the observations of Staub et al. (1967), Schultz (1959) and Guyton and Lindsey (1959).

References

In addition to the references cited in the text, the following books may be consulted:

Daly and Hebb (1966), Fishman (1963), Fishman and Hecht (1968), Folkow and Neil (1971), Giuntini (1970), Nagaishi (1972) von Hayek (1960), West (1974, 1977).

Much of the material presented in this chapter is taken from the papers by the author and Dr. Sobin, especially Fung and Sobin (1977, a, b).

Banister, J. and Torrance, R. W. (1960). The effects of the tracheal pressure upon flow: Pressure relations in the vascular bed of isolated lungs. *Q. J. Exp. Physiol.* **45**: 352–367.

Benjamin, J. J., Murtagh, P. S., Proctor, D. F., Menkes, H. A. and Permutt, S. (1974). Pulmonary vascular interdependence in excised dog lobes. *J. Appl. Physiol.* **37**: 887–894.

Bergel, D. H. and Milnor, W. R. (1965). Pulmonary vascular impedance in the dog. *Circ. Res.* **16**: 401–415.

Bhattacharya, J. and Staub, N. C. (1980). Direct measurement of microvascular pressure in the isolated, perfused dog lung. *Science* **210**: 327–328.

Bhattacharya, J., Overholser, K., Gropper, M. and Staub, N. C. (1982). Comparison of pressures measured by micropuncture and venous occulsion in Zones III and II of the isolated dog lung. *Federation Proc.* **41**: 1685. (Abstract).

Brody, J. S., Stemmler, E. J. and duBois, A. B. (1968). Longitudinal distribution of vascular resistance in the pulmonary arteries, capillaries, and veins. *J. Clin. Invest.* **47**: 783–784.

Bruderman, I., Somers, K., Hamilton, W. K., Tooley, W. H. and Butler, J. (1964). Effect of surface tension on circulation in the excised lungs of dogs. *J. Appl. Physiol.* **19**: 707–712.

Caro, C. G., Harrison, G. K. and Mognoni, P. (1967). Pressure wave transmission in the human pulmonary circulation. *Clin. Sci.* **23**: 317–329.

Cramer, H. (1946). *Mathematical Method of Statistics*, Princeton University Press, Princeton, N.J.

Cumming, G., Henderson, R., Horsfield, K. and Singhal, S. S. (1969). The functional morphology of the pulmonary circulation. In *the Pulmonary Circulation and Interstitial Space*. (A. P. Fishman and H. H. Hecht, eds.) Univ. of Chicago Press, Chicago, IL, pp. 327–338.

Daly, I. de B., and Hebb, C. (1966). *Pulmonary and Bronchial Vascular Systems*. Williams & Wilkins, Co.

Dawson, S. V. and Elliott, E. A. (1977). Wave-speed limitation on expiratory flow—a unifying concept. *J. Appl. Physiol.* **43**(3): 398–515.

De Bono, E. F. and Caro, C. G. (1963). Effect of lung inflation pressure on pulmonary blood pressure and flow. *Amer. J. Physiol.* **205**: 1178–1186.

Fishman, A. P. (1963). Dynamics of the pulmonary circulation. In *Handbook of Physiology*, Sec. 2. *Circulation*, Vol. II (W. H. Hamilton and P. Dow, eds.). Amer. Physiol. Soc., Washington, D.C. pp. 1667–1743.

Fishman, A. P. (1972). Pulmonary edema: The water exchange function of the lung. *Circulation*. **46**: 390–408.

Fishman, A. P. and Hecht, H. H. (eds.) (1968). *The Pulmonary Circulation and Interstitial Space*. Univ. of Chicago Press, Chicago, IL.

Folkow, G. and Neil, E. (1971). *Circulation*. Oxford Univ. Press, New York.

Fung, Y. C. (1969). Studies on the blood flow in the lung. In *Proceedings of the Second Canadian Congress of Applied Mechanics*, Waterloo, Canada, pp. 433–545.

Fung, Y. C. (1972). Theoretical pulmonary microvascular impedance. *Annals of Biomedical Eng.* **1**: 221–245.

Fung, Y. C. (1974). Fluid in the interstitial space of the pulmonary alveolar sheet. *Microvas. Res.* **7**: 89–113.

Fung, Y. C. (1981). *Biomechanics: Mechanical Properties of Living Tissues*. Springer-Verlag, New York.

Fung, Y. C. (1984). *Biodynamics: Flow, Motion, and Stress*. Springer-Verlag, New York. In press.

Fung, Y. C. and Sobin, S. S. (1969). Theory of sheet flow in lung alveoli. *J. Appl. Physiol.* **26**(4): 472–488.

Fung, Y. C. and Sobin, S. S. (1972a). Elasticity of the pulmonary alveolar sheet. *Circ. Res.* **30**: 451–469.

Fung, Y. C. and Sobin, S. S. (1972b). Pulmonary alveolar blood flow. *Circ. Res.* **30**: 470–490.

Fung, Y. C. and Sobin S. S. (1977a). Pulmonary alveolar blood flow. In *Bioengineering Aspects of Lung Biology* (J. B. West, ed.) Marcel Dekker, New York, pp. 267–358.

Fung, Y. C. and Sobin, S. S. (1977b). Mechanics of pulmonary circulation. In *Cardiovascular Flow Dynamics and Measurements*. (N. H. C. Hwang and N. A. Norman, eds.) University Park Press, Baltimore, MD, pp. 665–730.

Fung, Y. C., Sobin, S. S., Tremer, H., Yen, M. R. T. and Ho, H. H. (1983). Patency and compliance of pulmonary veins when airway pressure exceeds blood pressure. *J. Appl. Physiol. Resp. Envir. and Exer. Phy.* **54**: 1538–1549.

Gaar, K. A. Jr., Taylor, A. E., Owens, L. J. and Guyton, A. C. (1967). Pulmonary capillary pressure and filtration coefficient in the isolated perfused lung. *Am. J. Physiol.* **213**: 910–914.

Giuntini, C. (ed.) (1970). *Central Hemodynamics and Gas Exchange*. Minerva Medica, Torino, Italy.

Glazier, J. B., Hughes, J. M. B., Maloney, J. E. and West, J. B. (1969). Measurements of capillary dimensions and blood volume in rapidly frozen lungs. *J. Appl. Physiol.* **26**: 65–76.

Guyton, A. C. and Lindsey, A. W. (1959). Effect of elevated left atrial pressure and decreased plasma protein concentration on the development of pulmonary edema. *Circ. Res.* **7**: 649–657.

Hakim, T. S., Michel, R. P. and Chang, H. K. (1982). Partition of pulmonary vascular resistance in dog by arterial and venous occulsion. *J. Appl. Physiol.: Respirat. Environ. Exercise Physiol.* **52**: 710–715.

Horsfield, K. (1978). Morphometry of the small pulmonary arteries in man. *Circ. Res.* **42**: 593–597.

Hughes, J. M. B., Glazier, J. B., Maloney, J. E. and West, J. B. (1968). Effect of extra-alveolar vessels on distribution of blood flow in the dog lung. *J. Appl. Physiol.* **25**: 701–712.

Johnson, R. L., Jr., Spicer, W. S., Bishop, J. M. and Forster, R. E. (1960). Pulmonary capillary blood volume, flow and diffusing capacity during exercise. *J. Appl. Physiol.* **15**: 893–902.

Krahl, V. E. (1964). Anatomy of mammalian lung. In *Handbook of Physiology*. (W. O. Fenn & H. Rahn, eds.) Sec. 3, *Respiration*, Vol. 1, Amer. Physiology Society, Washington, D.C. pp. 213–284.

Lai-Fook, S. J. (1979). A continuum mechanics analysis of pulmonary vascular inter-dependence in isolated dog lobes, *J. Appl. Physiol. Respirat. Environ., Exercise Physiol.* **46**: 419–429.

Lee. J. S. (1969). Slow viscous flow in a lung alveoli model. *J. Biomech.* **2**: 187–198.

Lee, J. S. and Fung, Y. C. (1968). Experiments on blood flow in lung alveoli models. Paper No. 68-WA/BHF-2, American Society of Mech. Engineers. pp. 1–8.

Lloyd. T. C., Jr. (1967). Analysis of the relation of pulmonary arterial or airway conductance to lung volume, *J. Appl. Physiol.* **23**: 887–894.

Maloney, J. E., and Castle, B. L. (1969). Pressure-diameter relations of capillaries and small blood vessels in frog lung. *Respiration Physiology* **7**: 150–162.

Maseri, A., Caldini, P., Permutt, S. and Zierler, K. L. (1970). Frequency function of transit times through dog pulmonary circulation. *Circ. Res.* **26**: 527–543.

Miller, W. S. (1947). *The Lung*. Thomas, Springfield, IL.

Milnor, W. R. (1972). Pulmonary hemodynamics. In *Cardiovascular Fluid Dynamics*, (D. H. Bergel, ed.) Vol. 2, Academic Press, New York, Ch. 18, pp. 299–340.

Milnor, W. R., Bergel, D. H., and Bargainer, J. D. (1966). Hydraulic power associated with pulmonary blood flow and its relation to heart rate. *Circ. Res.* **19**: 467–480.

Milnor, W. R., Conti, C. R., Lewis, K. B. and O'Rourke, M. F. (1969). Pulmonary arterial pulse wave velocity and impedance in man. *Circ. Res.* **25**: 637–649.

Miyamoto, Y., and Moll, W. A. (1971). Measurements of dimensions and pathway of red blood cells in rapidly frozen lungs *in situ*. *Respir. Physiol.* **12**: 141–156.

Nagaishi, C. (1972). *Functional Anatomy and Histology of the Lung*. University Park Press, Baltimore, MD.

Patel, D. J., de Freitas, F. M. and Fry, D. L. (1963). Hydraulic input impedance to aorta and pulmonary artery in dogs. *J. Appl. Physiol.* **18**: 134–140.

Permutt, S., Bromberger-Barnea, B., and Bane, H. N. (1962). Alveolar pressure, pulmonary venous pressure, and the vascular waterfall. *Med. Thorac.* **19**: 239–260.

Permutt, S. and Riley, R. L. (1963). Hemodynamics of collapsible vessels with tone: the vascular waterfall. *J. Appl. Physiol.* **18**: 924–932.

Permutt, S., Caldini, P., Maseri, A., Palmer, W. H., Sasamori. T. and Zierler, K. (1969). Recruitment versus distensibility in the pulmonary vascular bed. In *The Pulmonary Circulation and Interstitial Space*. (A. P. Fishman and H. H. Hecht, eds.) Univ. of Chicago Press, Chicago, IL, pp. 375–387.

Pollack, G. H., Reddy, R. V. and Noordergraaf, A. (1968). Input impedance, wave travel, and reflections in the human pulmonary arterial tree: studies using an electrical analog. *IEEE Trans. Biomedical Eng.* **BME-15**, 151–164.

Purday, H. F. P. (1949). *An Introduction to the Mechanics of Viscous Flow*. Dover, New York, pp. 16–18.

Roos, A., Thomas, L. J., Jr., Nagel, E. L. and Prommas, D. C. (1961). Pulmonary vascular resistance as determined by lung inflation and vascular pressures. *J. Appl. Physiol.* **16**: 77–84.

Rosenquist, T. H., Bernick, S., Sobin, S. S. and Fung, Y. C. (1973). The structure of the pulmonary interalveolar microvascular sheet. *Microvascular Res.* **5**: 199–212.

Schultz, H. (1959). *The Submiscroscopic Anatomy and Pathology of the Lung*. Springer-Verlag, Berlin.

Singhal, S., Henderson, R., Horsfield, K., Harding, K. and Cumming, G. (1973). Morphometry of the human pulmonary arterial tree. *Circ. Res.* **33**: 190–197.

Skalak, R. (1969). Wave propagation in the pulmonary circulation. In *The Pulmonary Circulation and Interstitial Space*. (A. P. Fishman and H. H. Hecht, eds.) Univ. of Chicago Press, Chicago, IL, pp. 361–373.

Skalak, R., Wiener, F., Morkin, E. and Fishman, A. P. (1966). The energy distribution in the pulmonary circulation. Part I. Theory. *Phys. Med. Biol.* **11**(2): 287–294; Part II: Experiments, *ibid* **11**(3): 437–449.

Smith, J. C. and Mitzner, W. (1980). Analysis of pulmonary vascular interdependence in excised dog lobes. *J. Appl. Physiol: Respirat. Envir. Exercise. Physiol.* **48**(3): 450–467.

Sobin, S. S. and Tremer, H. M. (1966). Functional geometry of the microcirculation. *Federation Proceedings* **15**: 1744–1752.

Sobin, S. S., Tremer, H. M. and Fung, Y. C. (1970). The morphometric basis of the sheet-flow concept of the pulmonary alveolar microcirculation in the cat. *Circulation Res.* **26**: 397–414.

Sobin, S. S., Fung, Y. C., Tremer, H. M., and Rosenquist, T. H. (1972). Elasticity of the pulmonary alveolar microvascular sheet in the cat. *Circulation Res.* **30**: 440–450.

Sobin, S. S., Lindal, R. G. and Bernick, S. (1977). The pulmonary arteriole. *Microvas. Res.* **14**: 227–239.

Sobin, S. S., Lindal, R. G., Fung, Y. C. and Tremer, H. M. (1978). Elasticity of the smallest noncapillary pulmonary blood vessels in the cat. *Microvas. Res.* **15**: 57–68.

Sobin, S. S., Fung, Y. C., Lindal, R. G., Tremer, H. M. and Clark, L. (1980). Topology of pulmonary arterioles, capillaries, and venules in the cat. *Microvas. Res.* **19**: 217–233.

Sobin, S. S., Fung, Y. C. and Tremer, H. M. (1982). The effect of incomplete fixation of elastin on the appearance of pulmonary alveoli. *J. Biomechanical Eng.* **104**: 68–71.

Starling, E. H. (1915). *The Linacre lecture on the law of the heart, given at Cambridge, 1915.* Longmans, Green & Co., London, 1918. In *Starling on The Heart.* (C. B. Chapman and J. H. Mitchell, eds.) facs. reprints; Dawson, London, 1965, pp. 119–147.

Staub, N. C. (ed.) (1978). *Lung Water and Solute Exchange.* Marcel Dekker, New York.

Staub, N. C., Nagano, H. and Pearce, M. L. (1967). Pulmonary edema in dogs, especially the sequence of fluid accumulation in lungs. *J. Appl. Physiol.* **22**: 227–240.

Staub. N. C. and Schultz, E. L. (1968). Pulmonary capillary length in dog, cat, and rabbit. *J. Appl. Physiol.* **5**: 371–378.

Tancredi, R. and Zierler, K. L. (1971). Indicator-dilution, flow-pressure and volume-pressure curves in excised dog lung. *Fed. Proc.* **30**: 380 (Abstract).

von Hayek, H. (1960). *The Human Lung.* Hefner, New York.

Wagner, W. W., Jr., Latham, L. P., Gillespie, M. N. and Guenther, J. P. (1982). Direct measurement of pulmonary capillary transit times. *Science* **218**: 279–381.

Warrell, D. A., Evans, J. W., Clarke, R. O., Kingaby, G. P., and West, J. B. (1972). Pattern of filling in the pulmonary capillary bed. *J. Appl. Physiol.* **32**: 346–356.

Weibel, E. R. (1963). *Morphometry of the Human Lung.* Academic Press, New York.

Weibel, E. R. (1973). Morphological basis of alveolar-capillary gas exchange. *Physiol. Res.* **53**: 419–495.

Weiner, D. E., Verrier, R. L., Miller, D. T. and Lefer, A. M. (1967). Effect of adrenalectomy on hemodynamics and regional blood flow in the cat. *Am. J. Physiol.* **213**: 473–476.

West, J. B. (1974). *Respiratory Physiology—the Essentials.* Williams & Wilkins, Baltimore, MD.

West, J. B. (1977). *Regional Differences in the Lung.* Academic Press, New York.

West, J. B. (ed.) (1977) *Bioengineering Aspects of the Lung*, Marcel Dekker, New York.

West, J. B., Dollery, C. T. and Naimark, A. (1964). Distribution of blood in isolated lung: relation to vascular and alveolar pressure. *J. Appl. Physiol.* **19**: 713–724.

West, J. B. and Dollery, C. T. (1965). Distribution of blood flow and the pressure-flow relations of the whole lung. *J. Appl. Physiol.* **20**: 175–183.

West, J. B., Dollery, C. T., Matthews, C. M. E. and Zardini, P. (1965). Distribution of blood flow and ventilation in saline-filled lung. *J. Appl. Physiol.* **20**: 1107–1117.

Wiener, F., Morkin, E., Skalak, R. and Fishman, A. P. (1966). Wave propagation in the pulmonary circulation. *Circ. Res.* **19**: 834–850.

Yen, M. R. T. and Fung, Y. C. (1973). Model experiments on apparent blood viscosity and hematocrit in pulmonary alveoli. *J. Appl. Physiol.* **35**: 510–517.

Yen, M. R. T., Fung, Y. C. and Bingham, N. (1980). Elasticity of small pulmonary arteries in the cat. *J. Biomech. Eng., Trans. ASME* **102**: 170–177.

Yen, M. R. T. and Foppiano, L. (1981). Elasticity of small pulmonary veins in the cat. *J. Biomech. Eng., Trans. ASME* **103**: 38–42.

Yen, R. T., Zhuang, F. Y., Fung, Y. C. Ho, H. H., Tremer, H. and Sobin, S. S. (1983a). Morphometry of the cat's pulmonary venous tree. *J. Appl. Physiol.: Respirat. Environ. Exercise Physiol.* **55**: 236–242.

Yen, R. T., Zhuang, F. Y., Fung, Y. C., Ho, H. H. and Sobin, S. S. (1983b). Morphometry of the cat's pulmonary arteries. *J. Biomech. Eng.* In press.

Yen, R. T., Fung, Y. C., Zhuang, F. Y., and Zeng, Y. J. (1983c) "Comparison of theory and experiments of blood flow in cat's lung". Paper presented at the *First China–Japan–USA Conference on Biomechanics*, held in Wuhan, on May 9–13, 1983. To appear in a forthcoming book *Biomechanics in China, Japan, and USA*, Chinese Scientific Press., Beijing, China.

Zhuang, F. Y., Fung, Y. C., and Yen, R. T. (1983a). Analysis of blood flow in cat's lung with detailed anatomical and elasticity data. *J. Appl. Physiol.: Respirat. Environ. Exercise Physiol.* **55**: 1341–1348.

Zhuang, F. Y., Yen, M. R. T., Fung, Y. C. and Sobin, S. S. (1983b). How many pulmonary alveoli are supplied (drained) by an arteriole (venule)? *Microvas. Res.* In press.

Basic Field Equations

A.1 Introduction

In this appendix we list the basic equations of mechanics. We present these equations in order to exhibit the mathematical expressions of the basic laws of physics (conservation of mass, momentum, and energy) and to show the notations used in this book.

How easily the material presented here will be assimilated depends on the background of the reader. For some, a quick glance will be sufficient. For others, some hard study and further reading will be necessary. The author's book, *A First Course in Continuum Mechanics* (Fung, 1977), is one of the shortest and most convenient references for this purpose. Other larger treatises are listed at the end of this appendix.

The mechanical properties of materials are expressed in *constitutive equations*. The constitutive equations of biological materials are discussed in the author's book, *Biomechanics: Mechanical Properties of Living Tissues* (Fung, 1981). They are often quoted below without discussion.

A.2 Conservation of Mass and Momentum

Let us consider the motion of a solid or a fluid. Let x_1, x_2, x_3 or x, y, z be rectangular Cartesian coordinates. Let the velocity components along the x-, y-, z-axis directions be denoted by v_1, v_2, v_3 or u, v, w, respectively. Let p denote pressure, and σ_{ij} or (σ_{xx}, σ_{yy}, σ_{zz}, σ_{xy}, σ_{yx}, σ_{zz}) be the stress components. Throughout this book the index notation will be used. Unless stated otherwise, all indices will range over 1, 2, 3. The summation convention will be used: repetition of an index means summation over 1, 2, 3.

The basic equations of mechanics consist of the equation of continuity which expresses the law of conservation of mass, the equation of motion which expresses the law of conservation of momentum, the equation of balance of energy, and the constitutive equation and boundary conditions. A general derivation of the conservation equations is given in the author's *First Course*, (Fung, 1977, Chap. 10). This derivation makes use of the Gauss theorem and the concept of "material" derivatives. The Gauss theorem states that

$$\int_V \frac{\partial A}{\partial x_i} dV = \int_S A v_i dS \qquad (i = 1, 2, 3), \qquad (A.2:1)$$

where A is a quantity (a scalar, a vector, or a tensor) continuously differentiable in a convex region V which is bounded by a surface S that consists of a finite number of parts whose outer normals v_i form a continuous vector field. v_i is unit normal vector of S.

To discuss the concept of "material" derivative, consider

$$I(t) = \int_V A(\mathbf{x}, t) dV, \qquad (A.2:2)$$

where $A(\mathbf{x}, t)$ is a continuously differentiable function of spatial coordinates $\mathbf{x}(x_1, x_2, x_3)$ and time t, V is a regular region as defined above, occupied by a given set of material particles. The integration is extended over a given set of particles, so that when time changes and the particles change their position, the spatial region V changes with them. The rate at which $I(t)$ changes with respect to t is defined as the *material derivative of I* and is denoted by DI/Dt:

$$\frac{DI}{Dt} = \lim_{dt \to 0} \frac{1}{dt} \left[\int_{V'} A(\mathbf{x}, t + dt) dV - \int_V A(\mathbf{x}, t) dV \right], \qquad (A.2:3)$$

where V' is the volume occupied by the same set of particles at time $t + dt$. It is shown in *First Course* (Fung, 1977, p. 249) that

$$\frac{D}{Dt} \int_V A dV = \int_V \frac{\partial A}{\partial t} dV + \int A v_j v_j dS$$

$$= \int_V \left(\frac{\partial A}{\partial t} + v_j \frac{\partial A}{\partial x_j} + A \frac{\partial v_j}{\partial x_j} \right) dV \qquad (A.2:4)$$

$$= \int_V \left(\frac{DA}{Dt} + A \frac{\partial v_j}{\partial x_j} \right) dV,$$

where

$$\frac{DA}{Dt} = \left(\frac{\partial A}{\partial t} \right)_{\mathbf{x} = \text{const.}} + v_1 \frac{\partial A}{\partial x_1} + v_2 \frac{\partial A}{\partial x_2} + v_3 \frac{\partial A}{\partial x_3}, \qquad (A.2:5)$$

is the *material derivative of A*; i.e., the rate at which the quantity A associated with a particle is seen changing as the particle moves about in a velocity field. v_i is the velocity field, of course.

If A in the equation above is the velocity vector with components u, v, w, then DA/Dt is the acceleration vector, and $\partial A/\partial t$ is the transient acceleration, whereas the last three terms in Eq. (A.2:5) are the convective acceleration. Thus, the components of transient acceleration are

$$\frac{\partial u}{\partial t}, \quad \frac{\partial v}{\partial t}, \quad \frac{\partial w}{\partial t};$$

whereas the three components of the convective acceleration are

$$u\frac{\partial u}{\partial x} + v\frac{\partial u}{\partial y} + w\frac{\partial u}{\partial z}, \quad u\frac{\partial v}{\partial x} + v\frac{\partial v}{\partial y} + w\frac{\partial v}{\partial z}, \quad u\frac{\partial w}{\partial x} + v\frac{\partial w}{\partial y} + w\frac{\partial w}{\partial z}.$$

Now, consider the mass contained in a region V:

$$m = \int_V \rho dV. \tag{A.2:6}$$

Refer to Eq. (A.2:2). Iedntify A with ρ and I with m. The law of conservation of mass states that $Dm/Dt = 0$. Applying Eq. (A.2:4) we obtain the following *equation of continuity*, which expresses the law of conservation of mass:

$$\frac{\partial \rho}{\partial t} + \frac{\partial \rho v_j}{\partial x_j} = 0. \tag{A.2:7}$$

If the fluid density ρ is a constant, then the material is said to be *incompressible*. The *equation of continuity of an incompressible fluid* is

$$\frac{\partial v_j}{\partial x_j} = 0 \quad \text{or} \quad \frac{\partial u}{\partial x} + \frac{\partial v}{\partial y} + \frac{\partial w}{\partial z} = 0. \tag{A.2:8}$$

Next, consider the momentum of particles in V,

$$\mathscr{P}_i = \int_V \rho v_i dV. \tag{A.2:9}$$

Newton's law of motion states that the material rate of change of momentum is equal to the force acting on the body:

$$\frac{D}{Dt}\mathscr{P}_i = \mathscr{F}_i. \tag{A.2:10}$$

If the body is subjected to surface tractions $\overset{v}{T}_i$ and body force per unit volume X_i, the resultant force acting on the body is

$$\mathscr{F}_i = \int_S \overset{v}{T}_i dS + \int_V X_i dV. \tag{A.2:11}$$

Now $\overset{v}{T}_i = \sigma_{ji} v_j$. Applying Eqs. (6.2:1), (6.2:4), and (6.2:9)–(6.2:11), we obtain the *Euler's equation of motion*

$$\rho\frac{Dv_i}{Dt} = \frac{\partial \sigma_{ij}}{\partial x_j} + X_i. \tag{A.2:12}$$

If there is no heat input into the system and no heat source in the region, the equation for balance of energy is the same as balance of mechanical energy and work: it leads to no new independent equation.

When these equations are combined with the constitutive equation of the material, we obtain the basic equations of mechanics. We shall illustrate this by several examples in the following sections.

A.3 Navier–Stokes Equations for an Incompressible Newtonian Fluid

Consider an incompressible, Newtonian viscous fluid. Let us use the same notations for pressure, velocity, and coordinates for position as in the previous section. Let μ be the coefficient of viscosity which is a constant for a Newtonian fluid. Then the stress–strain rate relationship is given by

$$\sigma_{ij} = -p\delta_{ij} + \lambda V_{kk}\delta_{ij} + 2\mu V_{ij} \tag{A.3:1}$$

where δ_{ij} is the Kronecker delta,

$$V_{ij} = \frac{1}{2}\left(\frac{\partial v_i}{\partial x_j} + \frac{\partial v_j}{\partial x_i}\right) \tag{A.3:2}$$

is the *strain rate* tensor, and λ and μ are two material constants. Since the fluid is assumed to be incompressible, the condition of incompressibility

$$\frac{\partial v_i}{\partial x_i} = 0 \quad \text{or} \quad \frac{\partial u}{\partial x} + \frac{\partial v}{\partial y} + \frac{\partial w}{\partial z} = 0 \tag{A.3:3}$$

reduces Eq. (A.3:1) to the form

$$\sigma_{ij} = -p\delta_{ij} + 2\mu V_{ij}. \tag{A.3:4}$$

These are, of course,

$$\sigma_{xx} = -p + 2\mu\frac{\partial u}{\partial x},$$

$$\sigma_{yy} = -p + 2\mu\frac{\partial v}{\partial y}, \tag{A.3:5}$$

$$\sigma_{zz} = -p + 2\mu\frac{\partial w}{\partial z},$$

$$\sigma_{xy} = \mu\left(\frac{\partial u}{\partial y} + \frac{\partial v}{\partial x}\right), \qquad \sigma_{yz} = \mu\left(\frac{\partial v}{\partial z} + \frac{\partial w}{\partial y}\right), \qquad \sigma_{zx} = \mu\left(\frac{\partial w}{\partial x} + \frac{\partial u}{\partial z}\right).$$

Substituting these into Eq. (A.2:12), we obtain the Navier–Stokes equations

$$\frac{\partial u}{\partial t} + u\frac{\partial u}{\partial x} + v\frac{\partial u}{\partial y} + w\frac{\partial u}{\partial z} = X - \frac{1}{\rho}\frac{\partial p}{\partial x} + v\nabla^2 u, \tag{A.3:6}$$

$$\frac{\partial v}{\partial t} + u\frac{\partial v}{\partial x} + v\frac{\partial v}{\partial y} + w\frac{\partial v}{\partial z} = Y - \frac{1}{\rho}\frac{\partial p}{\partial y} + v\nabla^2 v,$$

$$\frac{\partial w}{\partial t} + u\frac{\partial w}{\partial x} + v\frac{\partial w}{\partial y} + w\frac{\partial w}{\partial z} = Z - \frac{1}{\rho}\frac{\partial p}{\partial z} + v\nabla^2 w,$$

(A.3:6)

where $v = \mu/\rho$ is the *kinematic viscosity* of the fluid, and ∇^2 is the *Laplacian operator*

$$\nabla^2 = \frac{\partial^2}{\partial x^2} + \frac{\partial^2}{\partial y^2} + \frac{\partial^2}{\partial z^2}.$$

(A.3:7)

Equations (A.3:3) and (A.3:6) comprise four equations for the four variables u, v, w, and p occurring in an incompressible viscous flow. To solve these equations, we need to specify appropriate boundary conditions. If the fluid is in contact with a solid, the boundary condition is that there is no relative motion between the solid and the fluid. The fluid adheres to the solid, whether the surface is wettable or not. The justification of this condition is discussed at some length in Fung (1977, p. 268 et seq.). If the fluid is in contact with another fluid, then at the interface the boundary conditions must be consistent with the interfacial surface tension, surface viscosity, and conditions of cavitation or its absence. See Fung (1977, p. 270).

A.4 Navier's Equation for an Isotropic Hookean Elastic Solid

If the material is an isotropic elastic body obeying Hooke's law, the stress–strain relationship can be expressed either as

$$\sigma_{ij} = \lambda e_{\alpha\alpha}\delta_{ij} + 2Ge_{ij}$$

(A.4:1)

or as

$$e_{ij} = \frac{1+v}{E}\sigma_{ij} - \frac{v}{E}\sigma_{\alpha\alpha}\delta_{ij}.$$

(A.4:2)

Here e_{ij} ($i, j = 1, 2, 3$) or e_{xx}, e_{yy}, e_{zz}, e_{xy}, e_{yz}, e_{zx} are strain components. λ, G, E, v are elastic constants. λ and G are called *Lamé's constants*, G is called the *shear modulus* or the *modulus of rigidity*, E is called the *Young's modulus* or *modulus of elasticity*, and v is called the *Poisson's ratio*.

On substituting Eq. (A.4:1) into the equation of motion (A.2:12), we obtain

$$\rho\frac{Dv_i}{Dt} = \lambda\frac{\partial}{\partial x_i}e_{\alpha\alpha} + 2G\frac{\partial e_{ij}}{\partial x_j} + X_i.$$

(A.4:3)

To proceed further we need to express Dv_i/Dt and e_{ij} in terms of the displacements of material particles. An elastic body has a "natural" state (of zero stress and zero strain). We measure elastic displacements of every point in the body relative to the natural state with respect to a set of inertial, rectangular, Cartesian coordinates. Let the displacement of a point located at x_i at time t be $u_i(x_1, x_2, x_3, t)$, $i = 1, 2, 3$. The acceleration Dv_i/Dt and the strain e_{ij} can be expressed in terms of u_i, but the expressions are non-linear and complex if u_i is finite and if the velocity is high. Simplicity can be achieved if we can assume u_i to be infinitesimal. Since there is a large class of important practical problems in which this infinitesimal displacement assumption holds well, we shall use this assumption to obtain some simple results. Finite deformation is discussed in Chapter 16 of the author's book *Foundations of Solid Mechanics* (Fung (1965)).

If $u_i(x_1, x_2, x_3, t)$ is infinitesimal, then, on neglecting small quantities of higher order, we have

$$e_{ij} = \frac{1}{2}\left(\frac{\partial u_i}{\partial x_j} + \frac{\partial u_j}{\partial x_i}\right), \tag{A.4:4}$$

$$v_i = \frac{\partial u_i}{\partial t}, \qquad \frac{Dv_i}{Dt} = \frac{\partial^2 u_i}{\partial t^2}. \tag{A.4:5}$$

To the same order of approximation, the material density is a constant:

$$\rho = \text{const.} \tag{A.4:6}$$

On substituting Eqs. (A.4:4) and (A.4:5) into (A.4:3), we obtain the well-known *Navier's equation*:

$$G\nabla^2 u_i + (\lambda + G)\frac{\partial e}{\partial x_i} + X_i = \rho\frac{\partial^2 u_i}{\partial t^2}, \tag{A.4:7}$$

where e is the divergence of the displacement vector u_i:

$$e = \frac{\partial u_j}{\partial x_j} = \frac{\partial u_1}{\partial x_1} + \frac{\partial u_2}{\partial x_2} + \frac{\partial u_3}{\partial x_3}. \tag{A.4:8}$$

∇^2 is the Laplace operator, see Eq. (A.3:7).

If we introduce the Poisson's ratio as in Eq. (A.4:2),

$$v = \frac{\lambda}{2(\lambda + G)}, \tag{A.4:9}$$

we can write Navier's equation (A.4:7) as

$$G\left(\nabla^2 u_i + \frac{1}{1 - 2v}\frac{\partial e}{\partial x_i}\right) + X_i = \rho\frac{\partial^2 u_i}{\partial t^2}. \tag{A.4:10}$$

Navier's equation is the basic field equation of the linearized theory of elasticity. It must be solved with appropriate initial and boundary conditions. Unfortunately, most biological soft tissues are subject to finite deformation in normal function. Therefore, very often the linearization cannot be justified. Frequently biomechanics has to deal with nonlinear theories. Nevertheless much can be learned from the linearized theory.

In the following sections we shall consider some examples in which the constitutive equation is more complex than Newtonian viscosity or Hooke's law.

A.5 Fundamental Equations of Hemodynamics

Blood is a non-Newtonian incompressible viscoplastic fluid. When it is not flowing, it behaves like an elastic solid. This solid has a small yield stress. When the yield condition is reached, the blood flows. Its flowing characteristics is non-Newtonian. The non-Newtonian features are more evident when the shear strain rate is small. At large shear strain rates the flow characteristics of blood can be approximated by a Newtonian constitutive equation. Thus, as it is discussed in *Biomechanics* (Fung, 1981, Chap. 3, Sec. 3.2), blood viscosity can be represented approximately by the following equations in three different regimes:

(a) Elastic regime, blood not flowing. This regime is defined by the yield condition. Since yielding is due to distortion and is unaffected by pressure or mean stress, we make use of the *stress deviation* tensor σ'_{ij} defined by the equation

$$\sigma'_{ij} = \sigma_{ij} - \tfrac{1}{3}\sigma_{kk}\delta_{ij} \qquad (A.5:1)$$

to describe the yield condition. The mean stress of σ'_{ij} is zero. The yield condition is stated in terms of the second invariant of the stress deviation tensor:

$$J'_2(\sigma') = \tfrac{1}{2}\sigma'_{ij}\sigma'_{ij}. \qquad (A.5:2)$$

The material yields if

$$J'_2(\sigma') = K. \qquad (A.5:3)$$

It remains elastic if

$$J'_2(\sigma') < K. \qquad (A.5:4)$$

For blood, the value of K is of the order of 4×10^{-4} dyn^2/cm^4 or 4×10^{-6} N^{2}m^{-4}, with exact number depending on the hematocrit. When Eq. (A.5:4) applies, blood obeys Hooke's law, Eq. (A.4:1).

(b) If $J'_2(\sigma') \geq K$, then flow ensues, and the second invariant of the strain rate tensor $J_2(v) \neq 0$. If $J_2(v) > c$, a certain constant which depends on the hematocrit, then blood obeys the Newtonian viscosity law, and the results of Sec. A.3 apply:

$$\sigma_{ij} = -p\delta_{ij} + \mu\left(\frac{\partial v_i}{\partial x_j} + \frac{\partial v_j}{\partial x_i}\right), \qquad \mu = \text{const.} \qquad (A.5:5)$$

Here

$$J_2(v) = \tfrac{1}{2} V_{ij} V_{ij}, \tag{A.5:6}$$

$$V_{ij} = \frac{1}{2}\left(\frac{\partial v_i}{\partial x_j} + \frac{\partial v_j}{\partial x_i}\right). \tag{A.5:7}$$

(c) If $J_2'(\sigma') \geq K$, and $J_2(v) \leq c$, then blood obeys the following constitutive equation:

$$\sigma_{ij} = -p\delta_{ij} + \mu(J_2)\left(\frac{\partial v_i}{\partial x_j} + \frac{\partial v_j}{\partial x_i}\right), \tag{A.5:8}$$

where

$$\mu(J_2) = \left[(\eta^2 J_2)^{1/4} + 2^{-1/2}\tau_y^{1/2}\right]^2 J_2^{-1/2} \tag{A.5:9}$$

and η and τ_y are constants known as the *Casson viscosity* and *yielding stress*, respectively. Hence, in the flow regime, we obtain, on substituting (A.5:5)–(A.5:9) into (A.2:12),

$$\rho\frac{Dv_i}{Dt} = X_i - \frac{\partial p}{\partial x_i} + \frac{\partial}{\partial x_k}\left(\mu\frac{\partial v_k}{\partial x_i}\right) + \frac{\partial}{\partial x_k}\left(\mu\frac{\partial v_i}{\partial x_k}\right). \tag{A.5:10}$$

Differentiating and using Eq. (A.2:8) under the assumption that blood is incompressible, we obtain

$$\rho\frac{Dv_i}{Dt} = X_i - \frac{\partial p}{\partial x_i} + \mu\frac{\partial^2 v_i}{\partial x_k \partial x_k} + \frac{\partial\mu(J_2)}{\partial x_k}\left[\frac{\partial v_k}{\partial x_i} + \frac{\partial v_i}{\partial x_k}\right]. \tag{A.5:11}$$

Written out *in extenso*, Eq. (A.5:11) is, on account of Eq. (A.2:5),

$$\begin{aligned}
\rho\left(\frac{\partial u}{\partial t} + u\frac{\partial u}{\partial x} + v\frac{\partial u}{\partial y} + w\frac{\partial u}{\partial z}\right) &= X - \frac{\partial p}{\partial x} \\
&+ \mu(J_2)\left(\frac{\partial^2}{\partial x^2} + \frac{\partial^2}{\partial y^2} + \frac{\partial^2}{\partial z^2}\right)u \\
&+ 2\frac{\partial\mu(J_2)}{\partial x}\frac{\partial u}{\partial x} \\
&+ \frac{\partial\mu(J_2)}{\partial y}\left(\frac{\partial v}{\partial x} + \frac{\partial u}{\partial y}\right) + \frac{\partial\mu(J_2)}{\partial z}\left(\frac{\partial w}{\partial x} + \frac{\partial u}{\partial z}\right),
\end{aligned} \tag{A.5:12}$$

and two more equations obtained from (A.5:11) by successively replacing u, v, w by v, w, u, and w, u, v; and x, y, z by y, z, x and z, x, y, respectively. If the derivatives of $\mu(J_2)$ are dropped, as is justified for blood when $J_2(v) > c$, then we obtain the Navier–Stokes equation, (A.3:2).

Equations (A.2:8) amd (A.5:12) comprise four equations for the four variables u, v, w, and p. What are the boundary conditions? In blood vessels, the endothelium of the blood vessel may be regarded as a solid surface, and the boundary conditions are *no-slip* and *continuity*, i.e., there are no relative tangential and normal velocities between the blood and the wall. The normal velocities of the fluid and wall are the same because the fluid and the wall move together. The no-slip condition is gathered from general experience of fluid mechanics.

Blood interacts biochemically with artificial surfaces. Glass, for example, causes red blood cells to deform; its surface should be "siliconized" by coating it with silicone before permitting it to contact blood. Stainless steel is traumatic to blood. Many plastics work well with blood. Some of them, such as polyethylene, silicone rubber, and teflon, are permeable to oxygen and CO_2 and are used in blood oxygenators.

Blood abhors free surfaces. If exposed to a gas for too long blood proteins denature on the free surface and trauma results. Therefore few problems of blood flow involve free surfaces. If a gas–blood interface does exist, then the effect of the surface tension at the interface (of the order of 45 dyn/cm), and of the surface viscosity (resistance to shear strain rate in the surface) must be taken into account.

A.6 Dynamic Similarity and Reynolds Number

Consider first a blood flow in which the shear rate is sufficiently high so that the Navier–Stokes equations apply. See Eqs. (A.5:5) and (A.3:6). Let us put the Navier–Stokes equation in dimensionless form. Choose a characteristic velocity V and a characteristic length L. For example, if we investigate the flow in the aorta, we may take V to be the average speed of flow and L to be the blood vessel diameter. Having chosen these character- istic quantitites, we introduce the dimensionless variables

$$x' = \frac{x}{L}, \qquad y' = \frac{y}{L}, \qquad z' = \frac{z}{L}, \qquad u' = \frac{u}{V},$$
$$v' = \frac{v}{V}, \qquad w' = \frac{w}{V}, \qquad p' = \frac{p}{\rho V^2}, \qquad t' = \frac{Vt}{L}, \tag{A.6:1}$$

and the parameter

$$\text{Reynolds number} = N_R = \frac{VL\rho}{\mu} = \frac{VL}{\nu}. \tag{A.6:2}$$

Equation (A.3:6) can then be put into the form

$$\frac{\partial u'}{\partial t'} + u'\frac{\partial u'}{\partial x'} + v'\frac{\partial u'}{\partial y'} + w'\frac{\partial u'}{\partial z'} = -\frac{\partial p'}{\partial x'} + \frac{1}{N_R}\left(\frac{\partial^2 u'}{\partial x'^2} + \frac{\partial^2 u'}{\partial y'^2} + \frac{\partial^2 u'}{\partial z'^2}\right) \tag{A.6:3}$$

and two additional equations obtainable from Eq. (A.6:3) by changing u' into v', v' into w', w' into u' and x' into y', y' into z', z' into x'. The body force is ignored. The $\partial\mu/\partial x_k$ term is dropped because μ is a constant. The equation of continuity (A.2:8) can also be put in dimensionless form:

$$\frac{\partial u'}{\partial x'} + \frac{\partial v'}{\partial v'} + \frac{\partial w'}{\partial z'} = 0. \tag{A.6:4}$$

Since Eqs. (A.6:3) and (A.6:4) constitute the complete set of field equations for an incompressible fluid, it is clear that only one physical parameter, the Reynolds number N_R, enters into the field equations of the flow.

To solve these equations for a specific problem we must consider the boundary equations. Consider two flows in two geometrically similar vessels. The vessels have the same shape but different sizes. If the vessels are stationary and rigid, the boundary conditions are identical (no-slip). Then the two flows will be identical (in the dimensionless variables) if the Reynolds numbers for the two flows are the same, because two geometrically similar bodies having the same Reynolds number will be governed by identical differential equations and boundary conditions (in dimensionless form). Therefore, flows about geometrically similar bodies at the same Reynolds numbers are completely similar in the sense that the functions $u'(x', y', z', t')$, $v'(x', y', z', t')$, $w'(x', y', z', t')$, $p'(x', y', z', t')$ are the same for the various flows. Thus the Reynolds number is said to govern the dynamic similarity.

The Reynolds number expresses the ratio of inertial force to the shear stress. In a flow the inertial force due to convective acceleration arises from terms such as ρu^2, whereas the shear stress arises from terms such as $\mu \partial u / \partial y$. The orders of magnitude of these terms are, respectively,

$$\text{Inertial force: } \rho V^2,$$

$$\text{Shear stress: } \frac{\mu V}{L}.$$

The ratio is

$$\frac{\text{Inertial force}}{\text{shear stress}} = \frac{\rho V^2}{\mu V / L} = \frac{\rho V L}{\mu} = \text{Reynolds number.} \tag{A.6:5}$$

A large Reynolds number signals a preponderant inertial effect. A small Reynolds number signals a predominant shear effect.

Another way to interpret this ratio is to look at the equation of motion, (A.6:3), which expresses the balance of forces:

$$\Delta \text{ inertial force} = \Delta \text{ pressure force} + \Delta \text{ viscous forces,} \tag{A.6:6}$$

where the symbol Δ may be read as the "net change of."

If all the dimensionless derivatives $\partial u'/\partial t$, $\partial u'/\partial x'$, $\partial^2 u'/\partial x'^2$, etc., are of the same order of magnitude, then it is evident that the Reynolds number N_R determines whether the last group of terms is important compared with the rest of terms. If N_R is much larger than 1, then the viscous force terms can be neglected. If N_R is much smaller than 1, then the viscous force terms are predominant.

If the shear rate in a blood flow is smaller than certain number (say, 200 sec^{-1}), then we must use Eq. (A.5:11). Introducing the dimensionless variables listed in Eqs. (A.6:1) and again ignoring body forces, Eq. (A.5:11) becomes

$$\frac{\partial u'}{\partial t'} + u\frac{\partial u'}{\partial x'} + v\frac{\partial u'}{\partial y'} + w\frac{\partial u'}{\partial z'} = -\frac{\partial p'}{\partial x'} + \frac{1}{N_R}\left(\frac{\partial^2 u'}{\partial x'^2} + \frac{\partial^2 u'}{\partial y'^2} + \frac{\partial^2 u'}{\partial x'^2}\right)$$

$$+ 2\frac{\partial}{\partial x'}\left(\frac{1}{N_R}\right)\frac{\partial u'}{\partial x'} + \frac{\partial}{\partial y'}\left(\frac{1}{N_R}\right)\left(\frac{\partial v'}{\partial x'} + \frac{\partial u'}{\partial y'}\right) + \frac{\partial}{\partial z'}\left(\frac{1}{N_R}\right)\left(\frac{\partial w'}{\partial x'} + \frac{\partial u'}{\partial z'}\right).$$

$$\text{(A.6:7)}$$

In this case the Reynolds number $N_R = VL\rho/\mu$ is no longer a constant in the whole flow field because the viscosity $\mu(J_2)$ varies from place to place. The flow is affected not only by the Reynolds number, but also by the dimensionless gradient of the Reynolds number,

$$\frac{\partial}{\partial x'}\left(\frac{1}{N_R}\right), \qquad \frac{\partial}{\partial y'}\left(\frac{1}{N_R}\right), \qquad \frac{\partial}{\partial z'}\left(\frac{1}{N_R}\right). \qquad \text{(A.6:8)}$$

Dynamic similarity of two geometrically similar flows requires identification of the Reynolds number and the gradient of the Reynolds number, i.e., the Reynolds number at corresponding points in the two flows must be the same.

A.7 Basic Equations for an Elastic Solid

In Sec. A.5, we indicated how the Navier–Stokes equation can be modified for a non-Newtonian fluid such as blood. In this section we shall see how Navier's equation can be modified for solids that do not obey Hooke's law.

A major decision must be made in solid mechanics whether the deformation can be limited to infinitesimal strain or not. If it can, then the problem can be greatly simplified. If it cannot, then the problem is in general highly nonlinear because the strains are nonlinear functions of the derivatives of the displacements.

Consider first the small deformation. In this case, the strain tensors defined by Green and Almansi (see Fung (1981, Sec. 2.3, p. 30)) are equal, and both become Cauchy's infinitesimal strain tensor:

$$\varepsilon_{ij} = \frac{1}{2}\left[\frac{\partial u_j}{\partial x_i} + \frac{\partial u_i}{\partial x_j}\right]. \qquad \text{(A.7:1)}$$

Here u_i are the components of displacement of a material particle at x_i, and the first partial derivatives of u_i are assumed to be so small that the squares and products of these derivatives are negligible.

If the body is elastic, then the stresses must be functions of the strains. If the functions are analytic, they can be expanded in power series of the strains, and then it is seen that the stress–strain relationship must be linear, because all higher-order terms can be neglected under the assumption of infinitesimal strain. The most general form of constitutive equation for infinitesimal strain is, therefore,

$$\sigma_{ij} = C_{ijkl}\varepsilon_{kl}, \tag{A.7:2}$$

where C_{ijkl} are the elastic constants. This is a generalized Hooke's law. The isotropic case given in (A.4:1) is a special case. On substituting (A.7:2) into (A.2:12), we obtain the equation of motion:

$$\rho \frac{Dv_i}{DE} = C_{ijkl} \frac{\partial \varepsilon_{kl}}{\partial x_j} + X_i. \tag{A.7:3}$$

With Eqs. (A.7:1) and (A.4:5), Eq. (A.7:3) is reduced to

$$\rho \frac{\partial^2 u_i}{\partial t^2} = \frac{1}{2} C_{ijkl} \frac{\partial}{\partial x_j} \left(\frac{\partial u_k}{\partial x_l} + \frac{\partial u_l}{\partial x_k} \right) + X_i. \tag{A.7:4}$$

This is a generalized form of the Navier equation.

Now, turn to finite deformation. In this case, we must carefully distinguish the location of material particles before and after deformation. Referring to a set of rectangular Cartesian coordinates, let a particle located initially at (a_1, a_2, a_3) be displaced to (x_1, x_2, x_3) after deformation. Then the Green's strain is defined as (see Fung (1981, Sec. 2.3)).

$$
\begin{aligned}
E_{ij} &= \frac{1}{2}\left(\delta_{\alpha\beta}\frac{\partial x_\alpha}{\partial a_i}\frac{\partial x_\beta}{\partial a_j} - \delta_{ij}\right) \\
&= \frac{1}{2}\left(\frac{\partial u_j}{\partial a_i} + \frac{\partial u_i}{\partial a_j} + \frac{\partial u_\alpha}{\partial a_i}\frac{\partial u_\alpha}{\partial a_j}\right),
\end{aligned} \tag{A.7:5}
$$

where δ_{ij} is the Kronecker delta. The displacement vector is

$$u_i = x_i - a_i. \tag{A.7:6}$$

If the material is elastic or pseudo-elastic in finite deformation, a strain energy function $\rho_0 W(E_{11}, E_{12}, \dots)$ exists whose derivative yields the Kirchhoff's stress tensor S_{ij}:

$$S_{ij} = \frac{\partial(\rho_0 W)}{\partial E_{ij}}. \tag{A.7:7}$$

The Kirchhoff stress S_{ij} is related to the Cauchy stress σ_{ij} by the relation

$$\sigma_{ij} = \frac{\rho}{\rho_0}\left[S_{ij} + \left(\delta_{i\beta}\frac{\partial u_j}{\partial a_\alpha} + \delta_{j\alpha}\frac{\partial u_i}{\partial a_\beta} + \frac{\partial u_i}{\partial a_\alpha}\frac{\partial u_j}{\partial a_\beta} \right) S_{\alpha\beta} \right]. \tag{A.7:8}$$

Here ρ and ρ_0 are the density of the material in the deformed and initial states, respectively. The equation of motion (A.2:12) is valid with σ_{ij} representing Cauchy stress:

$$\rho \frac{Dv_i}{Dt} = \frac{\partial \sigma_{ij}}{\partial x_j} + X_i. \tag{A.7:9}$$

The particle acceleration is given by the material derivative of the velocity:

$$\frac{Dv_i}{Dt} = \frac{\partial v_i}{\partial t} + v_j \frac{\partial v_i}{\partial x_j}. \tag{A.7:10}$$

The particle velocity is given by the material derivative of the displacement:

$$v_i = \frac{\partial u_i}{\partial t} + v_j \frac{\partial u_i}{\partial x_j}. \tag{A.7:11}$$

The conservation of mass is given by the equation of continuity

$$\frac{\partial \rho}{\partial t} + \frac{\partial(\rho v_i)}{\partial x_i} = 0. \tag{A.7:12}$$

Equations (A.7:5) through (A.7:12) define the finite deformation of an elastic body.

If the viscoelastic features of the tissue are important, we must replace Eqs. (A.7:7) and (A.7:8) with a constitutive equation for viscoelasticity. For active contraction of muscle, the muscle constitutive equation must be used.

These field equations must be solved in conjunction with appropriate boundary conditions. The interplay of anatomy, physiology, and biomechanics in defining the boundary conditions and field equations is the main theme of this book.

A.8 Viscoelastic Bodies

Most linearly viscoelastic bodies have the following constitutive equation:

$$\sigma_{ij}(\mathbf{x}, t) = \int_{-\infty}^{t} G_{ijkl}(t - \tau) \frac{\partial}{\partial \tau} E_{kl}(\mathbf{x}, \tau) d\tau, \tag{A.8:1}$$

where G_{ijkl} is the tensor of relaxation functions, σ_{ij} and E_{kl} are strains, t and τ are time, and the integration over τ is from the beginning of motion to the time t. The equation of motion is obtained by substituting Eq. (A.8:1) into Eq. (A.2:12).

Biological materials usually have very complex viscoelastic properties. Most living soft tissues, however, may be represented approximately by a *quasi-linear* constitutive equation, as follows (see *Biomechanics* (Fung, 1981, Chaps. 7–12)):

$$\sigma_{ij}(\mathbf{x}, t) = \int_{-\infty}^{t} G_{ijkl}(t - \tau) \frac{\partial \sigma_{kl}^{(e)}(\mathbf{x}, \tau)}{\partial \tau} d\tau, \tag{A.8:2}$$

where $\sigma^{(e)}$ is the *pseudo-elastic stress* (see *Biomechanics* (Fung, 1981, Sec. 7.7, pp. 238–242)) and is a function of the strain, which in turn is a function of $\mathbf{x}$ and t. If a *pseudo-strain-energy-function* $\rho_o W$ exists, then

$$\sigma_{kl}^{(e)} = \frac{\partial \rho_o W}{\partial E_{kl}}, \tag{A.8:3}$$

where $\rho_o W$ is a function of the strain components E_{11}, E_{22}, E_{12}, $\ldots$, symmetric with respect to the symmetric shear strains $E_{ij} = E_{ji}$. For arteries, skin, mesentery, cartilage, etc., $\rho_o W$ may be represented by a simple exponential function:

$$\rho_o W = ce^Q, \tag{A.8:4}$$

where c is a constant and Q is a quadratic form:

$$Q = a_{rs} E_r E_s. \tag{A.8:5}$$

Here a_{rs} are constants and E_1, E_2, $\ldots$, E_6 represent E_{11}, E_{22}, E_{33}, E_{12}, E_{23}, E_{31}, respectively. If Eq. (A.8:3) applies, then Eq. (A.8:2) becomes, if we designate $\sigma_1, \sigma_2, \ldots \sigma_6$ for $\sigma_{11}, \sigma_{22}, \sigma_{33}, \sigma_{12}, \sigma_{23}, \sigma_{31}$,

$$\sigma_i(\mathbf{x}, t) = \int_{-\infty}^{t} G_{im}(t - \tau) \frac{\partial^2 (\rho_o W)}{\partial E_n \partial E_m} \frac{\partial E_n(\mathbf{x}, \tau)}{\partial \tau} d\tau. \tag{A.8:6}$$

Further, if Eqs. (A.8:4) and (A.8:5) apply, then

$$\sigma_i(\mathbf{x}, t) = \int_{-\infty}^{t} G_{im}(t - \tau) ce^Q \left(\frac{\partial Q}{\partial E_m} \frac{\partial Q}{\partial E_n} + \frac{\partial^2 Q}{\partial E_m \partial E_n} \right) \frac{\partial E_n(\mathbf{x}, \tau)}{\partial \tau} d\tau. \tag{A.8:7}$$

A substitution of Eq. (A.8:7) into Eq. (A.2:12) yields the equation of motion.

In the equations above, the strains are tacitly assumed to be small. If they are finite, then it is necessary to distinguish σ_{ij} from S_{ij} as it is indicated in Sec. A.7.

If the material is incompressible, then there may exist in the material a pressure that is independent of the deformation of the body. See Sec. A.3, Eq. (A.3:1). Thus, for an incompressible fluid we should add a term $-p\delta_{ij}$ to the right hand side of Eqs. (A.8:1) and (A.8:2). The pressure p will be determined by the equations of motion and boundary conditions.

A.9 Cylindrical Polar Coordinates

If the structure and properties of the material, loading, and boundary conditions are all axially symmetric, then the field of flow or deformation may also have axial symmetry, and it would be advantageous to use cylindrical polar coordinates. The equations presented in the preceding sections can be transformed into cylindrical coordinates. The transformation is discussed in books on fluid and solid mechanics or tensor analysis. We shall quote the results below with references to where they can be found in Fung (1977).

The coordinate system and the notation of stresses are shown in Figs. A.9:1 and A.9:2 (Fung, 1977, pp. 78, 84). The notations of displacement

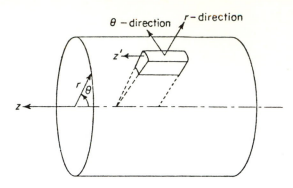

Figure A.9:1 Cylindrical polar coordinates.

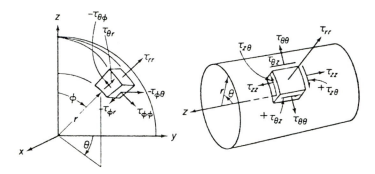

Figure A.9:2 Stress components in cylindrical polar coordinates.

vectors are shown in Fig. A.9:3. The strain components expressed in terms of the displacements are (Fung, 1977, p. 138)

$$\varepsilon_{rr} = \frac{\partial u_r}{\partial r},$$

$$\varepsilon_{\theta\theta} = \frac{u_r}{r} + \frac{1}{r}\frac{\partial u_\theta}{\partial \theta},$$

$$\varepsilon_{r\theta} = \frac{1}{2}\left(\frac{1}{r}\frac{\partial u_r}{\partial \theta} + \frac{\partial u_\theta}{\partial r} - \frac{u_\theta}{r}\right),$$

$$\varepsilon_{zr} = \frac{1}{2}\left(\frac{\partial u_r}{\partial z} + \frac{\partial u_z}{\partial r}\right),$$ \hfill (A.9:1)

$$\varepsilon_{z\theta} = \frac{1}{2}\left(\frac{1}{r}\frac{\partial u_z}{\partial \theta} + \frac{\partial u_\theta}{\partial z}\right),$$

$$\varepsilon_{zz} = \frac{\partial u_z}{\partial z}.$$

$$u_x = u_r \cos \theta - u_\theta \sin \theta,$$
$$u_y = u_r \sin \theta + u_\theta \cos \theta,$$
$$u_z = u_z.$$

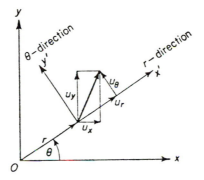

Figure A.9:3 A displacement vector and its components in cylindrical polar coordinates.

These are infinitesimal strains. Finite strains are nonlinear functions of the derivatives of displacements. Note that we have used a tensor notation for strain, and the shear strain component $\varepsilon_{r\theta}$, ε_{rz}, $\varepsilon_{z\theta}$ are one-half those ordinarily given as $\gamma_{r\theta}$, γ_{rz}, $\gamma_{z\theta}$ in most books.

The equations of equilibrium,

$$\frac{\partial \sigma_{ij}}{\partial x_j} = 0, \tag{A.9:2}$$

are transformed into the following three equations:

$$\frac{\partial \sigma_{rr}}{\partial r} + \frac{1}{r}\frac{\partial \sigma_{r\theta}}{\partial \theta} + \frac{\sigma_{rr} - \sigma_{\theta\theta}}{r} + \frac{\partial \sigma_{rz}}{\partial z} = 0,$$

$$\frac{1}{r}\frac{\partial \sigma_{\theta\theta}}{\partial \theta} + \frac{\partial \sigma_{r\theta}}{\partial r} + \frac{2\sigma_{r\theta}}{r} + \frac{\partial \sigma_{r\theta}}{\partial z} = 0, \tag{A.9:3}$$

$$\frac{\partial \sigma_{zz}}{\partial z} + \frac{1}{r}\frac{\partial \sigma_{z\theta}}{\partial \theta} + \frac{\partial \sigma_{zr}}{\partial r} + \frac{\sigma_{rz}}{r} = 0.$$

If there is motion, let v_i and a_i denote the velocity and acceleration, respectively; then the equations of motion,

$$\frac{\partial \sigma_{ij}}{\partial x_j} + X_i = \rho \frac{Dv_i}{Dt} = \rho a_i, \tag{A.9:4}$$

are transformed into:

$$\rho a_r = \frac{\partial \sigma_{rr}}{\partial r} + \frac{1}{r}\frac{\partial \sigma_{r\theta}}{\partial \theta} + \frac{\sigma_{rr} - \sigma_{\theta\theta}}{r} + \frac{\partial \sigma_{rz}}{\partial z} + F_r,$$

$$\rho a_\theta = \frac{1}{r}\frac{\partial \sigma_{\theta\theta}}{\partial \theta} + \frac{\partial \sigma_{r\theta}}{\partial r} + \frac{2\sigma_{r\theta}}{r} + \frac{\partial \sigma_{r\theta}}{\partial z} + F_\theta, \qquad (A.9:5)$$

$$\rho a_z = \frac{\partial \sigma_{zz}}{\partial z} + \frac{1}{r}\frac{\partial \sigma_{z\theta}}{\partial \theta} + \frac{\partial \sigma_{zr}}{\partial r} + \frac{\sigma_{rz}}{r} + F_z,$$

where F_r, F_θ, F_z are body force per unit volume in the direction of r, θ, and z, respectively. The components of acceleration,

$$a_x = \frac{\partial v_x}{\partial t} + v_x \frac{\partial v_x}{\partial x} + v_y \frac{\partial v_x}{\partial y} + v_x \frac{\partial v_x}{\partial z}, \qquad (A.9:6)$$

etc., are transformed into

$$a_r = \frac{\partial v_r}{\partial t} + v_r \frac{\partial v_r}{\partial r} + \frac{v_\theta}{r}\frac{\partial v_r}{\partial \theta} - \frac{v_\theta^2}{r} + v_z \frac{\partial v_r}{\partial z},$$

$$a_\theta = \frac{\partial v_\theta}{\partial t} + v_r \frac{\partial v_\theta}{\partial r} + \frac{v_\theta}{r}\frac{\partial v_\theta}{\partial \theta} + \frac{v_r v_\theta}{r} + v_z \frac{\partial v_\theta}{\partial z}, \qquad (A.9:7)$$

$$a_z = \frac{\partial v_z}{\partial t} + v_r \frac{\partial v_z}{\partial r} + \frac{v_\theta}{r}\frac{\partial v_z}{\partial \theta} + v_z \frac{\partial v_z}{\partial z}.$$

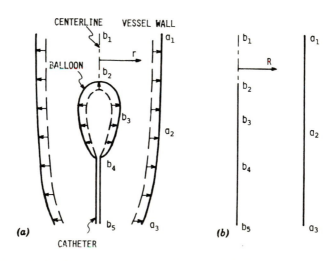

Figure A.9:4 A sketch of a cardiac assist device with balloon pumping in aorta. (a) Domain of flow in cylindrical coordinates. (b) Domain of flow in transformed coordinates.

Finally, the equation of continuity, (A.2:7), becomes

$$\frac{1}{r}\frac{\partial}{\partial r}(\rho r v_r) + \frac{1}{r}\frac{\partial \rho v_\theta}{\partial \theta} + \frac{\partial \rho v_z}{\partial z} + \frac{\partial \rho}{\partial t} = 0. \qquad (A.9:8)$$

Corresponding expressions in spherical polar coordinates can be found in Fung (1977, p. 329), and in many other textbooks.

Figure A.9:4 shows the boundary conditions of a practical problem in biomechanics: the flow of blood with the assistance of a pumping balloon. The shape of the boundary is complicated. Hung (1981) shows that for numerical calculations it is convenient to transform the radial coordinates r into a dimensionless radius R:

$$R = \frac{r - b(z, t)}{a(z, t) - b(z, t)} = \frac{r - b}{a - b}, \qquad (A.9:9)$$

in which $a(z, t)$, $b(z, t)$ represent the instantaneous radius of the aorta and that of the balloon, respectively. In the transformed plane, the domain of the flow is fixed, as shown in Fig. A.9:4(b). This transformation, of course, sends the Navier–Stokes equation into a very complex form. According to Hung (1981), it is still simpler to deal with the complicated field equation than with the variable boundary geometry.

A.10 Turbulent Flow

Turbulence is a yet unsolved problem in fluid mechanics, but because of its importance to biomechanics (see Chap. 2), we list a set of equations that are frequently used. For simplicity, let us consider a steady, turbulent, axisymmetric flow of an incompressible, Newtonian fluid. Let a polar coordinates system be used and let u, v be the velocity components in the axial (z) and radial (r) directions, respectively. Define the *vorticity* Ω and the *stream function* ψ as

$$\Omega = \frac{\partial V}{\partial z} - \frac{\partial U}{\partial r}, \qquad (A.10:1)$$

$$\frac{1}{r}\frac{\partial \psi}{\partial r} = \rho U, \qquad \frac{1}{r}\frac{\partial \psi}{\partial z} = -\rho V, \qquad (A.10:2)$$

where ρ is the fluid density. The velocities u, v consist of the mean values U, V and the turbulent components u' and v':

$$u = U + u', \qquad v = V + v'. \qquad (A.10:3)$$

If an overbar " $\overline{}$ " indicates an average with respect to time, then $\overline{u'} = \overline{v'} = 0$, but the mean square values $\overline{u'^2}$ and $\overline{v'^2}$ do not vanish. We define ρk as the *kinetic energy of turbulence*;

$$\rho k = \tfrac{1}{2}\rho(\overline{u'^2} + \overline{v'^2}) \qquad (A.10:4)$$

TABLE A.10:1 Coefficients a, b, c, and d

ϕ	a	b	c	$d*$
ψ	0	$(\rho r^2)^{-1}$	1	$-\Omega/r$
Ω/r	r^2	r^2	0	0
k	1	$\mu_{\text{eff}}/\sigma_k$	1	$\mu_t G - \rho\varepsilon$
ε	1	$\mu_{\text{eff}}/\sigma_\varepsilon$	1	$c_1\varepsilon\mu_t G/k - \rho c_2\varepsilon^2/k$

$$* \quad G = 2\left[\left(\frac{\partial U}{\partial z}\right)^2 + \left(\frac{\partial V}{\partial r}\right)^2 + \left(\frac{V}{r}\right)^2\right] + \left(\frac{\partial V}{\partial z} + \frac{\partial U}{\partial r}\right)^2.$$

and ε as the *volumetric dissipation rate* of turbulent kinetic energy:

$$\varepsilon = C_D k^{3/2}/L, \tag{A.10:5}$$

where C_D is an empirical constant, and L is a length scale proportional to the mixing length. The *turbulent viscosity* is calculated from the relationship

$$\mu_t = C_\mu \rho k^2/\varepsilon \tag{A.10:6}$$

in which C_μ is an empirical constant.

Gosman et al. (1969) and Launder and Spalding (1974) show that the governing equation can be put in the following form:

$$a\left[\frac{\partial}{\partial z}\left(\phi\frac{\partial\psi}{\partial r}\right) - \frac{\partial}{\partial r}\left(\phi\frac{\partial\psi}{\partial z}\right)\right] - \frac{\partial}{\partial z}\left[br\frac{\partial(c\phi)}{\partial z}\right] - \frac{\partial}{\partial r}\left[br\frac{\partial(c\phi)}{\partial r}\right] + rd = 0. \tag{A.10:7}$$

Here ϕ denotes the conserved general property such as ψ, Ω/r, k and ε. The coefficients a, b, c, and d are listed in Table A.10:1.

The *effective viscosity* u_{eff} is the sum of the *turbulent* viscosity and the *molecular* (or *laminar*) viscosity:

$$\mu_{\text{eff}} = \mu_t + \mu_L. \tag{A.10:8}$$

The normal and shear stresses for the incompressible axisymmetric flow are

$$\tau_{rr} = -2\mu_{\text{eff}}\partial U/\partial r, \quad \tau_{\theta\theta} = -2\mu_{\text{eff}}U/r, \quad \tau_{zz} = -2\mu_{\text{eff}}\partial V/\partial z, \tag{A.10:9}$$

$$\tau_{rz} = \tau_{zr} = -\mu_{\text{eff}}(\partial V/\partial r + \partial U/\partial z). \tag{A.10:10}$$

Yang and Wang (1982) applied these equations to solving the problem of turbulent flow through a prosthetic heart valve. They give the following values for the empirical constants:

$$\sigma_k = 1.0, \quad \sigma_\varepsilon = 1.3, \quad c_D = 1.0, \quad c_\mu = 0.082, \quad c_1 = 1.45, \quad c_2 = 2.0,$$

which were obtained through numerical experiments and combined rotational-swirling flows.

Problems

A.1 Design an experiment to test the no-slip boundary condition of blood flow in a blood vessel.

A.2 Blood drips at the end of a pipette connected to a reservoir as in a blood transfusion apparatus. Let the pipette be vertical and let the drops form under gravity. It is important to know the size of each drop and the rate at which it is formed. A controlling factor is the surface tension. Measuring the drop size is a way of measuring the surface tension between blood and air. Describe mathematically the boundary conditions that apply to the surface of the drop. Also, formulate the field equations.

A.3 The inner wall of a blood vessel (endothelium) is easily injured by mechanical stress or heat. Platelets are activated by the injured endothelium cells, white blood cells begin to attach to the endothelium, and a thrombus is gradually formed. Derive the governing field equations for the blood and the thrombus, and all the relevant boundary conditions.

A.4 A plastic surgeon cuts out a piece of skin and sutures the remainder together. In analyzing the stresses in the skin as a result of the surgery, what are the boundary conditions at the suture? What are the field equations for the skin?

A.5 In a membrane blood oxygenator, blood flows between two sheets of silastic membranes which are exposed to concentrated oxygen. Design a possible oxygenator, and write down all the equations necessary in order to analyze the flow of blood in the oxygenator.

A.6 The bone is an orthotropic elastic solid. Derive the field equations and boundary conditions for an diarthrodial joint.

A.7 In the derivation of the equations in Sec. 2.3, the fluid is assumed incompressible. How should these equations be modified to account for fluid compressibility so that they are applicable to a gas?

A.8 Write down all the field equations and boundary conditions necessary for solving the problem of propagation of pulse wave in arteries.

A.9 Do the same for the ventilation in airways.

A.10 Think of some problems, either in biology or in engineering, in which gas–fluid interfaces exist and in which surface tension on the interfaces is important. Formulate such a problem mathematically.

A.11 Think of and formulate mathematically some problems, real or hypothetical, in which surface viscosity plays an important role.

A.12 Consult a book on anatomy; sketch a knee joint. It is filled with viscoelastic synovial fluid. The ends of bone are covered with articulate cartilage, which is a porous, compressible tissue. Give a mathematical formulation of the problem of joint lubrication as one walks or runs.

A.13 A surgeon has to excise a certain dollar-sized circular patch of skin from a patient with a skin tumor. A circulat patch was cut off and the edges sewed together. What would be the stress and strain distribution in the skin after surgery? What is the tension in the suture? Formulate an approximate theory for the solution.

Note: In the theory of functions of a complex variable, a transformation from $z = x + iy$ to $w = u + iv$ by

$$w = z + \frac{1}{z}$$

transforms a circle to a straight line segment. Would this knowledge be helpful?

A.14 Consider the skin surgery problem of Problem A.13 again. There will be a large stress (and strain) concentration at the ends of the line of suture if the surgery was done as stated in Problem A.13. To minimize the stress concentration, a diamond-shaped area of skin is excised and the edges sewed together. Formulate the mathematical problem and explain why is the stress concentration reduced?

A.15 Consider the skin problem again. Design a better way of excising a piece of diseased skin from the point of view of minimizing stress concentration. In skin surgery there is a technique called z-plasty. Explain why is it a good technique.

A.16 In some soft tissues there is a natural direction along which collagen fibers are aligned. Healing will be faster if a cut is made in such a direction as compared with a cut perpendicular to this direction. Explain this qualitatively and formulate a mathematical theory for this.

References

Caro, C. G., Pedley, T. J. and Seed, W. A. (1974). Mechanics of circulation. In *Cardiovascular Physiology*, (Goyton, A. C., ed.). Medical and Technical Publishers, London, Chap. 1.

Fung, Y. C. (1965). *Foundations of Solid Mechanics*. Prentice-Hall, Englewood Cliffs, NJ.

Fung, Y. C. (1977). *A First Course in Continuum Mechanics*, 2nd edn., Prentice–Hall, Englewood Cliffs, N.J.

Fung, Y. C. (1981). *Biomechanics: Mechanical Properties of Living Tissues*. Springer-Verlag, New York, Heidelberg, Berlin.

Gosman, A. D., Pun, W. M., Runchal, A. K., Spalding, D. B. and Wolfstein, M. (1969). *Heat and Mass Transfer in Recirculating Flows*. Academic Press, London.

Hung, T. K. (1981). Forcing functions in Navier–Stokes equations. *J. Engineering Mechanics Division. Trans. Amer. Soc. Civil Engineers* **107**, No. EM 3, 643–648.

Launder, B. E., and Spalding, D. B. (1974). Numerical computation of turbulent flows. *Comput. Meth. Appl. Mech. Eng.* **3**: 269–289.

Yang, W. J. and Wang, J. H. (1983). Turbulent flows through a disk-like prosthetic heart valve. *J. Biomech. Eng.*, **105**: 263–267.

Yih, C. S. (1977). *Fluid Mechanics*. West River Press, Ann Arbor, MI.

Author Index

Subject Index